ATTENTION DEFICIT HYPERACTIVITY DISORDER IN CHILDREN AND ADOLESCENTS

Edited by **Somnath Banerjee**

Attention Deficit Hyperactivity Disorder in Children and Adolescents
http://dx.doi.org/10.5772/50252
Edited by Somnath Banerjee

Contributors

Hojka Gregoric Kumperscak, Debby Zambo, Rahn Kennedy Bailey, Ejike Kingsley Ofoemezie, Chen, Smadar Celestin-Westreich, Leon-Patrice Celestin, Nitin Patel, Paul Glaser, Marian Soroa, Nekane Balluerka, Arantxa Gorostiaga, Yanling Ren, Zaytoon Amod, Adri Vorster, Kim Lazarus, Alban Burke, Amanda Edge, Esra Ozdemir Demirci, Merve Cikili, Didem Behice Oztop, Rabia Durmus, Sarina Grosswald, Antigone Papavasiliou, Irene Nikaina

Published by InTech

Janeza Trdine 9, 51000 Rijeka, Croatia

Publishing Process Manager Iva Simcic
Technical Editor InTech DTP team
Cover InTech Design team

Additional hard copies can be obtained from orders@intechopen.com

Attention Deficit Hyperactivity Disorder in Children and Adolescents, Edited by Somnath Banerjee
p. cm.
ISBN 978-953-51-1086-6

For EU product safety concerns:
IN TECH d.o.o., Prolaz Marije Krucifikse Kozulić 3, 51000 Rijeka, Croatia,
info@intechopen.com or visit our website at intechopen.com.

Meet the editor

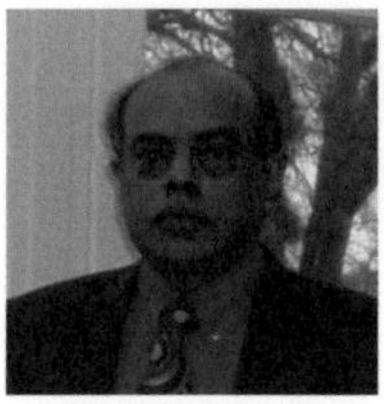

Dr Somnath Banerjee is a Community Paediatrician in UK. His interests are ADHD and Epilepsy in children. He Chairs ADHD team meetings in his Trust. Dr Banerjee received the annual Trust Award 2004 for the 'Best Clinical Audit Project'. He has presented various papers/ posters and conducted workshops on ADHD in National and International conferences. He has been involved with various Pan-European researches on ADHD drugs. Dr Banerjee has contributed chapters in many medical books. He is the co-founder of Kent ADHD Network and Convenor; George Still Forum (National Paediatric ADHD Network Group), a special interest group of Royal College of Paediatrics and Child Health in UK.

Contents

Preface XI

Section 1 Introduction 1

Chapter 1 **ADHD Through Different Developmental Stages 3**
Hojka Gregoric Kumperscak

Chapter 2 **Neurodevelopmental Pathways of Childhood ADHD into Adulthood: Maturational Lag, Deviation, or Both? 21**
Alban Burke and Amanda Edge

Chapter 3 **Difficulties in Recognizing ADHD in an Urban Population and Treatment Satisfaction with a Short and a Long Acting Stimulant 51**
Antigone Papavasiliou, Irene Nikaina, Anna Spyridonidou and Eleanna Nianiou

Chapter 4 **Is ADHD a Stress-Related Disorder? Why Meditation Can Help 71**
Sarina J. Grosswald

Section 2 Role of Endocrine Hormones 93

Chapter 5 **The Potential Role of Neuroendocrine in Patients with Attention-Deficit/Hyperactivity Disorder 95**
Liang-Jen Wang and Chih-Ken Chen

Chapter 6 **Dopamine and Glutamate Interactions in ADHD: Implications for the Future Neuropharmacology of ADHD 109**
Erin M. Miller, Theresa C. Thomas, Greg A. Gerhardt and Paul E. A. Glaser

Section 3 Assessment and Diagnosis 139

Chapter 7 **Clinical Phenomena of ADHD 141**
Nitin Patel

Chapter 8 **Review of Tools Used for Assessing Teachers' Level of Knowledge with Regards Attention Deficit Hyperactivity Disorder (ADHD) 151**
Marian Soroa, Arantxa Gorostiaga and Nekane Balluerka

Section 4 Drugs in ADHD 179

Chapter 9 **Effects of Methylphenidate in Children with Attention Deficit Hyperactivity Disorder: A Comparison of Behavioral Results and Event–Related Potentials 181**
Ren Yan-ling and Dong Xuan

Chapter 10 **The Impact of Attention Deficit/Hyperactivity Disorder in African-Americans; Current Challenges Associated with Diagnosis and Treatment 193**
Rahn Kennedy Bailey and Ejike Kingsley Ofoemezie

Section 5 Outcome 213

Chapter 11 **Attention-Deficit/Hyperactivity Disorder (ADHD) as a Barrier to Learning and Development within the South African Context: The Perspective of Teachers 215**
Zaytoon Amod, Adri Vorster and Kim Lazarus

Chapter 12 **ADHD Children's Emotion Regulation in FACE© – Perspective (Facilitating Adjustment of Cognition and Emotion): Theory, Research and Practice 243**
Smadar Celestin-Westreich and Leon-Patrice Celestin

Chapter 13 **A Comparison Between Life Quality and Weight-Height Measurements of Patients, Under Stimulant and Non-Stimulant Treatment due to Attention-Deficit and Hyperactivity Disorder, and Healthy Population 285**
Esra Ozdemir Demirci, Merve Cikili Uytun, Rabia Durmus and Didem Behice Oztop

Section 6 Ethical Issues 305

Chapter 14 **Ethical Concerns Raised by Neuroscience, Labeling, and Intervening in the Lives of Individuals with ADHD 307**
Debby Zambo

Preface

A few topics in child mental health have sparked continued interest and controversy. Attention Deficit Hyperactivity Disorder (ADHD) is one of them. ADHD is a developmental disorder of behavioural inhibition and self-regulation. Since its first description by George Frederick Still in 1902, this clinical diagnosis had many name changes as well as changes in the diagnosis criteria. Despite many researches the exact cause of ADHD is still not known. Epidemiological studies have estimated its prevalence between 5% and 10%. Many of our colleagues doubt if it even exists as an entity. There are stories in TV and media about its over-diagnosis and treatment with drugs that are life-threatening.

Despite this hue and cry, the diagnosis and management approach have very little changes over last 30 or 40 years. Despite some fine tuning in diagnosis and management, we still rely on clinical judgement to make the diagnosis and management plan. Children/ Adolescents with ADHD perceive the world differently from others. Awareness and understanding of this increasingly recognised entity is the need of the hour.

ADHD is primarily a condition of brain dysfunction, involving many sites in the brain. There is much more to ADHD than just hyperactivity. This book aims to encourage further reading and research in ADHD. ADHD is a combination of "nature" versus "nature". The topics covered in the book plan to improve quality of lives in children with ADHD and in their family members. This book is intended to provide an overview rather than act as an exhaustive guide. It is hoped that many readers among mental health professionals all over the world will find this book to contribute in the field of ADHD. Finally this book would not have been possible without the able guidance of Ms Mirna Cvijic, the commissioning editor.

Dr Somnath Banerjee
MBBS, DCH, MRCPCH, MSc community Paediatrics, FRCPCH
Community Paediatrician
East Kent Hospitals University NHS Foundation Trust
Dover, Kent, UK

Section 1

Introduction

Chapter 1

ADHD Through Different Developmental Stages

Hojka Gregoric Kumperscak

Additional information is available at the end of the chapter

http://dx.doi.org/10.5772/53963

1. Introduction

Persistent and severe impairment of psychological development resulting from a high level of inattentive, restless and impulsive behaviour is classified according to the fourth Diagnostic and Statistical Manual of Mental Disorders (DSM-IV) as attention-deficit/hyperactivity disorder (ADHD) [1] and according to the Tenth International Classification of Diseases (ICD-10) as hyperkinetic disorder (HD) [2]. In both classifications the behaviours to be recognized are very much the same, they differ mostly in the ways the symptoms are weighted and combined into categories. The diagnostic criteria are in general broader in DSM-IV, which is why ADHD is a more common diagnosis. The ICD-10 diagnosis of HD is a narrower category, where nearly all cases of HD fulfil the diagnostic criteria for ADHD [3].

Hyperactivity is the most noticeable symptom group in ADHD. Children are running and climbing excessively, often in very inappropriate situations. They often fidget with their hands or feet when they should seat still. They are always on the go and often act as if driven by a motor. Inattention is the second markmal of ADHD. Children often fail to give close attention to details and make careless mistakes in their schoolwork or in other activities. They do not seem to listen when spoken to directly, they often do not follow through instructions and they fail to finish their schoolwork or other duties. Also, they have difficulties organizing their tasks and activities. They are easily distracted by extraneous stimuli and they tend to be forgetful in their daily activities. The third group of symptoms is impulsivity. Children have difficulty waiting their turn and interrupt or intrude on others.

The term *hyperactivity* in this chapter is restricted to mean the combination of symptoms that define overactive behaviour. The term *ADHD symptoms* is used to refer to the combination of hyperactive, impulsive and inattentive symptoms.

The onset of the disorder is in early childhood, nearly always before the age of 5 and frequently even earlier. It often persists into adolescence and adult life [4]. Up to 65% of children with ADHD continue to experience symptoms as adults, however they manifest differently in different age periods. Hyperactivity, for instance, is seldom a problem in adults. It diminishes through adolescence and causes minimal or manageable problems in adulthood. Impulsivity, on the other hand, can even increase in adolescence but diminishes slightly through adulthood. The majority of ADHD problems in adults is caused by inattention. Adults with ADHD are disorganized, inaccurate, frequently experiencing difficulties in their relationships, at work and with finances [5,6].

Early recognition and treatment of ADHD is crucial, since longitudinal studies indicate that inattentive and restless behaviour is a developmental risk. Untreated ADHD is also a risk for a range of other mental disorders such as conduct disorder, oppositional defiant disorder, depression, and substance abuse or addiction. Many children with ADHD present with school difficulties including poor classroom participation and associated learning disabilities in reading, written expression, or mathematics. As a result, they receive low grades, are retained in a grade level or do not complete the school at the level they started with [4-6].

Untreated ADHD is not only a burden for a person with the disorder and its family, but also for a society in many aspects. For example, young adults with ADHD are more likely to be apprehended for violations of traffic laws and to be cited more often for such violations [7].

The treatment of ADHD must be comprehensive and individually tailored. Psychological interventions, educational change, medication, education and support for parents and/or teachers should be available. Multimodal interventions are usually indicated [4-6]. Most children whose problems are severe enough to receive an ICD-10 diagnosis of HD will need a medication [3]. There are clear guidelines about ADHD treatment including pharmacotherapy, which, however, will not be discussed further in this chapter. The most prescribed group of medication are psychostimulants and atomoxetine [8,9].

2. History

ADHD is not some new diagnosis made-up in these times when there is an increasing need for children to sit longer and learn more. Already back in 1844 H. Hoffman wrote a story about fidget Philip, and in 1890 W. James talked about the attention disorder as a deficit of inhibitory control. In 1932 Kramer and Pollnow introduced the term hyperkinetic syndrome. Only 4 years later (in 1937) the first psychostimulant was available. Strauss and Lethinen used the term minimal cerebral dysfunction to refer to the same symptomatic condition. World Health Organisation (WHO) introduced in ICD-8 hyperkinetic syndrome of childhood, to change it in 1992 to hyperkinetic disorder. American Psychiatric Association (APA), on the other hand, introduced in 1980 the term attention deficit disorder and 7 years later Attention-deficit/hyperactivity disorder (ADHD) [4-6].

Originally, ADHD was thought to be a transient phenomenon because of the tendency for symptoms (especially hyperactivity) to diminish as children reached adolescence. It is now clear that the disorder persists into adolescence and into adulthood, but manifests differently in each developmental stage [6].

3. DSM and ICD categorization

The DSM-IV classification is mostly used in North America and UK, while the ICD-10 is more commonly used in Europe. DSM-V is to come in a year. There was a tendency to bring definitions of ADHD and HD closer together, and indeed the criteria for the identification of inattentive, hyperactive and impulsive symptoms are almost identical (see diagnostic criteria in Table 1). However, there are still significant differences in the number of criteria in each domain required for a diagnosis, the role of inattention, the definition of pervasiveness and the handling of comorbidity. The diagnosis of ADHD requires the presence of six inattentive or six hyperactive-impulsive symptoms, or both. The diagnosis of HD requires at least six inattentive and three hyperactive as well as one impulsive symptom. Both – ICD-10 and DSM-IV – stress that the symptoms must be present by age 7 and in at least two settings (home/school) [1,2].

In DSM-V, the age by which the symptoms should be present is to be changed from 7 to 12 years [10]. One of the reasons for this change is the concern about appropriate criteria for adults. Population survey data indicated that in adults with ADHD, only half recalled onset by age 7 but 95% recalled the onset by age 12 [11].

Because of heterogeneity of symptoms in ADHD, three different subtypes are distinguished in the DSM-IV classification [1]:

- Attention-deficit/hyperactivity disorder, **combined type**: if both criteria A1 and A2 are met for the past 6 months
- Attention-deficit/hyperactivity disorder, **predominantly inattentive type (ADD):** if criterion A1 is met but criterion A2 is not met for the past 6 months
- Attention-deficit/hyperactivity disorder, **predominantly hyperactive-impulsive type**: if criterion A2 is met but criterion A1 is not met for the past 6 months.

HD is a narrower category than ADHD, and it appears that nearly all cases of HD fulfil the diagnostic criteria of ADHD [3]. Most of the children fulfilling the ADHD diagnostic criteria are not particularly impaired [6]. On the other hand, children with HD constitute the most severe 20% of those with ADHD [6]. Both diagnostic schemes (DSM and ICD) have their advantages and disadvantages. When assessing an individual child, first the fulfilment of the ADHD criteria is checked, and if the latter are met, the HD criteria fulfilment is checked as next. If the diagnostic criteria for HD are met, medication will be included in the treatment approaches available [3].

Essential components of a full assessment process include a clinical interview, medical examination and administration of rating scales to patients, parents and teachers. There are broad-band instruments that evaluate general behavioural and psychosocial functioning, among most used one being the Strengths and Difficulties Questionnaire (SDQ), Achenbach scales and Conners' Rating Scales (CRS) [8].

A. Either (1) or (2):
(1) six (or more) of the following symptoms of inattention have persisted for at least 6 months to a degree that is maladaptive and inconsistent with developmental level:
Inattention
(a) often fails to give close attention to details or makes careless mistakes in schoolwork, work, or other activities (b) often has difficulty sustaining attention in tasks or play activities (c) often does not seem to listen when spoken to directly (d) often does not follow through on instructions and fails to finish schoolwork, chores, or duties in the workplace (not due to oppositional behavior or failure to understand instructions) (e) often has difficulty organizing tasks and activities (f) often avoids, dislikes, or is reluctant to engage in tasks that require sustained mental effort (such as schoolwork or homework) (g) often loses things necessary for tasks or activities (e.g., toys, school assignments, pencils, books, or tools) (h) is often easily distracted by extraneous stimuli (i) is often forgetful in daily activities
(2) six (or more) of the following symptoms of hyperactivity/impulsivity have persisted for at least 6 months to a degree that is maladaptive and inconsistent with developmental level:
Hyperactivity
(a) often fidgets with hands or feet or squirms in seat (b) often leaves seat in classroom or in other situations in which remaining seated is expected (c) often runs about or climbs excessively in situations in which it is inappropriate (in adolescents or adults, may be limited to subjective feelings of restlessness) (d) often has difficulty playing or engaging in leisure activities quietly (e) is often "on the go" or often acts as if "driven by a motor" (f) often talks excessively
Impulsivity
(g) often blurts out answers before questions have been completed (h) often has difficulty awaiting turn (i) often interrupts or intrudes on others (e.g., butts into conversations or games)
B. Some hyperactive-impulsive or inattentive symptoms that caused impairment were present before age 7 years.
C. Some impairment from the symptoms is present in two or more settings (e.g., at school [or work] and at home).
D. There must be clear evidence of clinically significant impairment in social, academic, or occupational functioning.
E. The symptoms do not occur exclusively during the course of a pervasive developmental disorder, schizophrenia, or other psychotic disorder and are not better accounted for by another mental disorder (e.g., mood disorder, anxiety disorder, dissociative disorder, or a personality disorder).

Table 1. Diagnostic criteria according to DSM-IV for attention-deficit/hyperactivity disorder [1].

http://dx.doi.org/10.5772/53963

4. ADHD through different developmental stages

The only constant of ADHD symptoms is that they are changing in each particular child. Not only from day to day, but also with development. In pre-school children, hyperactivity is most obvious and impairing. Inattention becomes more salient once a child confronts school demands. In adolescence and adulthood, hyperactivity diminishes, and inattention and impulsiveness become most impairing, especially in social situations.

4.1. ADHD in children

4.1.1. Epidemiology

The prevalence of ADHD depends on the diagnostic measures used. In [12] survey, 10% of the children in one elementary school in North Carolina had been given the diagnosis of ADHD and 7% were taking medication [12]. An epidemiological study found a cumulative incidence of ADHD in the elementary and secondary school population of 7.5% [13]. The rate of lifetime childhood diagnosis of ADHD in another study [14] was 7.8%, 4.3% were treated with medication [14]. Prevalence for HD is of course smaller, it is 1–3% for children aged 6–14 years [4].

The ratio males : females is around 3 : 1, the prevalence is highest among school-aged boys, and lowest in girls. But the prevalence in girls is more stable across the age [6].

4.1.2. Clinical picture

Hyperactivity is the most obvious and impairing symptom in children. At playing, hyperactive children are more often off-task and spend less time on a particular activity than their non-hyperactive peers [6]. Hyperactive children are more active through the day [6]. Many children without ADHD are occasionally hyperactive to some extent and this normal hyperactivity should not be confused with the more severe and persistent hyperactivity seen in ADHD children. In ADHD hyperactivity is frequent, severe and persistent and most importantly it interferes with a child's peer and parental relationships, impeding their school performance and undermining their psychological well- being [6]. Not to forget that there must be six symptoms from the hyperactivity domain present plus the criterion C (two or more settings) plus criterion D (clear evidence of clinically significant impairment in social, academic, or occupational functioning) to fulfil DSM-IV diagnostic criteria for ADHD [1].

Lack of hyperactivity, on the other hand, does not mean that a child does not have ADHD. Inattentiveness is the most overlooked symptom, especially in pre-school children and in particular in girls. Inattentive children are quiet, day-dreaming, sitting in the last row of the classroom without bothering/disturbing anyone. They have "dreamy" symptoms, typical for attention deficit disorder (ADD) [15] such as:

- difficulties in following instructions and organizing tasks
- tendency to avoid tasks

• forgetfulness and tendency to lose things

Among ADHD subtypes, combined type seems to be the most common (43%), and also the most severe and persistent one [15]. On the other hand, in [16] study the ADD type emerged as the most prevalent. This study also revealed lower male : female ratios in ADHD diagnoses than other studies, which implies that females and the ADD subtype could be underdiagnosed and/or undertreated [16].

Many children with ADHD present with school difficulties including failure to complete their homework, poor test preparation and test-taking skills, poor organizational skills, poor understanding of material, poor classroom participation and failure to ask teachers for needed help, disruptive behaviour in the classroom, and truancy. Children with ADHD who are constantly singled out by their teachers and parents to "sit down" and "be quiet," eventually have a negative perception (low self-esteem) of themselves. By age 10, these children are often behind their peers in terms of social and academic skills [17].

The social and academic impairments of children with ADHD cause stress within the family. Parents can become worried and anxious. Confronted with frustration, anger and self-blame can present with lower self-esteem as parents and as a family. The family seeks a social isolation, often self-imposed. It is difficult to determine if these effects are a result of parenting a child with ADHD or if the parental psychopathology is contributing to the child's psychological reaction and disorder [6,17].

As ADHD is among most heritable of psychiatric disorders with a high risk for familial aggregation, it is quite common that ADHD children have parents with the same disease. This fact further complicates the assessment, treatment and the course of disease. ADHD parents may have impairment across a variety of domains, including parenting [18], which could be the reason why many needed changes in a daily life of a child and family cannot/are harder to be indorsed. 20% to 40% are likely to have the disorder themselves [19]. Families of children with ADHD display higher rates of alcoholism, substance abuse and depression than families of children with Down's syndrome [20].

4.1.3. Comorbidity

Over 50% of children with ADHD have also comorbid disorders [4-6]. 35–50% have oppositional-defiant disorder, 25% conduct disorder, 15% are depressed and 25% have anxiety disorder [6]. Learning disorder occurs in 15–40% of children, particularly among ADD. Language impairment is present in 15–75% of children with ADHD [21,22].

Epilepsy is commoner in ADHD children compared with general population. 36% of children with epilepsy met DSM-IV criteria for ADHD. Neither seizure type nor focus of electroencephalographic (EEG) discharge predict the occurrence of ADHD, but there is a tendency for ADHD to occur more frequently in those with generalized seizures [23].

http://dx.doi.org/10.5772/53963

4.1.4. Course and prognosis

As normal children develop better impulse control, attention focus, other executive functions, and ability to remain calm as they mature, so do those with ADHD, just at slower pace, lagging behind their age mates – usually never reaching them [5]. Various factors have been suggested as predictors of persistence of ADHD symptoms into adolescence and adulthood (among them family history of ADHD, childhood severity of ADHD, psychiatric comorbidity and psychological adversity, impact of treatment) [15]. Among all the factors, studies have found that the childhood ADHD severity is a strongest predictor of persistence of ADHD into adolescence and adulthood [5,24].

Regarding the impact of treatment (intensity and type) on ADHD outcome, the MTA study found that neither the type nor intensity of 14 months of treatment for ADHD in childhood (at age 7.0–9.9 years old) does not predict functioning six-to-eight years later. Rather, early ADHD symptom trajectory regardless of treatment type is prognostic. This finding implies that children with behavioural and sociodemographic advantage, with the best response to any treatment, will have the best long-term prognosis [24]. The same study also found that as a group, however, despite initial symptom improvement during treatment that is largely maintained post-treatment, children with combined-type ADHD exhibit significant impairment in adolescence [24].

Across the life span, unmanaged ADHD can contribute to problems in social and academic settings that coincide with the child's developmental level. These are:

- Disruptive behaviour
- Oppositional defiant disorder
- Poor academic performance and learning delay
- Low self-esteem
- Poor social skills
- Parent-child relationship difficulties
- Physical injury

A review study found that children treated with stimulants for as long as 2 years showed improvement in ADHD symptoms, comorbid oppositional defiant disorder and academic and school functioning [25].

4.2. ADHD in adolescents

4.2.1. Epidemiology

ADHD does not remit with the onset of puberty. Follow-up studies show that a majority (60–85%) of children with ADHD will continue to meet criteria for the disorder during teenage years (ages 13-18 years) [26].

4.2.2. Clinical picture

At adolescence, symptoms of hyperactivity and impulsivity related to ADHD tend to diminish in intensity and are replaced with an inner restlessness, unableness to relax and feelings of unhappiness when not occupied [5]. Impulsivity presents in adolescents as interruptions of others, quick decisions, multitasking and feeling down when not occupied and feeling up when something is happening [5]. Inattention presents as disorganization, poor time management, not listening to what is being said and as forgetfulness.

The [15] study found variations within ADHD subtypes in children and adolescents in the clinical population. Combined subtype is the most common one in childhood (43%), but in adolescence ADD subtype is more common (64%) [15].

Symptoms of ADHD in adolescence most often manifest during instructional or vocational situations. ADHD adolescents show signs of procrastination and disorganization with schoolwork. 46.3% of them did not complete high school and 29.3% retained a grade level at least once and 10.6% have been suspended from school. Feelings of tension, apprehension, the need for reassurance, irritability, negative self-image, and physical complaints are reported in more than 70% of ADHD patients [7, 27].

4.2.3. Comorbidity

ADHD in adolescence, especially if not treated can result in further complication (school suspension and/or expulsion, social exclusion, poor motivation, teen pregnancy, driving accidents) and comorbid disorders (substance abuse or dependence, mood disorders, conduct disorders) [7, 17, 28].

Adolescents with (untreated) ADHD are more prone to substance abuse than their peers. In a [29] study the cumulative incidence of substance abuse disorders throughout adolescence was compared in 56 medicated ADHD patients, 19 non-medicated ADHD patients, and 137 non-ADHD control subjects. The analysis was restricted to male subjects older than 15 years of age. Substance abuse disorder was defined as any diagnosis of any of the following: alcohol abuse/dependence (A/D), marijuana A/D, hallucinogen A/D, stimulant A/D, and cocaine A/D [29]. Non-medicated ADHD patients were at a significantly higher risk for substance abuse than either controls or medicated ADHD patients during the follow-up period of 4 years. However, there was no significant difference between medicated ADHD patients and controls. Medication was found to be associated with an 85% reduction in the risk of substance abuse in ADHD patients [29].

ADHD and substance use disorder (SUD) may share also biological factors. Familial association between ADHD and SUD is strong, which suggests that two disorders may share genetic or other familial factors. The offspring of SUD parents are at greater risk not only for SUD, but also for inattention, impulsivity, aggressiveness, hyperactivity and ADHD [28].

4.2.4. Course and prognosis

It remains difficult to predict persistence of ADHD into adulthood. Controlling for severity and excluding treatment, none of the other variables (sociodemographics, childhood adversity, traumatic life experiences and comorbidity) significantly predicted persistence, even though they were significantly associated with childhood ADHD [30]. Many studies reported adult persistence was much greater for inattention than for hyperactivity/impulsivity [6,30].

4.3. ADHD in adults

4.3.1. Epidemiology

Being diagnosed with ADHD as an adult actually means that the condition has been present since childhood, it just was not recognized or diagnosed at that time. Many follow-up studies consistently documented the persistence of ADHD into adulthood, but the level of persistence has been inconsistent across studies [4-6, 31].

The first reason is the methodological, which includes changes in informant (patient's parents versus adult patient), use of different instruments to diagnose ADHD in adults, comorbidity and diagnostic criteria [31]. Diagnostic criteria are designed for school-aged children with regard to the number of symptoms required to meet the diagnostic threshold, which can be developmentally inappropriate for adults. Adults can suffer significant impairment even though they have fewer than six of nine symptoms needed for the diagnosis. The second reason is that differences in reported remission rates reflected the definition used for remission rather than disorder's course [31].

The persistence of the full syndrome of ADHD in adulthood has been found to be between 2–8% when self-report is used [31]. When parent report is used, the prevalence increases to 46% [28]. The [30] study reported that 1 in 3 childhood ADHD still met DSM-IV criteria when aged 18- to 44-years [30]. In [32] study 40% of 18- to 20-year-old "grown up" ADHD patients met full criteria for ADHD, but 90% had at least five symptoms of ADHD [32].

Taking all studies together, the rates of syndromatic remission of ADHD in adults are quite in agreement; from 60% [32] to 65%–70% [33]. But majority of subjects continue to struggle with substantial number of ADHD symptoms and high levels of dysfunction despite a sizable rate of syndromatic remission by age 20 [32].

4.3.2. Clinical picture

ADHD symptoms in adults manifest quite differently from the way they manifest in children. Hyperactivity is not impairing any more. It is rare to see ADHD adults fidgeting and/or running around. But some adult ADHD patients seem jittery and have trouble sitting still. Some complain of having "ants in their pants" and may experience an irritating need to pace [34]. Adults can learn through time to manage to settle their hyperactivity through exercise or hard physical work. But if they are temporarily immobilized (broken leg, somatic illness) and are suddenly deprived of a coping method, their hyperactivity can present as aggression and/or agitation [34].

Symptoms of inattentiveness and impulsivity in adults manifest as [34]:

- forgetfulness, particularly if it involves remembering tasks or jobs that need to be done. They are often losing household items.
- unableness to keep track of several things at once
- difficulties in keeping promises or commitments to others
- making decisions impulsively, or on the spur of the moment, without thinking about the consequences
- frequently misjudge how much time they have – or need – to do something. They express difficulty with being on time.
- being unable to tear themselves away from something enjoyable to shift to a more urgent, important task
- they describe themselves having quick temper and low tolerance for frustration

Adults with (untreated) ADHD are at greater risk for further complications compared with general population: changing jobs and partners, unstable relationships, financial problems, involvedness in car accidents, injuries, crime, and substance abuse. 16-year follow-up study found that men who had ADHD as boys were significantly more likely to be financially dependent on their parents, less likely to graduate from college, and had a lower social class than controls. These functional deficits are likely to be aggravated by the higher levels of neuropsychological impairment, which was observed on psychometric tests and on behavioural measures of executive dysfunction [35].

In Norway study, only 22.2% adult ADHD patients had ordinary work as their source of income, compared with 72% in the general population [36]. Approximately 48% had junior high school as their highest degree of education, compared with 29.8% in the general Norwegian population. Thus, more than half had an educational level not suited for most domains in the work market. Only 8.9% had a college or university degree, compared with 20.8% in the general population. 33% of ADHD patients were receiving disability pension and 38% temporary social benefits. Maybe the most interesting founding in this study was the fact that only 17.4% of participants with adult ADHD had been treated with central stimulants by the age of 18. Results are suggesting that early recognition and drug treatment of ADHD might protect against occupational impairment in adulthood [36].

Young adult drivers with ADHD were found to be nearly twice as likely to be cited for unlawful speeding and to be cited more than three times as often as young adult subjects in the control group. Drivers with ADHD had more than 5 times as many traffic citations on their records than did controls [7].

http://dx.doi.org/10.5772/53963

4.3.3. Comorbidity

As in children and adolescents, adult ADHD is often present with comorbid disorders, which makes an accurate diagnosis even more difficult. Studies suggest that up to 90% of adult patients with ADHD have one or more comorbid psychiatric disorders [37]. The most common comorbid disorders in adults are anxiety disorders, affective disorders, substance abuse and antisocial personality disorder. In [36] study, the most prevalent comorbid disorders were lifetime depression (37.8%), substance abuse (28.1%) and alcohol abuse (23.3%), 14.6% had anxiety disorder. More than 19% had received a diagnosis of personality disorder. Interesting in this study was that more women then men had comorbid borderline personality disorder [36]. It is important to know that comorbid psychiatrics disorders emerge early on in development in childhood and adolescence [38].

Bipolar disorder coexists with adult ADHD in 6–20% cases. Many ADHD symptoms can be mistakenly attributed to and overlooked because of bipolar disorder [37]. Interesting results were found in [39] study, namely that ADHD brings significant impairment to bipolar patients, especially in adaptation and social functioning, compared with bipolar patients without comorbid ADHD. Even more interestingly, the authors failed to detect a significant impact of substance abuse on those same functional outcomes. This stresses out importance of making an accurate diagnosis of ADHD also in patients where the symptomatology (impulsiveness, multitasking, not finishing work, changing partners etc.) can be incorporated in another diagnosis (bipolar disorder) [39].

The high prevalence of comorbidity complicates the diagnostic process as well as treatment and some studies indicate that high rates of comorbidity in adult ADHD contribute negatively to the treatment outcome [40].

Follow-up periods into adulthood showed that stimulant treatment in childhood also was beneficial for social skills and self-esteem. Higher doses and longer treatment period predicted less comorbidity and better social functioning [25].

ADHD in adults have striking similarities with paediatric samples regarding psychiatric and cognitive impairment [41]. Some study suggest that the effect of stimulants is similar in paediatric and adult samples, which is a reason to believe that adult patients also will have long-term positive outcome [42].

5. Case report

8-year-old boy was admitted to Child and Adolescent Psychiatry Unit because he had been experiencing increasing behavioural problems in the school during the last 3 months. He also showed slowness in mental tasks, was very impulsive, self-willed, irritable and displayed enhanced verbal and physical aggression. *History of problems* revealed delayed schooling because of expressive language disorder. He was in the first grade of the primary school at admission, while his peers where in the second grade. His mother presented a list of complaints as if they were copied from the ADHD diagnostic criteria – he was always "on the go", running and climbing whenever possible, when needed to sit still he was fidgeting, he talked excessively, blurted out answers, he could not await his turn, he intruded on others, did not listen to what was being said, lost things daily, was easily distracted and his school work was a disaster.

Developmental history revealed a risk pregnancy with malpresentation (not head down position of a fetus). He was the third child, prematurely born, with icterus and apnoeic attacks. He was lagging in motor development (he walked independently at the age of 20 months) and in language development (spoke the first words at the age of 3, he visited speech and language therapist).

Family history was interesting since his father had symptoms of ADHD in his youth. One of his two brothers uttered the first words at the age of five. *General assessment at admission* showed clumsiness and stuttering. *Further observations* showed that he was easily distracted, had lapses in attention, was overactive, impulsive and impatient. He usually acted without thinking, behaved inappropriately, was verbally and physically aggressive towards co-patients and medical staff, testing the limits all the time and showing stubbornness. He also seemed unhappy, sad and angry with sudden changes in mood.

Neuropsychological tests found organic-cerebral dysfunction, psychomotor and visuospatial disturbances and profound attention deficit with hyperactivity. His IQ at the time of testing was borderline due to severe inattention and hyperactivity. He presented with diminished inhibition, showed personally and emotionally less mature compared with his peers and he has been found as quite egocentric. *Basic laboratory tests* (including thyroid levels) and EEG were normal.

The boy fulfilled DSM-IV diagnostic criteria for ADHD – combined type. Because of his changing mood and aggressive periods which were new in his behaviour, bipolar disorder was considered as a possible *differential diagnosis or comorbid disorder*. His hyperactivity existed ever since he was born and was not episodic (which is typical for hyperactivity in bipolar disorder). He was easily distracted and mostly did not finish his tasks – but not because of flight of ideas, thought racing or delusions as seen in manic episodes. He was impulsive, blurting answers and interrupting – again not because of pressured speech or impulsive poor judgment as seen in manic episodes. His school performance was bad because of his inattention and not because of the loss of interest – as seen in depressed episodes of bipolar disorder. He was never grandiose and had never any appetite or weight changes often seen in bipolar patients. He was diagnosed as *ADHD combined type with comorbid oppositional-defiant and expressive language disorder*. He received psychostimulants, we educated his parents and his school teachers about the disorder and advised them about the behavioural management techniques. He continued visiting the speech therapists. He responded well to all introduced measures and we followed him for about a year when he moved to another city.

Nine years later (as 17-year-old) he was admitted again to our child and adolescent psychiatry ward. Parents complained about severe behavioural problems lasting for two years. He threatened with suicide several times, had constant difficulties with authority, was disregarding his safety and was involved in a series of injuries and accidents. He changed three secondary schools, without finishing the first year in any of them. He was staying at home during the day, but went out in the evening taking his parent's money. When he took 2000 EUR, they started suspecting drug abuse for the first time

He acted quite aloof at admission. He sat quietly and admitted that he was smoking marihuana regularly for 3 years. He also tried ecstasy and cocaine several times – for the last time the weekend before. He drank alcohol regularly when he was in a company of others, otherwise he was too anxious. He had been playing poker for 3 years twice a week. He complained about his inner restlessness, which disappeared when he was on drugs or at least when he drank something. He revealed that he had rather poor peer relationships – actually he had no friends. He was unable to concentrate in school but had no problems concentrating at poker game or at other pleasure activities (computer games, TV). He felt that he was a loser; obviously he would not finish the school and he thought of suicide quite often.

He had been taking the medication for ADHD for two years (from the age of 8 till the age of 10), but stopped during the summer holidays. As he was no longer as hyperactive as before, his parents decided that he did not need it anymore. With a lot of help of his parents and instructors he somehow managed to finish the primary school, but at great cost – he struggled with extremely low self- esteem.

He was depressed and suicidal; anxious and tense but opponent to parents and medical staff at admission.

Neuropsychological tests at second hospitalization found organic-cerebral dysfunction, psychomotor and visuospatial disturbances as at the first testing. Actual IQ was discrepant with above average on verbal and lower borderline on non-verbal scale. Tests revealed executive deficits with diminished inhibition, planning, controlling and anticipation. Depressive symptomatic was also found.

He was fulfilling the DSM-IV diagnostic criteria for *ADHD – inattentive type and for major depressive disorder.* Again, bipolar disorder was considered as possible diagnosis, but was excluded due to a constant pattern of inattention, impulsive and hyperkinetic problems, without any episodic changes in ADHD or affective symptoms. He was treated with atomoxetine and antidepressants and he attended the program for addicted/at risk adolescents for a year. He managed to finish the first year of the secondary school. Then he stopped taking the medication and attending the program and started with marihuana and occasionally used other drugs again.

5.1. Discussion

Reported case describes prototypic ADHD child regarding the symptomatic and its changing over development, family attitude to medication and family stress, comorbidity in childhood and adolescence, and the course of disease.

It often happens that parents endure with hyperactivity symptoms and seek help only when school performance is critical. In severe ADHD cases, which also fulfil more strict ICD-10 diagnostic criteria for HD, the problems in school performance and behaviour are obvious already in the first grade of primary school and are so severe that parents are faced with the necessity for special assessment and treatment. Comprehensive treatment that includes education and support to parents and teachers, and also pharmacotherapy is very effective. As in presented case, children manage developmental tasks quite well as long the treatment is provided. Hyperactivity symptoms diminish with development and many parents understand this as a signal that the child has grown up of the ADHD and they stop with the treatment.

But in majority of ADHD cases, the symptoms only present differently but continue to interfere further in adolescent/adult life as inner restlessness, tension and irritability. Patients have low school/work performance, are disorganized, have difficulties in social relationships, often abuse drugs, and are engaged in car accidences. As a further burden, the majority of them also have comorbid disorders such as depression, anxiety, bipolar disorder and personality disorder. The stress on family grows and the vicious circle of self-blame, avoidance of social contacts and low self-esteem repeats. In such cases, comprehensive treatment enables better schoolwork, settles inner restlessness and tension, resulting in lower need for drug abuse.

6. Conclusion

ADHD disorder is predominantly diagnosed in childhood, persisting into adolescence and adulthood in majority of cases. With development the symptoms change, which is the reason why many of the adolescent and adult ADHD patients stay unrecognised. High comorbidity in adolescence and adulthood is the second reason for ADHD unrecognition after childhood. The fact is that it is quite difficult to consider ADHD when patients complain about depressive symptoms, drug abuse or have a personality disorder. But with careful personal history which also involves patient's childhood (interview with patient's parents) and with the help of specialized ADHD questionnaires, ADHD can be properly diagnosed.

Comprehensive treatment is crucial in any developmental period. It is essential not only for reducing the core ADHD symptoms, but also for preventing many consequences of untreated ADHD and for ensuring better quality of life for patients and their families.

Author details

Hojka Gregoric Kumperscak

Address all correspondence to: hojka.gregoric@guest.arnes.si

Department of Paediatrics, Child and Adolescents Psychiatry Unit, University Clinical Centre Maribor, Maribor, Slovenia

http://dx.doi.org/10.5772/53963

References

[1] American Psychiatric Association. [1994]. Diagnostic and statistical manual of mental disorders. 4th ed. Washington: the Association.

[2] Classification of mental and behavioural disorders (ICD-10]. World Health Organization, Geneva, 1993.

[3] Taylor E, Dopfner M, Sergeant J et al. European clinical guidelines for hyperkinetic disorder – first upgrade. Eur Child Adolescesc Psychiatry 2004;13 I/7-I/30.

[4] Remschmidt H. Kinder- und Jugendpsychiatry. Stuttgart: Geirg Thieme Verlag; 2005.

[5] Martin A, Volkmar FR. Lewis's child and adolescent psychiatry. New York: Wolters Kluwer, Lippincott Williams&Wilkins; 2007.

[6] Rutter M, Bishop D, Pine D et al. Rutter's child and adolescent psychiatry. Massachusetts: Wiley-Blackwell; 2008.

[7] Barkley RA, Murphy KR, Kwasnik D. Motor vehicle driving competencies and risks in teens and young adults with attention deficit hyperactivity disorder. Pediatrics 1996;98:1089-1095.

[8] National institute for health and clinical excellence. Attention deficit hyperactivity disorder. Diagnosis and management of ADHD in children, young people and adults. London: the British psychological society and the royal college of psychiatrists; 2009.

[9] Pliszka S, Bernet W, Bukstein O, Walter HJ et al. Practical parameter for assessment and treatment of children and adolescents with attention deficit hyperactivity disorder. J Am Acad Child Adolesc Psychiatry 2007; 46[7]:894-921.

[10] APA DSM-5. A 10 attention deficit/hyperactivity disorder. http://www.dsm5.org/ProposedRevisions/Pages

[11] Barkley RA, Brown TE. Unrecognized attention-deficit/hyperactivity disorder in adults presenting with other psychiatric disorders. CNS Spectr 2008; 13[11]: 977-984.

[12] Rowland AS, Umbach DM, Stallone L et al. Prevalence of medication treatment for attention deficit hyperactivity disorder among elementary school children in Johnston County, North Carolina. Am J Public Health 2002;92:231-234.

[13] Bararesi WJ, Katusic SK, Colligan RC et al. How common is attention deficit hyperactivity disorder? Incidence in a population-based birth cohort in Rochester. Minn Arch Pediatr Adolesc Med 2002; 156:217-224.

[14] Centers for disease control and prevention. Prevalence of diagnosis and medication treatment for attention deficit hyperactivity disorder – United States 2003. MMWR Morb Mortal Rep Wkly 2003;54[34]:842-847.

[15] Hurting T, Ebeling H, Taanila A et al. ADHD symptoms and subtypes: relationship between childhood and adolescent symptoms. J Am Acad Child Adolesc Psychiatry 2007; 46[12]:1605-1613.

[16] Ramtekkar UP, Reiersen AM, Todorov A et al. Sex and age differences in attention deficit hyperactivity disorder symptoms and diagnoses: implications for DSM-V and ICD-11. J Am Acad Child Adolesc Psychiatry 2010; 49[3]:217-228.

[17] Barkley RA. Attention Deficit Hyperactivity Disorder. In: Murphy KR, Galdon M. (eds.) A Handbook for Diagnosis and Treatment 2nd Edition. New York: Guildford Publications 1998. p197-203.

[18] Macek J, Gosar D, Tomori M. Is there a correlation between ADHD symptoms expression between parents and children? Neuro Endocrinol Lett 2012; 33[2]:201-6.

[19] Murphy KR, Barkley RA. Parents of children with attention deficit hyperactivity disorder: psychological and attentional impairment. Am J Orthopsychiatry 1996;66:93-102.

[20] Roizen NJ, Blondis TA, Irwin M et al. Psychiatric and developmental disorders in families of children with attention deficit hyperactivity disorder. Archives of Pediatrics & Adolescent Medicine 1996; 150[2]:203-8.

[21] Cohen NJ, Vallance DD, Barwick M et al. The interface between ADHD and language impairment: an examination of language, achievement and cognitive processing. J child Psychology Psychiatr 2000; 41: 353-362.

[22] Tannock R. Attention deficit disorders with learning disorders. In: Brown TE (ed.) Attention deficit disorder and comorbidities in children, adolescents and adults. Wachington DC: American Psychiatric Press; 2000.p231-295.

[23] Dunn DW, Austin JK, Harezlak J et al. ADHD and epilepsy in childhood. Dev Med Child Neurol 2003; 45:50-54.

[24] Molina BSG, Hinshaw SP, Swanson JM et al. The MTA at 8 Years: Prospective Follow-Up of Children Treated for Combined Type ADHD in a Multisite Study. J Am Acad Child Adolesc Psychiatry. 2009 May; 48[5]: 484–500.

[25] Hechtman L, Greenfield B. Long-term use of stimulants in children with attention deficit hyperactivity disorder. Safty, efficacy and long-term outcome. Pediatr Drugs 2003; 5:787-795.

[26] Barkley RA. Against the status qou: revising the diagnostic criteria for ADHD. J Am Acad Child Adolesc Psychiatry 2010; 49[3]:205-207.

[27] Greenhill LL. Diagnosing attention-deficit/hyperactivity disorder in children. J Clin Psychiatry 1998;59(Suppl 7]:31-41.)

[28] Medscape psychiatry & mental health. ADHD and substance use disorders. Biological risk. http://www.medscape.org/viewarticle/542601_2/ (accessed November 2006].

http://dx.doi.org/10.5772/53963

[29] Biederman J, Wilens T, Mick E et al. Pharmacotherapy of attention-deficit/hyperactivity disorder reduces risk for substance use disorder. Pediatrics 1999;104[2]:e20. http://www.pediatrics.org/cgi/content/full/104/2/e20.

[30] Kessler RC, Adler LA, Barkley R. Patterns and predictors of attention deficit hyperactivity disorder persistence into adulthood: results from the national comorbidity survey replication. Biologic psychiatry 2005;57:1442-1451.

[31] Barkley RA. ADHD – long term course, adult outcome and comorbid disorders. In: Jensen PS, Cooper JR (eds.) Attention deficit hyperactivity disorder. State of the science, best practice. Kingston, NJ: Civic research institute; 2002. p4-1-4-12.

[32] Biederman J, Mick E, Faraone SV. Age-dependent decline of symptoms of attention deficit hyperactivity disorder: impact of remission definition and symptom type. Am J Psychiatry 2000; 157:816-818.

[33] Hill JC, Schoener EP. Age-dependent decline of attention deficit hyperactivity disorder. Am J Psychiatry 1996;153:1143-1146.

[34] Young JL. ADHD Grown up. A guide to adolescent and adult ADHD.NY, London: W.W.Norton&Company; 2007.

[35] Biederman J, Petty CR, Woodworth KY et al. Adult outcome of attention deficit hyperactivity disorder: a controlled 16-year follow-up study. J Clin Psychiatry 2012; 73: 941-950.

[36] Gjervan B, Torgersen T, Nordahl HM et al. Functional impairments and occupational outcome in adults with ADHD. J Attention Disorders 2011;XX(X):1-9.

[37] Nutt DJ, Fone K, Asherson P et al. Evidence-based guidelines for management of attention deficit hyperactivity disorder in adolescents in transition to adult services and in adults: recommendations from the British association for psychopharmacology. J Psychopharmacol 2007; 21:10-41.

[38] Biederman J, Monuteaux MC, Mick E et al. Young adult outcome of attention deficit hyperactivity disorder: a controlled 10-year follow-up study. Psychol Med 2006;36[2]: 167-179.

[39] Sentissi O, Navarro JC, De Oliveira H. Bipolar disorder and quality of life: impact of ADHD and substance abuse in euthymic patients. Psychiatry Res 2008;30:36-42.

[40] Jensen PS, Martin D, Cantwell DP. Comorbidity in ADHD: implications for research, practice, and DSM-V. J Am Acad Child Adolesc psychiatry 1997; 36:1065-1079.

[41] Biederman J, Faraone SV, Monuteaux MC et al. Gender effects on attention deficit hyperactivity disorder in adults, revised. Biol Psychiatry 2004;55:692-700.

[42] Faraone SV, Spencer T, Aleardi M et al. Meta-analysis of the efficacy of methylphenidate for treating adult attention deficit hyperactivity disorder. J Clin Psychopharm 2004;24:24-29.

Chapter 2

Neurodevelopmental Pathways of Childhood ADHD into Adulthood: Maturational Lag, Deviation, or Both?

Alban Burke and Amanda Edge

Additional information is available at the end of the chapter

http://dx.doi.org/10.5772/53865

1. Introduction

The DSM-5 [1], which should be published in 2013, will in all likelihood have a category named Neurodevelopmental Disorders, under which ADHD will resort. This shift in nosology lays the foundation of the argument that will be put forward in this chapter, therefore the following points need to be emphasised and warrants further discussion. Firstly, this categorisation is based on shared aetiology, rather than shared symptoms or shared developmental stage (as was the case with the DSM-IV-TR). Historically, disorders were classified according to shared aetiology (as was the case with DSMI and DSM-II), as opposed to shared symptomatology (as was the case with DSM-III and DSM-IVTR). The DSM-5 is to a greater, or lesser, extent a combination of these as it proposes a change to the categorisation, but not the symptoms of this disorder.

The second point is that the shared aetiology is a *neurobiological based aetiology*. The name of the category implies that these disorders have a common, underlying, neurobiological cause. The question which arises is to what extent these disorders do have an underlying neurobiological cause, to what extent this is shared, and even to what extent these causes are shared within the sub-categories of disorders, for example ADHD. Grouping these disorders together implies a relatively homogenous group of disorders, and even further that the sub-categories are homogenous within themselves. The DSM-5 makes provision for 4 sub-categories of ADHD, i.e. the *Combined, Predominantly Inattentive, Inattentive (Restrictive)* and predominantly *Hyperactive/ Impulsive*, presentations. Does the grouping of these sub-categories necessarily imply that they share the same neurobiological aetiology? The argument that will be put forward in this chapter is that although they all share a neurobiological cause, this cause is not common and that the sub- categories may have subtle or gross, differences in these neurobiological factors.

The name of the category also implies a more fluid and dynamic process that starts in childhood and may, or may not, extend across the lifespan into adulthood. This is in sharp contrast to the more traditional, and rather rigid, distinction between adulthood and childhood pathologies. This category allows for the straddling between childhood and adulthood pathologies. An important point, which warrants emphasis, is that these disorders typically *originate in childhood,* which may then extend into adulthood. Again, in sharp contrast to the previous DSM classifications, the DSM-5 makes slightly more provision for ADHD in adulthood. As far as the specific criteria, as well as the sub-categories, are concerned, the criteria for ADHD in adulthood are rather superficial as it does not include the rather extensive research that has been done on the clinical manifestation of this disorder in adulthood, nor is it explicit enough in terms of possible sub-categories of this disorder in adulthood. This creates a picture of a rather homogenous disorder in adulthood which either influences, or is perpetuated by, research on this topic.

As much as many Mental Health professionals would like to accept that the diagnosis of ADHD in adulthood is a valid one, there is also still much scepticism about both the validity of this disorder, as well as the clinical picture / diagnostic criteria. Some authors [2] postulate that this scepticism may also be due to extensive, but poorly described, comorbid Axis I and Axis II disorders. Although some may consider ADHD and Personality Disorders (specifically Cluster B) to be co-morbid conditions, there are also those that would argue that these Personality Disorders are often misdiagnosed as ADHD, or *vice versa* [3]. The roots of the dilemma are twofold, i.e. that Personality Disorders are a separate and distinct set of disorders that do not have a biological underpinning and the arbitrary distinction between childhood and adult pathology. If one removes both these problematic issues, and rather view a disorder in terms of the aberrant development of behaviour, (neuro)cognition and emotion (as opposed to "personality") over time (rather than in life stages), a different picture, i.e. one of either maturational lag or maturational deviance, emerges. The neurodevelopmental disorders, such as ADHD, are associated with a unique temperament that is characterised by high novelty seeking, harm avoidance and low reward dependence [3]. The question that arises is whether the neurodevelopmental and personality disorders are the result of the same underlying neurological process, or whether they are parallel processes that may or may not have reciprocal effects on each other [4]. On a theoretical level, i.e. the maturational lag theory, these two categories of disorders may be considered together, if it is indeed that the maturational lag theory holds true for both of them.

2. Neurodevelopment of ADHD

The use of the concept neurodevelopment in the categorisation and organisation of disorders in the DSM-5 suggests that variant disorders can be arranged according to specific neurodevelopmental pathways. It is understood that the developmental pathway may account for the neurobiological underpinnings, and thus aetiological foundation of the syndrome observed. Two neurodevelopmental models, namely the *maturational lag model* and the *develop-*

mental deviation model, appear to be particularly relevant to the syndrome of ADHD. In this section evidence supporting these two views will be reported.

2.1. Maturational lag in ADHD

While some evidence has suggested that the ADHD brain develops in fundamentally different ways to typical ones, other results have argued that they are just the result of a lag in the normal timetable for development, which is known as the maturational lag model [5]. This model of ADHD is organised around the notion that that the behaviours of a child with ADHD is abnormal merely in reference to his or her age [5]. This direction in thinking was initially based on observations that children with ADHD behave similarly to younger children who are more active, impulsive and exhibit a shorter attention span [6]. According to this model [5], "if the child was younger, the findings would be regarded as normal" (p. 268). He further postulates that the neurological factors that limit the performance of a child with ADHD are synonymous to that which typically limits the performance of younger children. Hence, the maturational lag model [5] stipulates that an individual with ADHD presents with a relative delay in certain aspects of their neurological maturation, but that maturation will eventually 'catch up'. On average, the brain of ADHD children matured about three years later than those of their peers, with 50% of their cortex only reaching maximum thickness at age 10 years 6 months as opposed to 7 years and 6 months of those children without ADHD [7]. The lags in maturation seem to differ from one cortical area to the next, for example, the lag in the prefrontal cortex can be as high as 5 years. In other areas, the ADHD brain seems to mature faster than in a non-ADHD brain, an example being the primary motor cortex. These researchers draw the conclusion that their findings support the hypothesis of maturational lag, not maturational deviance.

Nearly 50 years of electrophysiological (EEG) research in the realm of ADHD suggest that children and adolescents who present with the disorder display abnormalities in their EEG [8]. The abnormalities observed are either organised according to the maturational lag or developmental deviation model. From an EEG perspective, the maturational lag model suggests that an individual with ADHD should present with cortical activity that is similar to that witnessed in younger children [9, 10], since an increase in slow wave activity (delta and theta) and decreased fast wave activity (alpha and beta) is typical in younger children [11]. A number of researchers [12-16] interpret their findings of increased slow wave activity in children and adolescents with ADHD during an eyes closed resting condition as evidence of a maturational lag. Additional EEG support for the maturational lag is presented in Table 1.

2.2. Maturational deviance in ADHD

The second neurodevelopmental model is that of the developmental deviation, also known as maturational deviance, which proposes that maturation is not necessarily lagging, but that it is not approaching normality or maturation, and that it is unlikely to do so at any stage during the lifespan. This model was built on EEG research where 90% of the ADHD sample presented with aberrances in their EEG activity [17]. Subsequently, the developmental deviation model of ADHD came into play, which suggests that ADHD results from abnormalities in CNS functioning [9]. It further denotes that the EEGs of children and adolescents with ADHD symptoms are not considered normal in children of any age and that it is also not likely to mature in a normal fashion [9]. Additional evidence for this model is provided by the adult ADHD (ADHD) studies which found that the presence of elevated slow wave activity, especially theta, persists into adulthood [18-19].

2.3. Summary and conclusion

The research referred to in this section was concerned with the investigation of cortical activity patterns in adults with ADHD via EEG methodologies. The research was specifically interested in the cortical activity patterns of adults with ADHD symptomatology at frontal, frontal midline and parietal sites seeing that these areas are often the most heavily implicated in ADHD. From existing literature, it can be concluded that there is evidence that supports both the maturational lag as well as the maturational deviance models (See Table 1).

EEG Based Model	Description of Model	EEG Findings	References
Maturational Lag	Individuals with ADHD symptoms present with cortical activity patterns that is similar to that witnessed in younger children	Increased relative and/or absolute slow wave activity and decreased relative and/or absolute fast wave activity Increased frontal relative and/or absolute theta Increased absolute and/or relative delta in temporal and parietal sites Decreased relative and/or absolute alpha and beta power in temporal and parietal sites	[8 -16, 20 – 27]
Developmental Deviation	ADHD symptoms result from abnormalities in CNS functioning. The EEGs of individuals with ADHD symptoms are not considered normal in individuals of any age and is not likely to mature in a normal fashion.	Increased absolute and/or relative theta activity in frontal and frontal midline sites. Decreased relative alpha activity in parietal and temporal sites. Decreased absolute and relative beta activity in frontal, parietal and temporal sites Elevated theta/beta and theta/alpha ratios	[9,19,26,28, 29]

Table 1. EEG support for the maturational lag and developmental deviation models

3. Personality disorders

Personality and psychopathology have, throughout the 20th century, been viewed as separate but related domains. Although they have been viewed as related domains, the exact relationship remains largely unclear. In 1980, within psychopathology, clinical syndromes were separated from personality disorders [34]. Splitting these domains highlighted the overlap between symptoms of clinical and personality disorders [34], which is also the foundation for on-going debates concerning the comorbidity between ADHD in adulthood and personality disorders. If one adopts a neurobiological / neurocognitive approach to personality, then the overlap between temperament, personality and personality disorders becomes more evident. Furthermore, given the mounting evidence that ADHD can persist from childhood into adulthood, it also follows that there should be more focus on the relationship between personality and ADHD [35]. Some authors [36] maintain that is important to describe ADHD in adulthood in terms of general personality structures as it could contribute to a better conceptualization of the disorder. Furthermore, there are suggestions that there is evidence that indicates that developmental factors may contribute to ADHD in ways that are separate from the associated behaviour problems. One could go further by saying that it is important to describe personality disorders (from a neurobiological perspective) in adults with ADHD, as this could aid in describing a possible shared aetiology. In fact one could go as far as to say that incomplete descriptions of Personality Disorders in ADHD continue to place pressure on the validity of the diagnosis in adulthood [2]. Although there have been a number of studies that have focused on the relationship between ADHD and personality, some authors [35] maintain that these studies have focussed on only a narrow range of personality constructs. Table 2 provides a summary of personality constructs that have been investigated in relation to ADHD, as well as how these characteristics may feature in personality disorders.

Construct	Characteristic of ADHD	Characteristic of Cluster B Personality Disorder
Sensation Seeking / External stimulation seeking	[38, 39]	Antisocial [49]
Behavioural disinhibition / Impulsivity	[40, 41]	Antisocial and Borderline [45] Borderline [46, 48, 51]
Self-regulation	[40]	Borderline, Antisocial and Histrionic [50] Axis II disorders [52]
Externalizing problem behaviours	[42]	Antisocial [50]
Emotional lability	[41]	Borderline [44] Antisocial and Borderline [45]
Low reward dependence	[43]	Antisocial [47]
Uncooperativeness	[43]	Borderline [46]

Table 2. Summary of personality constructs identified in ADHD and possible links with Cluster B disorders

There has traditionally been a great but, arguably unwarranted [43], emphasis on the prevalence of Cluster B personality disorder in adults with ADHD. This study, in effect wants to investigate whether there is some shared neurodevelopmental process in both of these sets of disorders. The argument is based on the following postulates:

- ADHD is a neurodevelopmental disorder and is the result of either maturational lag or maturational deviation

- In some cases ADHD does not continue beyond adolescence (which is in line with the maturational lag hypothesis), however
- ADHD may continue into adulthood, which cannot be explained fully by the maturational lag hypothesis.
- The is a reportedly high prevalence of personality disorders in adults with ADHD
- There is evidence of both maturational lag and deviation processes in personality disorders.

If these postulates are correct, the question that arises is whether these two disorders could be the result of the same neurodevelopmental process. Most, if not all, of the characteristics mentioned in Table 2 have an underlying neuropsychological or neurobiological correlate. These neurobiological correlates may be the result of either a maturational lag or maturational deviance process, depending on which personality disorder one focuses on. One way of distinguishing between these two hypotheses, would be to consider the course and prognosis of the different personality disorders. Regarding the Cluster B personality disorders, two interesting pictures evolve when reviewing course and prognosis, and these may, arguably be classified as maturational lag or maturational deviation.

3.1. Maturational lag

The roots of the development of Antisocial Personality Disorder can be traced to early adolescence (i.e. Conduct Disorder) which then follows an unremitting course, with a variable outcome. There is some evidence that suggests that the symptoms decrease with age [53]. The fact that the symptoms may decrease with age, is somewhat suggestive of a delayed maturation process [54]. A further indication of a maturational lag is the fact that there is excessive theta wave activity, while awake, which is akin to what is evident in younger children [54]. One explanation for this could be the temporal discounting paradigm which quantifies the ability to favour larger, delayed rewards over smaller, more immediate rewards. Temporal discounting matures with age, along with increased impulse control and self-regulation. This maturation seems to be associated with changes in activation of the ventromedial prefrontal cortex, anterior cingulate cortex, ventral striatum, insula, inferior temporal gyrus and posterior parietal cortex [55].

Although it is reported that adults with a histrionic personality disorder display less symptoms as they age [53], it is uncertain whether this is truly due symptoms diminishing due to maturation, or whether this is merely due to a decline in energy levels due to aging.

3.2. Maturational deviation

In the case of both borderline and narcissistic personality disorders, the disorders are stable over time showing neither intensifying or decline in symptoms [53]. Unlike antisocial personality disorder, the DSM does not make provision for early identification of these disorders; however, some research does provide some evidence for the early identification of specifically borderline personality disorder [56]. Although there is some evidence of epileptiform activity in borderline personality disorder [57], the prevalence is not high enough to substantiate that this disorder is due to abnormal brainwave activity. Abnormal brainwave activity is only one of the many possible neurobiological factors in this disorder and other factors such as neurotransmitter systems, the endogenous opioid system [58] and various sub-cortical areas have been included as possible contributing causes to this disorder. Despite numerous studies thyat have been done, the neurobiology of borderline personality disorder still remains largely unclear [58]. If there is evidence of neurobiological processes, and that symptoms do not appear to improve over time, one could deduce that these (narcissistic and borderline) are due to maturational deviation, rather than maturational lag.

3.2.1. Method

This study formed part of a much larger project, and this study itself was larger than what is reported here. The research question for this study is focused exclusively on maturational delay versus maturational deviation. Due to the fact that the existing literature seems to focus mainly on Cluster B personality disorders, and that EEG studies in relation to the research question focus mainly on resting state EEG recordings, this study does the same. Therefore, although there is more information available than reported here, it will be limited to what is pertinent to the research question only.

3.2.2. Participants

In order to address the research goals the study utilised purposive sampling methods to identify the ADHD sample. All participants had to be older than 18 years of age and as far as the other including characteristics are concerned, the researchers had to utilise their judgement to identify and select individuals from a target population that qualify for participation in the study, based on the sample characteristics [59]. During the initial phases of the sampling procedure the researchers verbally marketed the research undertaking to professional practitioners (mostly psychiatrists and psychologists). Furthermore participants who were selected on the basis of purposive sampling also nominated acquaintances whom they believed may qualify for participation in the research. In the initial phase the target population was broadly defined by observed ADHD type behaviours that may be explained by the syndrome and may be potentially differentially diagnosed from other clinical conditions.

Participants who were subject to the exclusion criteria were not included in the study. The list of exclusion criteria are informed by similar EEG studies [18, 60-62] which included:

- Psychoactive medication, with the exception of methylphenidate (ADHD related medication), in which case participants were asked to refrain from taking the medication for a minimum of 24 hours prior to the assessment.
- History of a neurological disorder, head injury or CNS infection.
- History of substance use disorder in the previous two months.
- Evidence of another Axis I or Axis II disorder.
- Current diagnosis of hypothyriodism.

All participants were subject to the clinical interview, and screened for a 'best estimate' diagnosis for ADHD by means of the ASRS-v.I.I. and also with the MCMI-III [63] for differential diagnosis of other clinical syndromes. The nature of these assessment tools and rationale for their use are discussed below. The recruitment of participants resulted in a group of 51 adults with ADHD and a group of 43 adults with no clear indications of a clinical disorder.

For the EEG study an initial 15 potential ADHD research participants were identified from the bigger pool, however, on further investigation 3 participants were excluded from further analysis on the basis that they met the criteria for another clinical condition. Subsequently 12 participants met the operational criteria to constitute the ADHD EEG study population. These participants were first subject to the EEG assessment before the age- and gender- matched non-ADHD sample was identified. The reason for this was to ensure that no further participants needed to be excluded and that the non-ADHD sample could be matched on the characteristics of the final ADHD sample. Two individuals were further excluded from the study population on the basis that the one participant experienced excessive drowsiness and another participant presented with significant muscle movement that may confound the obtained results. Subsequently, 10 participants were included in the research sample for the ADHD group. This sample met the necessary operational criteria for the inclusion in the study and produced an EEG reading that is acceptable according to the quality standards. The mean sample age for the ADHD group was 34.4 years. The female to male ratio was 3:1.

Following the identification of the research sample for the experimental group the study set out to identify an age- and gender- matched healthy non-ADHD group. Matched sampling for this group took place by purposively selecting participants from the initial pool of potential participants. The sampling of this group was matched exactly to gender and approximately within a four year range of the target age criterion. Subsequently the non-ADHD research sample that was identified exhibited a mean sample age of 33.6 years with a similar female to male ratio as the experimental group.

3.2.3. Measurement instruments

One of the main challenges in this study was to accurately identify adults with a diagnosis of ADHD. Due to the fact that ADHD, specifically in adulthood, is not a widely accepted diagnosis, or in other cases an over diagnosed disorder, one cannot rely only on formal diagnoses made by Mental Health Professionals. Added to this is the problem of a high rate of self-diagnosis of this disorder amongst adults [64], which brings into question relying only on self-report questionnaires to identify possible participants. For this reason, over and above the MCMI-III, a semi-structured interview and a self-report questionnaire were also included.

Semi-Structured Clinical Interview. The interview was conducted by any one of the trained clinical psychologists that formed part of the research team. The purpose of the interview was to ensure that participants met the sampling characteristics mentioned above and to make certain that none of the exclusion criteria were present in the respective population. The interview also obtained information regarding the biographical information of participants. Furthermore it served as a quick screening conformational tool by exploring the presence or absence of the criteria for ADHD in adulthood as proposed by a number of authors [65, 66].

Adult ADHD Self-Report Scale (ASRS). The ASRS is not a diagnostic tool but is used as a screening device to screen for signs and symptoms of adult ADHD. The Adult ADHD Self-Report Scale (ASRS) is a self-report 18 question questionnaire which screens adults for ADHD [67]. The ASRS is based on the criteria listed in the DSM IV, on ADHD [68]. Half of the questions focus on inattention and half of the questions focus on hyperactivity [69]. It is a paper pencil questionnaire which is self-scored and only takes 5 minutes to complete [67]. It has a five point Likert scale, where the testee ticks one of five responses, never, rarely, sometimes, often and very often [67]. The ASRS has demonstrated good reliability and validity in clinical and community samples [68]. The ASRS also has high-quality predictive power with values between 57 and 93%, showing that it can predict ADHD[70]. The ASRS proves good internal consistency with values between 0.75 and 0.89 [69]. Concordance was calculated by looking at the symptom responses of the ASRS and comparing the responses to clinical ratings, of which Cohen's k was used to assess this concordance [67]. The concordance however varied with a range of.16 to.81, which could be the result of error of measurement or the experience of the clinicians [67]. The total classification accuracy rated at 96%, however, the ASRS showed moderate levels of concurrent validity and sensitivity but high levels of specificity [69].

Millon Clinical Multi-axial Inventory-III. This test is primarily a self-report questionnaire that assesses a wide range of information about an adult's personality and emotional adjustment [71]. Furthermore this instrument was designed as a diagnostic tool that yields information about personality disorders as well as clinical syndromes [72]. The test consists of 175 questions that are forced-choice, true-false items [73]. The MCMI III has 28 sub-scales, of which are categorized into five different categories [71], i.e. Modifying Indices, Clinical Personality Patterns, Severe Personality Pathology, Clinical Syndromes, and Severe Syndromes. For the purposes of this study base rate scores below 75 were considered to be indications of no clinical significance, 75 – 84 as indicative of the presence of a personality trait, and 85 and higher as persistent personality traits [73].

The results for the internal consistency was :66 for the compulsive scales and 0.90 for major depression, and the Cronbach alpha's for the remaining 26 scales exceeded.80, showing strong internal consistency [73]. Test-retest reliability scores indicated the lowest score of.82 for debasement and the highest was.96 for somatoform, of which the median test-retest coefficient was.91, which shows stability of the instrument over time [71].

Construct and concurrent validity is tested by looking at how well the instrument performs in different populations and how much value it has in the real world [73]. The manner in which this is achieved was by comparing the MCMI to accepted standards achieved by other tests, comparing the scales on the MCMI to other scales on different tests [73]. It was identified that there is a high correlation between the scales of the MCMI-III and seven different tests, namely the symptom checklist-90, the Beck Depression Inventory, the State-Trait Anxiety Inventory, the General Behaviour Inventory, the Minnesota Multiphasic Personality Inventory (MMPI), the Michigan Alcoholism Screening Test and the MCMI-II [71]. The correlations on most of the scales where good, with some having negative scores, but these items were not related to the specific scales on the MCMI-III. Further evidence to assess how well the MCMI-III scales measure what they say they measure is by calculating the positive predictive power, which was remarkable showing a range of.30 to.80 [71]. The MCMI-III has proven construct validity and diagnostic validity, by comparing test items with other tests and by comparing clinical judgement with the results indicated from the scales on the MCMI-III [73].

Biopac MP Systems Hardware. The research question is concerned with the nature of the intracranial electrical currents of adults with ADHD symptomatology. Therefore EEG recording is appropriate for this study in that it records the electrical activity of cortical nerve cells in the brain [74]. It is noteworthy to mention that cortical activity is presented in waveforms and is measured in terms of amplitude and frequency [75]. Amplitude is expressed in microvolts (μV), EEG power is defined by the square of amplitude (μV^2) and frequency is defined as the number of oscillations, or cycles, within a given time frame, or epoch, and is measured in hertz (Hz) [76].

This study employed the Biopac MP Systems Hardware [77] for the assessment of cortical activity. The system is considered to be commercial EEG equipment utilised in the data acquisition and analysis for life science research. The recording technique utilised by this system is an ethically approved, non-invasive, safe and painless procedure [78]. In order to ensure the quality of research, the EEG methods employed in this study are informed by various other EEG studies that employed quantitative EEG techniques [75] as well as standardised guidelines for the technologic recording and quantitative analysis of EEG activity in the research context [79].

A final matter to consider in this section is the reliability and validity of EEG recordings. Various researchers report that EEG recordings are reliable, in that the intra-individual stability of EEG is stable over time (over a period of 10 to 90 days) [80,81]. The validity of EEG research depends on the concepts of sensitivity and specificity [76]. In ADHD research, sensitivity refers to the percentage of ADHD individuals who present with an abnormal EEG while specificity reveals the percentage of non-ADHD subjects who indicate a normal EEG [76]. In a literature review of several studies, it was concluded that EEG methods in ADHD research typically demonstrate good sensitivity (90% to 97%) and sound specificity (84%-94%)[76].

3.2.4. Procedure

All potential participants were required to complete the ASRS and MCMI for screening purposes. Based on the scores on these instruments they were allocated to different groups, or where they did not meet the criteria for any of the groups, were excluded from further studies. As explained previously, the sample for the EEG study was drawn from this pool. Potential participants were approached to participate in the EEG study.

Upon arrival to the research laboratory participants were requested to sit in the allocated chair. The researcher and EEG equipment was situated outside of the participants direct line of sight. Participants were then oriented to the Biopac MP Systems Hardware equipment, and was further provided with an opportunity to ask questions. The researcher enquired about whether participants adhered to the instruction to refrain from the aforementioned substances 24 hours before the assessment. Participants were informed that during the data

http://dx.doi.org/10.5772/53865

acquisition phase they will engaged in a three minute eyes-closed task. Participants were also instructed to remain as physically still as possible in order to limit muscle contamination throughout the entire assessment, and were requested to avoid speaking during the assessment as a further attempt to avoid contamination of results.

In the data acquisition phase subjects were fitted with an electrocap in accordance with the 10-20 International system of electrode placement. In order to tap the fronto-parietal attention network, electrodes were grouped into three areas: frontal (F3 and F4), frontal midline (Fz) and parietal (P3 and P4) sites (see Figure 1.). EEG signal for all subjects was recorded under an eyes-closed condition. Eye movements were monitored by electrodes placed on the outer canthus of each eye for horizontal movements and by electrodes above the eye for vertical movements. EEG signal was recorded using *Acq*Knowledge software and BIOPAC MP Systems hardware. Impedance was kept below 5Kohm (kΩ) and a sampling rate of 200Hz was applied. Continuous EEG data was reviewed off-line. Segments containing head and eye movement as well as muscle artefact were removed from further analysis. Subsequently, six two second epochs were extracted for the eyes-closed condition and for each of the cortical sites investigated and for the four frequency bands: delta (1-4Hz); theta (4-8Hz); alpha (8-13Hz); and Beta (13-20Hz). EEG data was Fast Fourier transformed (FFT) (Hanning window) and subsequently log transformed (In).

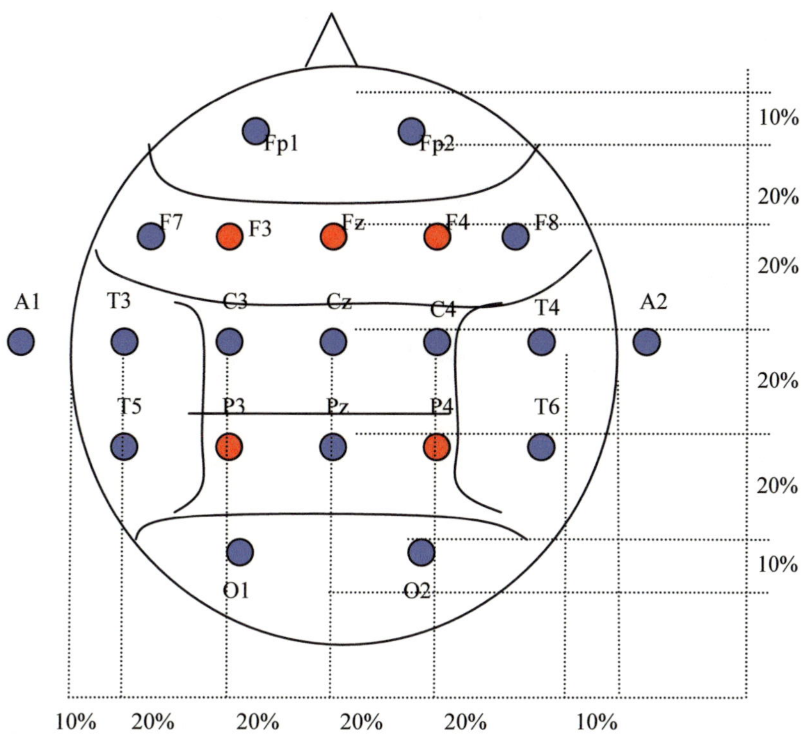

Figure 1. International 10-20 System of Electrode Placement (Adapted from [75])

3.2.5. Results

3.2.5.1. Personality disorder

In order to gain a meaningful picture of Personality Disorders in ADHD, and therefore a better picture of maturational lag versus maturational deviation, the data gained from the MCMI-III was used in different ways. Firstly the average base rate scores (interval scale) were compared between the groups, thereafter the scores were categorised into 3 categories (Ordinal scale), i.e. <75, 75-84 and 85>, where after the groups were compared, and lastly, based on the categorisation of the data, number of personality disorders per individual, per group are reported.

		Histrionic	Narcissistic	Antisocial	Borderline
ADHD (n=51)	Mean	50.6	58.5	61.4	55.4
	Std. Dev	23.6	21.7	14.3	21.7
	Min	0	15	35	0.0
	Max	95	110	90	92.0
Non-ADHD(n=43)	Mean	60.1	55.9	43.6	38.4
	Std. Dev	23.3	20.8	19.1	22.4
	Min	4	15	8	0.0
	Max	98	98	82	85.0

Table 3. Descriptive statistics for the 4 groups for the interpersonal sub-scales

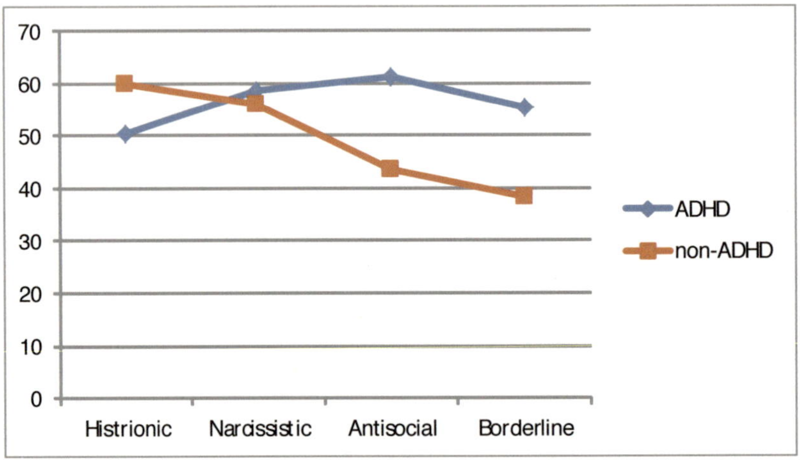

Figure 2. Mean scores of the 4 Cluster B Personality Scales for the 2 groups

http://dx.doi.org/10.5772/53865

In terms of the average base rate scores, Table 3 and Figure 2 reflected that the two groups were more or less equal in terms of Narcissism and that the non-ADHD group had a higher average score on the Histrionic, but significantly lower scores on both the Anti-Social and Borderline scales (See Tables 3 and 4). Of particular importance is that none of the average scores were higher than 75, indicating that neither of the two groups displayed typical persistent personality traits.

	Histrionic	Narcissistic	Antisocial	Borderline
Mann-Whitney U	861.0	980.5	502.5	612.5
Wilcoxon W	2187.0	1926.5	1448.5	1558.5
Z	-1.791	-.882	-4.521	-3.678
p	0.07	0.38	***0.000****	***.000****

Where: ***: p<0.001

Table 4. Differences between ADHD and Normal groups for the interpersonal sub-scales

Interpreting only the differences in base rate scores of the MCMI can be misleading, therefore the scores of individuals for each of the scales was categorised into one of three categories, i.e. Low (<75), High (75-84) or Significant (84>) (See Table 5).

		Low score	High score	Significant score	
		<75	75 - 84	85>	Total
		N	N	N	N
	ADHD	42	5	4	51
Histrionic	nADHD	30	4	9	43
	Total	72	9	13	
	ADHD	41	3	7	51
Narcissistic	nADHD	35	2	6	43
	Total	76	5	13	94
	ADHD	37	12	2	51
Anti-social	nADHD	39	4	0	43
	Total	76	16	2	94
	ADHD	40	8	3	51
Borderline	nADHD	41	1	1	43
	Total	81	9	4	94

Table 5. Number of participants per category of Cluster B Personality scores

When investigating the data in this way, the results indicate that there were significant differences between the 2 groups on all of the subscales (See Table 6).

	Histrionic	Narcissistic	Borderline	Anti-social
Chi-Square	79.43	96.53	118.5	98.64
Df	2	2	2	2
Significance	**.000*** **	**.000*** **	**.000*** **	**.000*** **
Where: ***: p<0.0001				

Table 6. Chi Square for differences between the 2 groups

Given these results, a frequency analysis was done to determine how many elevated scores (85>) an individual participant had (See Table 7).

Number of Personality Disorders	ADHD	nADHD
0	39 (76.5%)	39 (90.7%)
1	9 (17.6%)	4 (9.3%)
2	2 (3.9%)	0 (0.0%)
3	1 (2%)	0 (0.0%)
Total	51	43

Table 7. Number of Personality Disorders per group

These results, from a maturational deviation perspective are meaningful in that the majority of the ADHD participants (76%) did not show any evidence of a Cluster B Personality Disorder. If one assumes that ADHD is due to maturational lag, and that Cluster B Personality Disorders are also due to maturational lag, then these results seriously challenge this assumption. Given the fact that a higher percentage of ADHD (27.5%) showed indications of one or more Cluster B Personality Disorders than the non-ADHD group (9.3%), there seems to be evidence of a possible maturational deviation process.

3.2.5.2. EEG results

This part of the study focussed the brain's intracranial electrical currents and potentials, in other words cortical activity, of adults with ADHD, and those with no ADHD symptomatology. The patterns that are of particular concern are the activity (elevation or suppression) of the four frequency bands (delta, theta, alpha and beta).

The study focused on two domains of investigation: power spectral and ratio coefficients. Power spectral studies concerns the calculation of absolute and relative power estimates [20].

- Power spectral density or the power spectrum "… reflects the 'frequency content' of the signal or the distribution of signal power over frequency" [82, p. 806]. For the power spectral domain the analysis was concerned with two spectral parameters, i.e.:
- Relative power is determined by the amount of EEG activity in a frequency band divided by the sum of the other bands [75].
- Absolute power is the amount for one specific frequency band without its relationship to the other bands [79].
- Ratio coefficients refers to the ratio between power in different frequency bands [20].

These two domains of investigation were selected on the basis that they are the most common and often preferred means of investigation for ADHD studies [20]. The mean values obtained for the ADHD and non-ADHD group, per area of the brain investigated and per frequency cluster were employed in obtaining the values for the domains of investigation. The above-mentioned equations were applied and subsequently, the absolute, relative and power ratios were determined. Note that for this study frequency parameters are set as follows: delta (1-4Hz); theta (4-8Hz); alpha (8-13Hz); and Beta (13-20Hz). The Greek symbols employed to denote the different waves include: delta as δ; theta as θ; alpha as α; and finally beta as β. As far as the experimental condition is concerned, the abbreviation of EC is employed.

In order to address the research question a between-subjects analysis of diagnostic group differences was applied. Seeing that the small sample size was not representative of the greater population, nonparametric statistical procedures were employed [85]. Subsequently the Mann-Whitney U-test was applied with the use of SPSS software. The Mann-Whitney U test is the nonparametric alternative to an independent t-test. The Mann-Whitney U test is appropriate for the between-subjects analysis because it compares differences between two independent groups, in this case ADHD with non-ADHD [85].

In Table 8 the absolute mean power (μV^2) and Table 9 the relative mean power for the different frequency bands for the different cortical areas across the different conditions are reported. The table is formatted in this way as to compare the ADHD sample with the non-ADHD sample according to the four frequency clusters and according to the area of the brain investigated.

The results of the resting EEG reveal elevated ADHD relative theta activity at frontal midline sites. This finding is consistent with childhood and adolescent research that is suggestive of a maturational lag and developmental deviation profile. Increased relative theta activity is also indicated in the ADHD studies of [18,19] as well as Clarke et al. (2008b) at frontal midline sites. Although it was also expected that theta activity would be elevated in frontal sites, this was not confirmed in the present study. Moreover, the elevation or decrease of theta activity is not documented widely for parietal sites in ADHD literature. However, an interesting observation that was not indicated for the initial expectations for the current study is the presence of decreased absolute theta for the ADHD sample at parietal sites. The reduction of absolute theta at parietal sites is also not supported in the other six ADHD studies mentioned [10, 18, 19, 61,31,33].

The results of the resting EEG further reveal elevated theta/beta and theta/alpha ratios at frontal midline sites. These results are consistent with child and adolescent research that are suggestive of a developmental deviation profile. These results are also indicated in the ADHD studies of [18, 19, 33].

The resting EEG of the current study also indicates decreased relative beta power for the ADHD sample in the frontal midline area. These results are in line with child and adolescent research that are suggestive of a developmental deviation profile. Of the six ADHD studies [10, 18, 19, 31,33, 61] identified in the current author's literature search, none of the authors confirm such results. Also, although decreased beta power was expected for frontal and frontal midline sites, the finding was only apparent for the frontal midline area.

	ADHD	non-ADHD	Mann-Whitney U	Wilcoxon W	Z	Between group differences
						p
Frontal						
δ	0.0191	0.0210	35.5	90.5	-0.78	0.44
θ	0.0549	0.0588	38.0	93.0	-0.57	0.60
α	0.0444	0.0476	34.5	89.5	-0.86	0.40
β	0.0171	0.0178	38.5	93.5	-0.54	0.59
Midline						
δ	0.0106	0.0070	34.0	79.0	-0.91	0.40
θ	0.0304	0.0241	35.0	80.0	-0.82	0.45
α	0.0234	0.0206	38.5	83.5	-0.53	0.60
β	0.0082	0.0074	39.5	84.5	-0.454	0.66
Parietal						
δ	0.0171	0.0317	20.5	75.5	-2.01	**0.04***
θ	0.0459	0.0696	20.5	75.0	-2.05	**0.04***
α	0.0358	0.0513	21.0	76.0	-1.96	0.05
β	0.0129	0.0211	19.5	74.5	-2.09	**0.04***
Where: *: p<0.05						

Table 8. Absolute Mean Power (μV^2) for the ADHD (n=10) and the non-ADHD (n=9) Groups

	ADHD	non-ADHD	Mann-Whitney U	Wilcoxon W	Z	Between group differences
						p
Frontal						
δ	13.0985	13.5419	39.5	84.5	-0.45	0.50
θ	40.7944	40.6344	39.0	84.0	-0.49	0.66
α	33.4839	33.4904	40.0	85.0	-0.41	0.72
β	12.6232	12.3331	42.0	87.0	-0.25	0.80
Midline						
δ	12.6778	11.7963	34.0	79.0	-0.91	0.40
θ	41.9948	40.9362	0.00	45.0	-3.68	**0.000*****
α	33.6352	35.0017	11.0	64.0	-2.94	**0.004****
β	11.6922	12.2656	15.0	70.0	-2.45	**0.01****
Parietal						
δ	14.0345	16.4011	20.5	75.5	-2.01	**0.04***
θ	40.8777	40.1942	30.0	75.0	-1.23	0.24
α	33.1763	31.1389	29.0	74.0	-1.31	0.21
β	11.9112	12.2660	26.0	81.0	-1.55	0.13

Table 9. Relative Mean Power (μV^2) for the ADHD (n=10) and the non-ADHD (n=9) Groups

The results of the resting EEG further reveal decreased absolute alpha and beta activity for the ADHD sample at parietal sites. These findings are observed in child and adolescent research that are consistent with the maturational lag and developmental deviation profile. The results however have not been indicated in the six ADHD studies identified in the literature search.

	ADHD	non-ADHD	Mann-Whitney U	Wilcoxon W	Z	Between group differences (p)
Frontal						
θ:β	3.28	3.30	42.0	97.0	-0.25	0.84
θ:α	1.23	1.23	39.5	94.5	-0.45	0.66
Midline						
θ:β	3.69	3.33	6.0	51.0	-3.19	**0.001****
θ:α	1.28	1.17	2.0	47.0	-3.52	**0.000*****
Parietal						
θ:β	3.63	3.98	21.0	66.0	-1.96	0.05
θ:α	1.27	1.34	43.0	98.0	-0.16	0.91

Where ** p<.01 and *** p<.001

Table 10. Mean Power Ratio Values for the ADHD (n=10) and the nADHD (n=9) groups

3.2.5.3. Conclusion

The current study's results contribute to the neurobiological and pathophysiological information of ADHD and are important for the advancement of aetiological theorising in the field. Of particular relevance is the interpretation of data in accordance to the maturational lag and developmental deviation model. The abovementioned results are consistent with child and adolescent research that support both models. Hence this brings forth the question of which model more adequately describes the aetiological bases that may be related to the phenomenon of ADHD.

Given the overlap between the neurocognitive symptoms between ADHD and Personality Disorders (specifically Cluster B), the first part of the study investigated the prevalence of Personality Disorders in ADHD. The rationale for this was twofold, i.e. there is evidence to suggest that Cluster B disorders may be the result, as is the case with ADHD, of maturational lag, therefore, if this is true, all adults with ADHD should show signs of at least one Cluster B personality disorder. The results of the study indicated that the majority of the adults with ADHD did not show any significant signs of a Cluster B personality disorder. However, there were more ADHD adults showing signs of more than one personality disorder than those adults without ADHD. If one stays with the assumption that there is a neurocognitive component to personality disorders, this may be indicative of maturational deviation.

These findings seem to suggest that (1) ADHD cannot be viewed as a homogeneous disorder with the same underlying neurodevelopmental processes, and (2) childhood ADHD does not necessarily progress into a personality disorder (see Figure 6), therefore there is room for both an Axis I and Axis II diagnosis in adults with ADHD. One of the problems considering ADHD as a homogenous disorder is that it may suggest a single course with a single outcome. Research, however, suggests that there may be multiple outcomes, i.e. remission in adolescence or continuation into adulthood. If there is an assumption of multiple outcomes, it should firstly indicate that this is not a homogenous disorder, and secondly it implies that there are different etiological pathways as well. Before one can draw a final conclusiuon about these statements, it is important to also review the EEG results of the ADHD participants.

In order to further investigate the maturational lag vs. maturational deviation theory of ADHD, an EEG study, was done on a smaller sample. The maturational lag model suggests that ADHD behaviours are a consequence of a neurodevelopmental lag [8]. It further denotes that individuals with ADHD symptoms present with cortical activity patterns that are similar to that witnessed in younger children [8, 20]. Moreover it is accepted that cortical development is expected to 'catch up' and remit in adolescence [6]. The developmental deviation model denote that the cortical activity of individuals with ADHD symptoms are not considered normal at any age and is not likely to mature in a normal fashion [20].

http://dx.doi.org/10.5772/53865

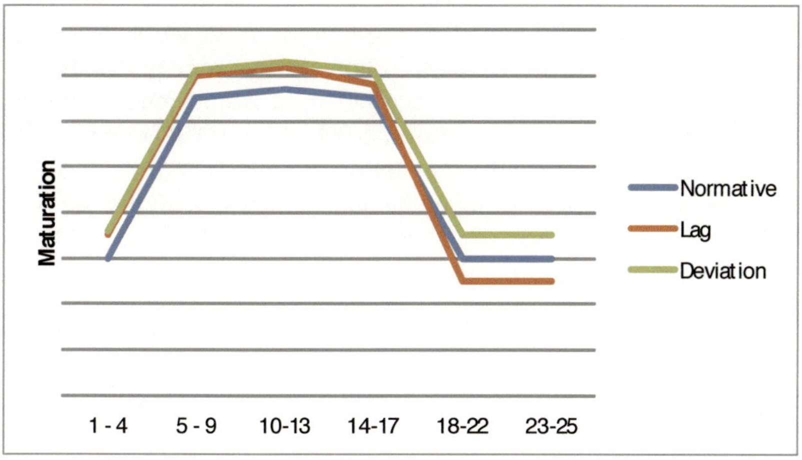

Figure 3. Comparison of normative, maturational lag and maturational deviation models of slow wave activity across developmental stages

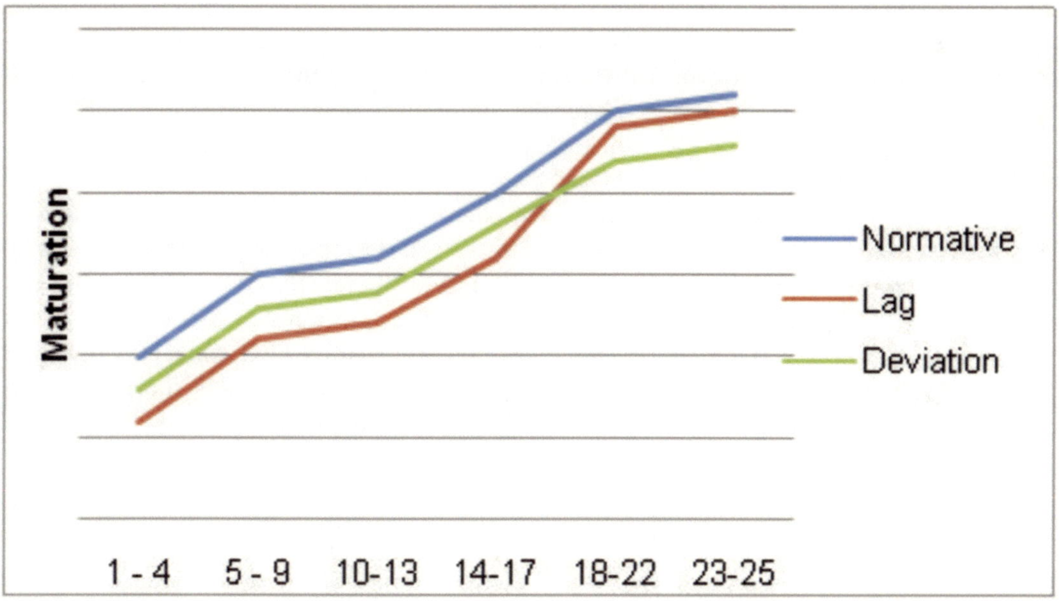

Figure 4. Comparison of normative, maturational lag and maturational deviation models of fast wave activity across developmental stages

As mentioned already, the results of the current study are in line with the ADHD results of [10, 18, 19, 33] who indicate elevated slow wave activity and increased theta/beta and theta/alpha ratios. Seeing that EEG aberrances are clearly indicated in adult samples, it does not confirm the maturational lag's assumption that cortical maturation will eventually 'catch up'

[6, 20]. Instead, the data suggests that ADHD symptoms do persist for some individuals into adulthood. The results further support the developmental deviation, which suggests that ADHD behaviours are related to the disorganisation of wave activity that deviates from normal development [17, 20]. The deviation is revealed in the results wherein the cortical activity patterns remain aberrant and have not normalised in the ADHD sample. Taken together, the results of the current study confirms [18] notion that since abnormalities of the EEG persists into adulthood for the ADHD sample, the data is indicative of a more *persistent* developmental deviation for some individuals with the disorder and that not all individuals who present with the disorder will eventually outgrow it.

Up to this point the results of the resting EEG suggests that the data obtained is more suggestive of a developmental deviation than a maturational lag. However, as mentioned already, the results of the current study indicates increased relative theta and consequently elevated theta/beta and theta/alpha ratios as well as decreased relative beta at frontal midline sites for the ADHD sample in comparison with controls. This profile displays an elevation in slow wave activity and a decrease in fast wave activity. Although this profile is clearly indicated in developmental deviation and maturational lag models, the maturational lag model provides the qualitative and aetiological information that links this profile with ADHD behaviours.

EEG support of the maturational lag model reveals in its findings cortical activity patterns that are similar to that witnessed in younger children [10, 20]. In accordance to Kinsbourne [5], the father of the model's ideas, the cortical activity patterns that limit the performance of younger children are synonymous to that which typically compromises the performance of individuals with ADHD symptomatology [10, 20]. Recent normative databases suggest that absolute and/or relative slow wave activity (delta and theta) is elevated in childhood and is the highest shortly before puberty, where after it declines by 60% and finally slows down in its decline after the age of 17 [83, 84] (see Figure 3). Following puberty, fast wave activity (alpha and beta) reportedly increases [86]. Finally, between the ages of 25 to 30 years the cortical thickening and thinning (myelination) stabilises and the process of growth spurts and oscillations in terms of cortical activity lessens and normalises [86]. In relation to normative EEG data it is evident that the increase in slow wave activity and decrease in fast wave activity would be more evident in younger children before puberty commences. Hence it appears that the ADHD type behaviours of the current ADHD sample may be aetiologically related to the patterns of cortical activity that typically limit the performance of younger children.

The abovementioned paragraphs elicit information that has implications for the interpretation and advancement of aetiological theorising according to EEG-based models of ADHD. The developmental deviation denotes that the EEG aberrances observed in individuals with ADHD symptoms are not normal in individuals of *any* age [20]. However, as indicated above, the cortical activity patterns observed in the ADHD sample is synonymous to that which is often observed in younger children. Hence, the data supports the assumption that cortical maturation deviates from normal development and that the deviation is more persistent; however, it does not support the notion that the resting EEG observed is not similar to patterns witnessed at *any* particular age. Also, the presence of this profile in ADHD EEG research does not automatically serve as evidence of a maturational lag. The reason for this

http://dx.doi.org/10.5772/53865

is because the observation of EEG activity, that is similar to that witnessed in younger children in one point in time, does not suggest that those patterns will eventually 'catch up'.

A further matter to consider in relation to the resting EEG of the current study is the posterior-anterior time course of cortical development. It is evident that the results of the current study yield EEG aberrances in parietal, frontal and frontal midline sites for the ADHD sample. As discussed previously, the posterior-anterior time course of cortical development suggests that the cortical activity in posterior regions mature more rapidly than frontal regions [87]. When cortical development follows this pathway, delta, theta and alpha develop first from birth in occipital regions and only appear later in parietal and central regions and finally in frontal regions [26].

The results of the current study indicate deviations in the EEG for the ADHD from the control group that are present in early-maturing (parietal area) and later-maturing (frontal and frontal midline area) sites. If maturation were seen to 'catch up' in the ADHD sample, then the greatest between- group differences would only have been indicated at frontal sites [26]. Hence, the data is not suggestive of development that is slow to 'catch up' but again suggests that development in the ADHD sample is indicating a more persistent deviation and disorganisation of wave activity [20, 30]. In Figure 5, a summary is provided of evidence for both a maturational lag and deviance model.

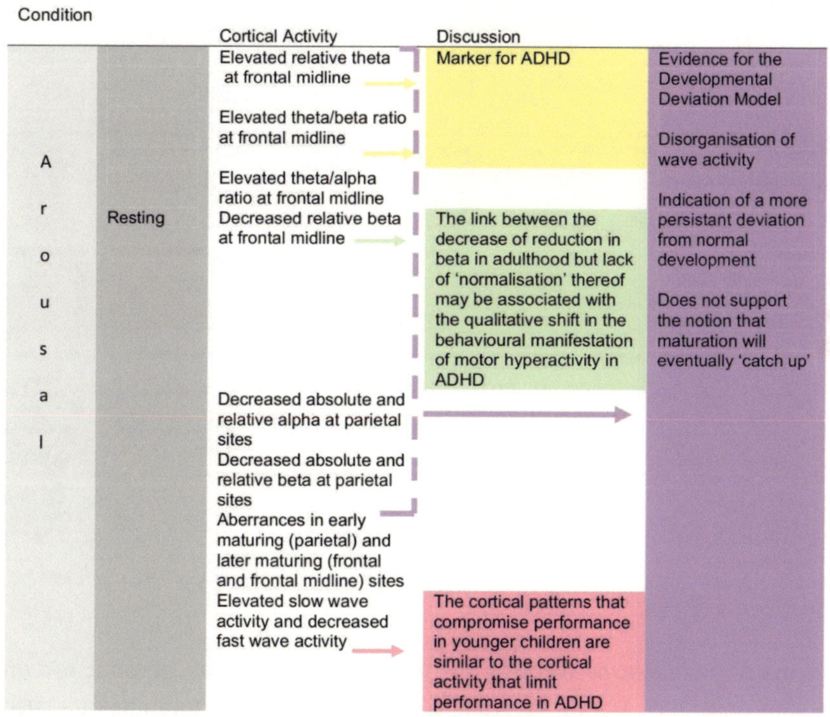

Figure 5. Cortical Activity Patterns of ADHD in Resting Conditions

It must be emphasised that this study was exploratory in nature, and in many ways it resulted in more questions than answers. What the study did do however, was to highlight some problems in our interpretation of quantitative data. The first of these is the problem of the *average*. The conclusion drawn from averages does not include a satisfactory explanation for the variance, i.e. in terms of maturational lag, as the findings suggest that there is a distinct possibility that some of these reach cortical maturity at the same rate as non-ADHD children (i.e. those at the higher end of the distribution), and that there are those who may reach this much longer after the 3 year average (i.e. those at the lower end of the distribution). At both ends of the distribution, it opens the possibility for maturational deviance as symptoms are present, but cannot be explained fully by the maturational lag theory (See Figure 6). In line with this above argument, even within studies, not all cortical areas are affected in the same way. This is, in essence, not problematic, however, formulating a general maturational lag model is, as it seems to imply that there is general maturational lag. Furthermore there are studies that report maturational lag, but include discrepant findings in cortical areas which are explained asymmetrical maturation. The question that arises is whether this should then be considered as maturational lag or maturational deviance.

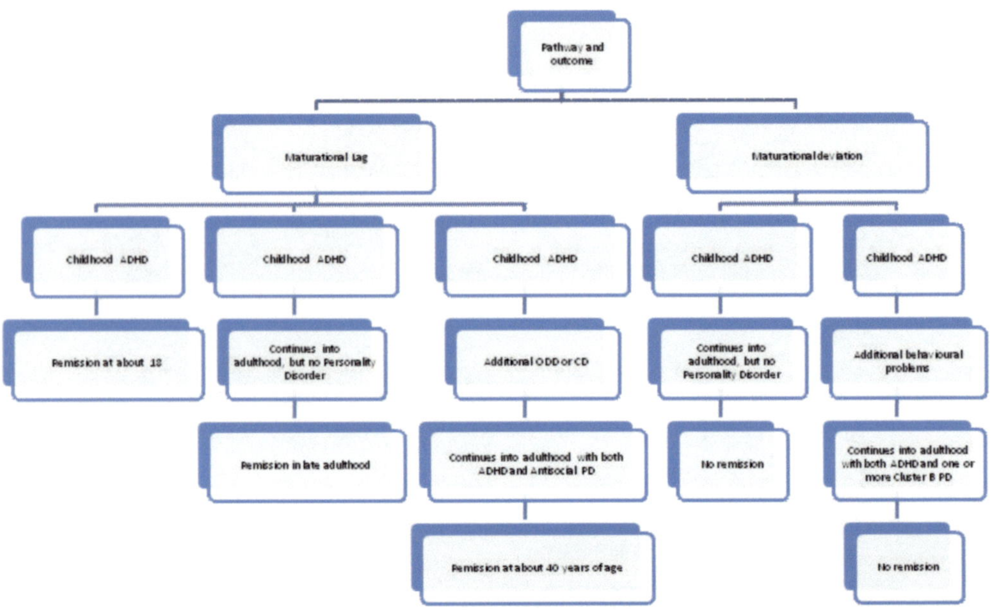

Figure 6. Multiple outcomes of ADHD in adulthood

A common theme which runs through all the studies, and may account for many of the comments above, is that ADHD is often considered to be a homogenous disorder. It is quite possible that maturational lag would best account for a certain sub-group, and deviance for others (See Figure 6). If we are going to gain more insight into the etiology of this disorder, we need to review our research methodologies. It is argued that many of the confounding / contradictory results is the way in which studies are conceptualised. In this regard, the sampling of participants needs to be more focused, as current studies seem to include mainly the combined sub-type of ADHD [6].If this were true, it would not be inaccurate to state that very little is known about brain maturation in children with the inattentive subtype. It is therefore imperative that sampling be done much more specifically and that subtypes are compared to each other. Furthermore, one needs to deviate from the common practice to exclude participants with both ADHD and comorbid conditions and rather group these participants together based on disorders that are alike in both symptomotology and theoretical etiology.

Author details

Alban Burke and Amanda Edge

Department of Psychology, University of Johannesburg, South Africa

References

[1] www.dsm5.org

[2] Miller TW, Nigg JT, Faraone, SV. Axis I and II comorbidity in adults with ADHD. Journal of Abnormal Psychology 2007; 116(3) 519-528.

[3] Anckarsäter H, Stahlberg O, Larson T, Hakansson C, Jutblad S-B, Niklasson L, Nyden A, Wentz E, Westergren S, Cloninger R, Gillberg C, Rastam M. The Impact of ADHD and Autism Spectrum Disorders on Temperament, Character, and Personality Development. American Journal of Psychiatry 2006; 163 1239-1244.

[4] Nigg JT, Goldsmith HH, Sachek J. Temperament and Attention Deficit Hyperactivity Disorder: The Development of a Multiple Pathway Model. Journal of Clinical Child and Adolescent Psychology 2004; 33(1) 42-53.

[5] Kinsbourne M. Minimal brain dysfunction as a neurodevelopmental lag. Annals of the New York Academy of Sciences 2004; 205 268-273.

[6] Rubia K. Neuro-anatomic evidence for the maturational delay hypothesis of ADHD. Proceedings of the National Academy of Sciences 2007; 104 19663-19664.

[7] Shaw P, Gogtay N, Rapoport J. Childhood psychiatric disorders as anomalies in neurodevelopmental trajectories, Human BrainMapping 2010; 31 917-925.

[8] Clarke, AR, Barry, RJ, Dupuy, FE, McCarthy, R, Selikowitz, M, Heaven, PCL. Childhood EEG as a predictor of adult attention-deficit/hyperactivity disorder. Clinical Neurophysiology 2011, 122 73-80.

[9] Barry, RJ, Clarke, RA, Johnstone, SJ. A review of electrophysiology in attention-deficit/hyperactivity disorder: I. qualitative and quantitative electroencephalography. Clinical Neurophysiology 2003; 114 171-183.

[10] [10] Clarke AR, Barry RJ, Heaven PCL, McCarthy R, Selikowitz M, Byrne M K. EEG in adults with attention-deficit/hyperactivity disorder. International Journal of Psychophysiology 2008; 70 176-183.

[11] Clarke AR, Barry RJ, McCarthy R, Selikowitz, M. Electroencephalogram differences in two subtypes of attention-deficit/hyperactivity disorder. Psychophysiology 2001; 38 212-221.

[12] Lubar JF, Bianchini K, Calhoun W, Lambert E, Brody, Z, Shabsin H. Spectral analysis of EEG differences between children with and without learning disabilities. Journal of Learning Disabilities 1985; 18 403-408.

[13] Lubar JF. Discourse on the development of EEG diagnostic and biofeedback for attention-deficit/hyperactivity disorders. Biofeedback Self Regulation 1991; 16 201-225.

[14] Mann CA, Lubar, JF, Zimmerman, AW, Miller, Muenchen RA. Quantitative analysis of EEG in boys with attention-deficit-hyperactivity disorder: Controlled study with clinical implications. Pediatric Neurology 1992; 8 30-36.

[15] Matsuura M, Okubo, Y, Toru M, Kojima T, He Y, Hou Y, Shen Y, Lee, CK. A cross-national EEG study of children with emotional and behavioural problems: a WHO collaborative study in the Western Pacific Region. Biological Psychiatry 1993; 34 59-65.

[16] Satterfield JH, Schell AM, Backs RW, Hidaka, KC. A cross-sectional and longitudinal study of age effects of electrophysiological measures in hyperactive and normal children. Biological Psychiatry 1984;19 973-990.

[17] Klinkerfuss GH, Lange PH, Weinberg, WA, O'Leary, JL. Electroencephalographic abnormalities of children with hyperkinetic behavior. Neurology 1965; 15 883 – 891.

[18] Bersnahan SM, Anderson, JW, Barry, RJ. Age-related changes in quantitative EEG in attention-deficit/hyperactivity disorder. Society of Biological Psychiatry 1999; 46 1690-1697.

[19] Bersnahan, SM, Barry, RJ. Specificity of quantitative EEG analysis in adults with attention deficit hyperactivity disorder. Psychiatry Research 2002; 112 133-144.

[20] Barry, RJ, Clarke, RA, McCarthy R, Selikowitz M, Rushby JA, Ploskova, E. EEG differences in children as a function of resting-state arousal level. Clinical neurophysiology 2004; 115 402-408.

[21] Chabot RJ, Serfontein G. Quantitative electroencephalographic profiles of children with attention deficit disorder. Biological Psychiatry 1996; 40 951-963.

[22] Clarke AR, Barry RJ, McCarthy R, Selikowitz M. EEG analysis in attention-deficit/hyperactivity disorder: a comparative study of two subtypes. Psychiatry Research 1998; 81 19-29.

[23] Clarke AR, Barry, RJ, Bond D, McCarthy R, Selikowitz M. Effects of stimulant medications on the EEG of children with attention-deficit/hyperactivity disorder. Psychopharmacology 2002; 164 277-284.

[24] Defrance JF, Smith S, Schweitzer FC, Ginsberg I, Sands S. Topographical analysis of attention disorders of childhood. International Journal of Neuroscience 1996;87 41-61.

[25] El-Sayed EM, Larsson JO, Persson HE, Rydelilus, P-A. Altered cortical activity in children with attention-deficit/hyperactivity disorder during attentional load task. Journal of American Academy of Child and Adolescent Psychiatry 2002; 41(7) 811-819.

[26] Hobbs MJ, Clarke AR, Barry, RJ, McCarthy, R, Selikowitz, M. EEG abnormalities in adolescent males with AD/HD. Clinical Neurophysiology 2007; 118 363-371.

[27] Schmidt, RG, Tirsch, WS, Reitmeir P. Correlation of developmental neurological findings with spectral analytical EEG evaluations in pre-school age children. Electroencephalography and Clinical Neurophysiology 1997; 103 516-527.

[28] Clarke AR, Barry RJ, McCarthy R, Selikowitz, M. Age and sex effects in the EEG: Differences in two subtypes of attention-deficit/hyperactivity disorder. Clinical Neurophysiology 2001; 112, 815-826.

[29] Hermens DF, Soei EXC, Clarke SD, Kohn, MR, Gordon E, Williams LM. Resting EEG theta activity predicts cognitive performance in attention-deficit hyperactivity disorder. Pediatric Neurology 2005; 32(4) 248-256.

[30] Alexander D M, Hermens DF, Keage, HAD, Clark CR, Williams LM, Kohn, MR, Clarke SD, Lamb C, Gordon E. Event-related wave activity in the EEG provides new marker of ADHD. Clinical Neurophysiology 2008; 119, 163-179.

[31] Loo KS, Sigi Hale T, Macion J, Hanada G, McGough JJ, McCracken JT, Smalley SL. Cortical activity patterns in ADHD during arousal, activation and sustained attention. Neuropsychologia 2009; 47 2114-2119.

[32] Tian L, Jiang T, Liang M, Zang Y, He Y, Sui M, Wang Y. Enhanced resting-state brain activities in ADHD patients: A fMRI study. Brain and Development 2008; 30 342-348.

[33] van Dongen-Boomsma M, Lansbergen M M, Bekker, E M, Kooij J-J S, van der Molen M, Kenemans JL, Buitelaar, J K. Relation between resting EEG to cognitive performance and clinical symptoms in adults with attention-deficit/hyperactivity disorder. Neuroscience Letters 2010; 469 102-106.

[34] Clark L A. Temperament as a Unifying Basis for Personality and Psychopathology. Journal of Abnormal Psychology 2005; 114(4) 505-521.

[35] Parker JDA, Majeski SA, Collin, VT. ADHD symptoms and personality: relationships with the five-factor model. Personality and Individual Differences 2004; 36 977-987.

[36] Valero S, Ramos-Quiroga A, Gomá-i-Freixanet M, Bosch R, Gomómez-Barros N, Nogueira M, Palomar G, Corrales M, Casas M. Personality profile of adult ADHD: The alternative five factor model. Psychiatry Research 2012; http://dx.doi.org/10.1016/j.psychres.2011.11.006

[37] Martel M, Nigg JT. Child ADHD and personality / temperament traits of reactive and effortful control, resiliency, and emotionality. Journal of Child Psychology and Psychiatry 2006; 47 (11), 1175-1183.

[38] White JD. Personality, temperament and ADHD: A review of the literature. Personality and Individual differences 1999; 27 589-598.

[39] Shaw GA, Gambria LM. Task unrelated thoughts of college students diagnosed as hyperactive in childhood. Developmental Neuropsychology 1993; 9 17-30.

[40] Barkley RA. Behavioral inhibition, sustained attention, and executive functions: constructing a unifying theory of ADHD. Psychological Bulletin 1997; 121 65-94.

[41] Shea T, Fisher, BE. Self ratings of mood levels and mood variability as predictors of Junior 1-6 impulsivity and ADHD classroom behaviors. Personality and Individual Differences 1996; 20 209-214.

[42] John OP, Caspi A, Robins RW, Moffit TE, Stouthamer-Loeber M. The 'little five": exploring the nomological network of the five-factor model of personality in adolescent boys. Child Development 1994; 65 160-178.

[43] Faraone SV, Kunwar A, Adamson J, Biederman, J. Personality traits among ADHD adults: implications of late-onset and sub-threshold diagnoses. Psychological Medicine 2009; 39(45) 685-693.

[44] Reich DB, Zanarini MC, Fitzmaurice G. Affective lability in bipolar disorder and borderline personality disorder. Comprehensive Psychiatry 2012; 53(4) 230-237.

[45] Beauchaine TP, Klein DN, Crowell SE, Derbridge C, Gatzke-Kopp L. Mutlifinality in the development of personality disorders: A Biology x Sex x Environment interaction model of antisocial and borderline traits. Development and Psychopathology 2009; 21(3) 735-770.

[46] Snyder S, Pitts WM, Pokorny, AD. Affective and behavioural features of DSM-III borderline personality disorder. Are they valid? Psychopathology 1985; 18(1) 3-10.

[47] Blonigen DM, Littlefield AK, Hicks BM, Sher, KJ. Course of Antisocial Behavior during Emerging Adulthood: Developmental Differences in Personality. Journal of Research in Personality 2010; 44(6) 729-733.

[48] Speranza M, Revah-Levy A, Cortese S, Falissard B, Pham-Scottez A, Corcos, M. ADHD in adolescents with borderline personality disorder. BMC Psychiatry 2010; 11 158.

[49] Ball SA, Carroll KM, Rounsaville BJ. Sensation Seeking, substance abuse, and psychopathology in treatment –seeking and community cocaine abusers. Journal of Consulting and Clinical Psychology 1994; 62(5) 1053-1057.

[50] Sarkar J, Adshead G. Personality disorders as disorganization of attachment and affect regulation. Advances in Psychiatric Treatment 2006; 12 297-305.

[51] Lampe K, Konrad K, Kroener S, Fast K, Kunert HJ, Herpertz SC. Neuropsychological and behavioural disinhibition in adult ADHD compared to borderline personality disorder. Psychological Medicine 2007; 37 1717-1729.

[52] Reimherr FW, Marchant BK, Williams ED, Strong RE, Halls C, Soni P. Personality disorders in ADHD Part 3: Personality disorder, social adjustment, and their relation to dimensions of adult ADHD. Annals of Clinical Psychiatry 2010; 22(2) 103-112.

[53] Sadock BJ, Sadock VA. Kaplan & Sadock's Synopsis of Psychiatry (9th Ed.). Philadelphia: Lippincott: Williams & Wilkins; 2003.

[54] von Krosigk B. Personality Disorders. In: Burke A. (ed.) Abnormal Psychology: A South African Perspective (2nd Ed.). Cape Town: Oxford University Press; 2012

[55] Christakou A, Brammer M, Rubia K. Maturation of limbic corticostriatal activation and connectivity associated with developmental changes in temporal discounting. Neuroimage 2011; 54(2) 1344-1354.

[56] Burke A, Austin, T-L. Early identification of Borderline Personality Disorder: A study of abused adolescent girls. Social Worker Practitioner-Researcher 2010; 22 (3) 381-401.

[57] Pincus JH, Tucker GJ. Behavioral Neurology (4th ed.). Oxford: Oxford University Press; 2002.

[58] Bandelow B, Schmahl C, Falkai P, Wedekind D. Borderline personality disorder: A dysregulation of the endogenous opioid system? Psychological Review 2010; 117(2), 623-636.

[59] Whitley BE. Principles of research in behavioural sciences (2nd ed.). New York: McGraw-Hill; 2002

[60] McLean A, Dowson J, Toone B, Young S, Bazins E, Robbins TW, Sahakian BJ. Characteristics neurocognitve profile associated with adult attention-deficit/hyperactivity disorder. Psychological Medicine 2004; 34 681-692.

[61] Clarke AR, Barry RJ, Heaven PCL, McCarthy R, Selikowitz M, Byrne MK. EEG coherence in adults with attention-deficit/hyperactivity disorder. International Journal of Psychophysiology 2008; 67, 35-40.

[62] Quinn CA. Detection of malingering in assessment of adult ADHD. Archives of Clinical Neuropsychology 2003; 18 379-395.

[63] Millon T. Millon Clinical Miltiaxial Inventory –III. Minneapolis: Computer Systems Inc.; 1994.

[64] Bates B. Worried Adults May Err in ADHD Self-Diagnosis. Clinical Psychiatry News 1999, 27(4) 24.

[65] Wender PH, Wolf, LE, Wasserstein J. Adults with ADHD. Annals New York Academy of Sciences 2001; 931 1-16.

[66] Goodman DW. ADHD in adults: Update for clinicians on diagnosis and assessment. Primary Psychiatry 2009; 16(11) 38-47.

[67] Kessler RC, Adler L, Ames M, Barkley RA, Birnbaum HG, Greenberg, PE, Johnston JA, Spencer T, Ustun TB. The world health organisation adult ADHD self-report scale (ASRS): A short screening scale for use in the general population. Psychological Medicine 2005; 35(2) 245-256.

[68] Garnier-Dykstra LM, Pinchevsky GM, Caldeira, KM, Vincent KB, Arria, AM. Self-reported adult attention-deficit/hyperactivity disorder symptoms among college students. Journal of American College Health 2010; 59(2) 133-136.

[69] Taylor A, Deb S, Unwin G. Scales for the identification of adults with attention deficit hyperactivity disorder (ADHD): A systematic review. Research in Developmental Disabilities 2011; 32 924-938.

[70] Adler LA, Ciranni M, Shaw DM, Paunikar P. ADHD screening and follow-up: Results from a survey of participants 2 years after and adult ADHD screening day. Primary Psychiatry 2010; 17(2) 32-37.

[71] Groth-Marnat G. Handbook of psychological assessment (3rd ed.). New York: John Wiley & Sons; 1997.

[72] Craig RJ. New directions in interpreting the Millon Clinical Multi-axial Inventory-III (MCMI-III). New Jersey: John Wiley & Sons; 2005.

[73] Millon T, Millon C, Davis R, Grossman S. MCMI-III Manual (4th Ed.). Minneapolis, MN: Pearson Education; 2009.

[74] Voeller KKS. Attention-deficit hyperactivity disorder (ADHD). Journal of Child Neurology 2004;19 798- 814.

[75] Kropotov JD. Quantitative EEG, event-related potentials and neurotherapy. London: Academic Press; 2009.

[76] Loo KS, Barkley RA. Clinical utility of EEG in attention deficit hyperactivity disorder. Applied Neuropsychology 2005: 12(2) 64-76.

[77] Biopac MP Systems Hardware [Apparatus and Software]. California, USA: SR Research; 2008.

[78] Zillmer, EA, Spiers, MV, Culbertson, WC. Principles of neuropsychology (2nd ed.). California: Thomason Wadsworth; 2008.

[79] Pivik RT, Broughton, RJ, Coppola R, Davidson RJ, Fox N, Nuwer MR. Guidelines for the recording and quantitative analysis of electroencephalographic activity in research contexts. Psychophysiology 1993; 30 547-558.

[80] Corsi-Cabrera M, Galindo-Vilchis L, Del-Rio-Portilla Y, Arce C, Ramos-Loyo J. Within-subject reliability and inter-session stability of EEG power and coherent activity in women evaluated monthly over nine months. Clinical Neurophysiology 2007; 118 9-21.

[81] Lansbergen MM, Schutter DJLG, Kenemans JL. Subjective impulsivity and baseline EEG in relation to stopping performance. Brain Research 2007; 1148 161-169.

[82] Dressler O, Schneider G, Stockmanns G, Kochs EF. Awareness and the EEG power spectrum: analysis of frequencies. British Journal of Anaesthetics 2004; 93(6) 806-9.

[83] Campbell IG, Feinberg I. Longitudinal trajectories of non-rapid eye movement delta and theta EEG as indicators of adolescent brain maturation. Proceedings of the National Academy of Science of the United States of America 2009; 106, 5177-5180.

[84] Kurth S, Ringli M, Geiger A, LeBourgeois M, Jenni OG, Huber R. Mapping of cortical activity in the first two decades of life: A high-density sleep electroencephalogram study. The Journal of Neuroscience 2010; 30(40) 13211-13219.

[85] Field A. Discovering statistics using SPSS (2nd ed.). London: Sage; 2005.

[86] Fox NA, Hane, AA, Pérez-Edgar K. Psychophysiological methods for the study of developmental psychopathology. In: Cicchetti D, Cohen DJ (Eds.), Developmental psychopathology: Developmental Neuroscience (2nd ed).. New Jersey: John Wiley & Sons; 2006. p 381-426.

[87] Ringli M, Huber R. Developmental aspects of sleep slow waves: Linking sleep, brain maturation and behaviour. In: Van Someren EJW, Van Der Werf YD, Roelfsema PR, Mansvelder HD, Lopes Da Silva FH(Eds). Progress in brain research: Slow brain oscillations of sleep, resting state and vigilance. London: Elsevier; 2011. p. 63-82

Difficulties in Recognizing ADHD in an Urban Population and Treatment Satisfaction with a Short and a Long Acting Stimulant

Antigone Papavasiliou, Irene Nikaina,
Anna Spyridonidou and Eleanna Nianiou

Additional information is available at the end of the chapter

http://dx.doi.org/10.5772/53791

1. Introduction

Attention deficit hyperactivity disorder (ADHD) is an established neuropsychiatric disorder in children and adolescents with paediatric or mental health services available across most of Europe. In spite of major improvements in the availability of services for the diagnosis of ADHD and several therapeutic options, including medications, psychosocial and psycho-educational therapies, families of children with ADHD experience considerable emotional and social burden [1-2]. The presence and severity of the child's ADHD is a significant predictor of heightened parental stress and the diagnosis of ADHD can result in impairments in the Quality of Life in patients and their families [3-4]. Yet, there is a rather limited number of studies exploring parental perceptions of the diagnosis and overall treatment of this disorder.

An American study determined that primary care physicians generally adhere to practices specified in the AAP guidelines [1] for the diagnosis and treatment of pediatric ADHD; some variations existed and improvements were possible. Poor access to mental health services, limited insurance coverage, and other potential system barriers to the delivery of ADHD care were noted [5]. An Australian study explored perceptions relating to the diagnosis, treatment and overall management of the disorder [6] in the families of 278 children with ADHD identified in a community sample of 11 184 children aged 10-12 years; only 66% of parents recalled the use of questionnaires or rating scales, drugs were tried in 82% and 66% of the children were still on them, behavioral intervention in 42% and alternative treatments, mostly elimination diet and/or fatty acid supplementation, were used in 71%. Overall, 55% of parents were satisfied or very satisfied with their child's care. The conclusion of this study was that adherence to recommended diagnostic guidelines was inadequate, behavioral intervention was underutilized and non-conventional therapies were widely used and considered helpful in one-third of the children who used them. A study conducted on 20 low socioeconomic status mothers with children 5-11 years of age with ADHD taking stimulants, aimed to examine the effect of a 5-week educational intervention on ADHD [7]. Parental satisfaction and parental sense of competency improved in mothers who participated in the educational intervention.

Psychosocial and psycho-educational interventions as well as pharmacological treatments are effective in reducing ADHD symptom frequency and severity [1]. Stimulant medications are recommended as a first-line modality for treating ADHD [8]. They proved effective in improving both ADHD core symptoms (inattention, hyperactivity and impulsivity) and the behavioral problems that frequently accompany the disorder (such as aggressive behavior, depressive mood, anxiety, tics, impaired social functioning and academic productivity) [9]. Remission of ADHD symptoms via medication provides the best possible chance for educational and social re-integration and improved functioning through the utilization of non-pharmacological interventions [10]. Methylphenidate (MPH), a stimulant, is available in immediate and extended release forms. Because the half-life of MPH in immediate-release formulations is short, twice or better thrice daily administration is needed in order to maintain the desirable therapeutic effect. This obviously creates many practical difficulties during school days; it affects the patient's emotions (embarrassment in taking medication at school), it interferes with medical privacy preservation, and contributes to poor compliance with the therapeutic regimen [10-11]. Once-daily MPH in extended release form is significantly more effective than short acting MPH based on multiple outcome measures including remission rate [10,12], with better compliance being a primary factor [13-16].

Satisfaction with medication or any therapeutic intervention is an important factor in the evaluation of overall treatment outcome in ADHD or any other disorder; it is predictive of better adherence and compliance to treatment, and prevents premature treatment termination [17]. It depends primarily on the effectiveness of the drug but it is also influenced by parental and patient expectations, demographic characteristics, social acceptability of the treatment, the relationship between patient/parents and physician as well as the physician's knowledge, competence and ability to communicate with patients and their families [18]. Cultural factors are also very important in the acceptability of the treatment [19]. Furthermore, use of stimulant medication combined with frequent reviews (at least 6 monthly) was more likely to be associated with overall management satisfaction [6].

The goals of this paper were a. to explore family experiences in seeking diagnosis and treatment of ADHD in an urban community and b. to investigate acceptance and compliance of stimulant medication and specifically the two preparations of MPH available in our country, one in immediate and one in extended-release form (Ritalin and Concerta).

2. Patients and methods

Two independent samples of children fulfilling DSM-IV criteria for ADHD and their families were recruited to test the study goals. Diagnosis was based on the clinical presentation of the child and on specific standardized diagnostic tools and was established by a specialized group of physicians (pediatrician, pediatric neurologist, pediatric psychiatrist), school and clinic psychologist and special educator. Relevant patient characteristics such as demographic characteristics (age, sex), ADHD type, previous treatments, concomitant disorders, along with information on the prescribed treatment were recorded.

Study group 1. Thirty three families with children who fulfilled DSM-IV criteria for ADHD, 5-16 years old, who consecutively visited our outpatient department for the first time received an open ended questionnaire, consisting of 6 main questions and 12 sub-questions that investigated family impressions and experience in dealing with this disorder. More specifically, we asked about a. reasons for seeking help, b. source of referral (self-referred, schools, special educators, physicians, psychologists), c. obstacles they confronted in reaching diagnosis and treatment (difficulty in reaching specialized care, difficulty in dealing with education problems). A DSM-IV derived inattention/hyperactivity scale was used in order for parents to rate their children for 18 DSM-IV category A symptoms, on a 4-point scale [20]. This form was used in the follow up visits of our patients in order to document response to treatment. Therapeutic options were then offered including the use of short acting MPH, with a dosage schedule that called for 5 mg qam or bid at the onset and dosage titration to less than 2.0 mg/kg/day or 60 mg per day [21]. Patients were also offered a psychotherapeutic program focusing in social capabilities practice. Their parents were involved in counseling sessions and were encouraged to participate in support and advice groups, aiming at strengthening the net of care around the patients. Other treatment options were speech therapy, occupational therapy and special education as needed per individual child. The therapy that was actually used as well as the efficacy of the medication was subsequently explored by a different physician 6 months after the initial visit. The safety of the prescribed medication was also explored at that time.

Study group 2. Eighty four patients ≤ 18 years old, who were also followed as outpatients in the Pediatric Neurology Department, were included in the current study group. Inclusion criteria were a. ADHD diagnosis and b. the decision to begin treatment with long acting MPH. Doses were calculated according to body weight with the final dose less than 2.0 mg/kg/day or 72 mg/day [21]. All patients had been also offered psychosocial and psychoeducational intervention programs and their parents were involved in counseling sessions as well as support and advice groups. Previous treatment with short acting MPH was not an exclusion criterion in this study.

Six months after treatment initiation, a telephone interview was scheduled by a physician other than the one who prescribed the treatment, in order to determine their satisfaction level from the newly introduced treatment. A four level Likert scale was used for this purpose (0= no satisfaction at all, 1=modest satisfaction, 2=moderate satisfaction, 4=great satisfaction) and free comments on their impressions were encouraged and recorded. The safety of the treatment was also explored.

3. Statistical analysis

Continuous variables were tested for normalcy with the Kolmogorov - Smirnov test. Normal variables were then presented as mean values (± standard deviation). Categorical variables were expressed either as percentages or as absolute numbers.

Study group 1. Descriptive statistics based on the parents' answers are reported.

Study group 2. In order to determine the prognostic factors which could affect the satisfaction level from the treatment with long standing methylphenidate a logarithmic regression model was applied with the variable coding the level of satisfaction, used as dependent variable modified to include only two categories (median to great satisfaction versus no to mild satisfaction). As independent variables in the model we used variables coding patients' characteristics (age, sex, ADHD type) and features of the treatment under study (previous treatment with short acting MPH and the response rate to this previous therapy), that may affect the level of satisfaction or that may be important confounding factors. Continuous variables that were introduced in the model were previously centered.

4. Results

Table 1 displays a summary of the characteristics of the two study groups.

Study group 1. The parents of 33 children (20 boys and 13 girls), 6-16 years old (10 years 3 months ± 2 years 10 months) reported the following: a. The reasons reported for seeking help were: 48.5 % increasing difficulties at home and poor school performance, 21.2 % school recommendation, 18.2 % other developmental problem (such as speech delay) and 12.1% parents' concern about child's behavior. b. Only 3% of our patients were referred by their peadiatrician, while 36.3% were self-referred, 27.3% were referred by a state mental health clinic, 21.2% by a psychologist/speech-therapist or occupational therapist, and 12.2% by a school teacher. c. Over half of the 33 families included in this study group had difficulties in reaching specialized help; more specifically, 33.3% encountered ignorance about ADHD-appropriate medical services, 27.3% reported no difficulty, 21.2% encountered lack of appropriate medical services, 12.1%, large waiting lists in hospitals and mental health services and 6.1%, other problems. Almost 50% of them reported ignorance and unwillingness on the part of school teachers to provide help with their children: 45.5 % of the school teachers were ignorant and not helpful, 30.5 % were ignorant but helpful and supportive to the child in the classroom and only 24 % were informed and helpful.

As for their impressions about the disorder, parents' considerations about the cause of ADHD were as follows: 30.3% reported ignorance, 24.3% believed that there was inheritance, 21.2% attributed it to a complication in pregnancy-delivery, 15.2%, to problems in school / family environment, 6%, to some psychological problem and 3%, to a complication due to a disease. Treatment with short acting MPH (Ritalin) was proposed to 91% and 79% of this patient population received Ritalin; of them 95% described benefit in attention and behavior (73% reported major improvement in the ADHD core symptoms, 23% reported little but important improvement). Continuation of treatment was accepted by 63%. Reasons for not accepting continuation of methylphenidate were fear of addiction and unspecified side effects. The medicine was well tolerated by the majority of them with only one having to interrupt the treatment because of gastrointestinal symptoms (vomiting). Other side effects (reported by 38% of the parents) were decreased appetite, sleepiness, tics, nervousness and headache.

http://dx.doi.org/10.5772/53791

Study group 2. Eighty four children, 66 boys and 18 girls, with a mean age of 13 years (± 3 years) were offered treatment with long standing methylphenidate (Table 1). Thirteen of them stopped prematurely or never started treatment and as consequence they were excluded from the statistics. In the subsequent analysis, 71 children who received treatment were finally included (55 males / 16 girls). According to their initial symptoms patients were categorized into three ADHD types: inattentive type 33,4% (ν=23), hyperkinetic/impulsive type 64,8% (ν=46) and mixed type 2,8% (ν=2). The age at diagnosis was 8 years and 4 months (SD = ± 3 years 3 months). Mean age at treatment onset was 10 years 8 months (± 3 years). Fifty of our patients (70.42%) had been previously treated with short acting MP. However, data about response to that treatment were available for 47 patients; with 34 out of them having responded well to that treatment (27 had a good response and 7 a very good response).

	Study group1	Study group 2
Age	10 years 3 months ± 2 years 10 months	10 years 8 months ± 3 years
Male/female	20/13	55/16
ADHD type (inattention / hyperactive/ combined)	13/5/15	23/46/2
Previous treatment (yes/no)	0/33	50/21

Table 1. Demographic and clinical characteristics of the two study groups

At the time of treatment initiation with the long acting MPH (Concerta), most of our patients (ν=47) were given an initial dose of 18 mg, that was subsequently titled to higher doses. A higher initial dose (36 mg) was given to 33 patients (46.48%) who had high body weight. Lowering this initial dose became necessary in only one patient.

Concerning parent satisfaction level, the majority of them (80.28%) reported moderate to full satisfaction, 36.6% moderate satisfaction and 43.7% full satisfaction. The most frequent effect was observed in the attention domain (improvement in 97.18% of the children), followed by the effect in hyperkinetic behaviour (improvement in 63.38% of the children). Impulsivity was not controlled in the majority of the patients (improvement in 19.72% of them). Almost half of the patients reported improvement in two of the ADHD domains (n=34, 47,89%), 12 patients (19,9%) improved in all three domains and only one reported no improvement in any of the domains of the disorder. Thirty eight of the patients previously treated with short acting MPH (80.85%) reported moderate to full satisfaction with the long acting formulation. Only one of the parents who were not satisfied with short acting MPH (n=13) continued to be dissatisfied with the long acting one. Eight patients with good response (2-3) to the short acting MPH, however, were not satisfied with the long-acting MPH.

The logistic regression analysis applied in order to reveal prognostic factors affecting parental satisfaction level showed that only age at treatment initiation with long acting MP was an independent prognostic factor (OR=1.38, 95%CI=1.04 –1.83, p=0.025). Treatment initiation at an older age resulted in higher probability (by 38%) of moderate to full parental satisfaction from the treatment, with the type of ADHD, sex and the previous treatment with short acting MP treated as confounding factors (p=0,423 p=0,963 and p=0.299, respectively). Similar results were also reported when the analysis was restricted to the subset of patients who were previously treated with the short acting regimen. In this analysis we also examined the response rate to the previous medication as an important prognostic factor. Age at treatment with long acting MPH onset was again the only significant determinant of parental satisfaction (OR= 1.49, 95%CI= 1.05-2.11 p=0.026). ADHD type, sex and response to Ritalin (moderate to full response vs no response to modest response) were not significant covariates (p=0.929, 0.543 and p=0.320, respectively).

5. Discussion

Families of children with ADHD frequently experience considerable emotional and financial stressors [21-23]. These harmful effects of ADHD on patients and families affirm the need for effective treatment and make it a public health concern [24]. Children with ADHD require more than 1.5 times more primary care visits, 9 times more outpatient mental health visits, and 3 times more prescriptions per year, compared to children without ADHD [25]. It was estimated that the total annual health care costs for children with ADHD is more than twice that of children without the disorder, and these costs become significantly larger when a child with ADHD is diagnosed with a comorbid condition [25-27]. It is also noted that the direct cost of treatment for this disorder has increased considerably during the last years. The increase in expenditure for the treatment of ADHD may be due to increasing demand for diagnostic and therapeutic services and improved availability of such services. [28-30].

The first important finding of this study was that only one fourth of the families studied (Study group 1) reported an easy accessibility to appropriate services for the diagnosis and therapy of ADHD in their children. Several barriers to the diagnosis of the disorder have been previously reported. It is interesting to note that, although parents usually realize that something is wrong with their child, especially if symptoms are severe, they are not always seeking medical advice. In 2003, Bussing et al demonstrated that whereas 88% of high risk for ADHD elementary school students were recognized as having a problem, only 39% had been evaluated [31]. Few years later, in 2006, Sayal et al, in another study exploring barriers to the identification of ADHD, found that the main barrier to care for ADHD is the limited presentation of these problems to primary care [32]. Although most of the parents contacted (80%) recognized that their child had a problem, only few had consulted primary care physicians or had sought help from specialist health services while some had been in contact with professionals in educational services. On the other hand, Leslie and coworkers suggested the existence of a pattern of delayed diagnosis, mostly associated with failure to recognize ADHD by parents/ caregivers [33]. This pattern was more common among youths with complicated clinical and/or environmental factors or primarily symptoms of inattention. Delayed diagnosis was reported especially in girls with ADHD, due to the predominance of symptoms of inattention rather than hyperactivity/impulsivity as compared to boys [34-35] and due to the lower frequency of conduct disorder, aggression, or delinquency [35-38]. Parental recognition

http://dx.doi.org/10.5772/53791

of problems and their perception of hyperactivity as a symptom of a disorder, rather than a childhood feature, were reported as to the most significant factors influencing contact with medical services [32, 39].

Recognition of the disorder by primary care physicians, though, was related to both child and parent factors (especially the first). Non-recognition of ADHD in the primary care setting was the main barrier to further accessing specialist services [39]; when the parent was unaware or reticent about the possibility of requesting a referral, then the diagnosis could be missed. Therefore, parental request for referral and thus parental recognition of hyperactive behaviour as problematic plays a crucial role in accessing primary care as well as specialist services [39]. Race has been one of the factors contributing to barriers in diagnosis; Caucasian children had twice the odds of being brought to attention than other racial groups, with boys having a 5-fold increased possibility of being evaluated [32]. Ethnic minorities had a lower rate of diagnosis and treatment for the disorder. Those racial/ethnic disparities in service use are the result of a combination of access barriers and individual, cultural, and societal factors [40]. After the diagnosis of ADHD was established, Hispanic families used the fewest services, single-mother families used the most of them and families with boys with ADHD used more services as compared to families with girls with ADHD [38]. Surprisingly, economic status of the family was not a stable prognostic factor of accessibility and usage of specialized services. In the study of Kendall et al income was not a significant factor in any services used or services requested, whereas in the study of Bussing et al poverty status was associated with lower treatment rates and with the most pervasive barriers [31, 41].

Another striking finding of this study was that only 3% of patients were referred to specialized care by a pediatrician; this points to the need for better education of paediatricians on ADHD and dissemination of existing knowledge and guidelines on diagnosis and treatment. According to clinicians' perceptions about ADHD, the diagnostic process is considered complicated, time-consuming and experience requiring, while published guidelines were viewed as vague [42]. Referral rate by school teachers was also quite low (approximately 12%); we believe that lack of appropriate education of the teachers on ADHD seems to be the most important factor. In a survey aiming at exploring perceptions of ADHD with a focus on gender differences, many teachers reported that they have received little or no education in ADHD as part of their curriculum (with only 10% of schools providing significant training for teachers on ADHD), while few reported having received significant training [43]. Moreover, half of the interviewed teachers revealed that even when they suspected that a child suffered of ADHD, they hesitated to inform his/hers parent or guardian. The years of experience with hyperactive children, the number of hyperactive pupils in their classrooms, and the level of perceived self-efficacy of the teachers seems to have a positive correlation with their knowledge about ADHD, which is focusing more on symptoms and diagnosis [44]. Lack of educational support and teachers' understanding of ADHD were also identified as problems, in the study of Concannon and Tang [6].

Concerning perceptions about the etiology of ADHD, one third of the parents we contacted had complete ignorance about causes of ADHD, almost 20% believed that environmental and psychological factors had a causal relationship and the remainder attributed the disorder to a medical condition/disease or to inheritance. Perceptions about ADHD causes have evolved during the recent years in different communities. Almost two decades before, the disorder was attributed to poor diet, antisocial conduct, lack of discipline, emotional problems at school and in interpersonal relations [45]. Yet, even today an impressing reluctance to accept the biomedical explanation of ADHD exists, especially in developing countries. Psychological problems, socio-environmental factors, learning and memory difficulties, inappropriate parenting and disciplinary practices [46-49] continue to be seen as possible causes. Guilt and self-blame, accusations towards the spouse and concerns about the volitional or non-volitional nature of the problem, still, prevail in parents' beliefs. In a study conducted in Greece, parents were more likely to report intentionality in boys with ADHD than in girls whereas biological dysfunction was considered as a more likely etiology in girls than in boys [50].

In this study, we explored attitudes towards ADHD treatment among the families that participated. In the first part of this study, 79% of the parents accepted MPH treatment following medical advice but only 63% finally continued the therapy. The respective percentage of the second study group for treatment initiation/6-month continuation was 84.5%, which is considerably increased compared to the first one; this difference could be attributed to the evolution of time, (study 1 preceded chronologically study 2). Yet, both rates are quite high. Hoare et al, reported that 88.1% of their sample wanted their child to continue treatment more than 21 days (the initial trial period) and 63 % completed the 1-year trial (extension phase) [51]. In contrast, Chen et al reported that approximately 30% of young people received MPH treatment within one year after diagnosis, and virtually none remained in treatment beyond 12 months [52]. Sample study composition may be responsible for the discrepancy among our results and those of Hoare et al in one hand and the results of Chen et al in the other hand. In the study of Chen et al, only newly diagnosed, and thus treatment naive, children were enrolled, whereas in our study more than half of the participants had previously used the short acting MPH regimen and in the study of Hoare and coworkers, all participants had changed from the short to the long acting MPH medication. It is reported that, despite high response rates to the pharmacotherapy (approximately 70% or more when patients were strictly complying with the treatment) [53-55], parents and teachers consider non-pharmacological therapies or the combination of pharmacological and non-pharmacological therapies to be more acceptable [54, 56-59]. Leslie et al suggested three types of parental reactions to medication proposal: a pattern of preference towards non medication treatment as their initial choice; a reluctant receipt of an ADHD diagnosis and/or treatment pattern, mainly seen among the low-income, Spanish-speaking families; and a rapid engagement in medication use pattern, characterized by directed movement to and maintenance of medication use [33].

Treatment decisions in ADHD are usually the result of a shared process between families, children, and the clinician [42]. Parents and clinicians conceptualize ADHD differently and they should negotiate a shared understanding of ADHD. Parents' terms reflected ADHD's effects on the child and family, while clinicians often mentioned school. Treatment discussions should be tailored to encompass families' varied emotional and educational needs [60]. Recognition of a medical etiology for the disorder was the most influential factor reported in willingness to accept drugs and/or combination treatment [58-59]. On the other hand, the main reasons for hesitating to start medication were concerns about side effects, worries about the stigma associated with ADHD or its treatment and concerns about medication (the belief that the medication would lead to drug addiction in adulthood) [43, 46]. Factors associated with earlier initiation of MPH treatment were older age, sex (with parents of girls being more willing to start medication), lower socioeconomic status, diagnosis of the disorder while school was in session, diagnosis from a physician specializing in pediatrics or psychiatry, and diagnosis in a district hospital/clinic [43, 52]. Patients more severely ill and/or having co-morbidities had also a greater possibility of receiving treatment [61] In a study aiming to evaluate predictors of long-term adherence to treatment with methylphenidate the authors reported that the presence of associated disorders, younger age, female gender, and single-parent families were predictors for continuing medication for 36 months (study duration) [62]. On the contrary, older age, medication concerns, the absence of associated disorders and serious side effects appeared to increase the risk of discontinuation of the treatment or loss to follow up [52, 62, 63, 65]. Generally, ADHD medication adherence and persistence seems to be suboptimal, with patients using non-stimulant medication being more compliant compared to stimulant users. Since ADHD can be effectively treated with medications, health professionals should be proactive in identifying patients with poor adherence and intervene to address barriers to medication adherence and persistence [66]. In this study, the reasons for treatment discontinuation were side effects and fears of addiction to treatment.

Side effects reported in this study included mostly gastrointestinal and central nervous system symptoms. This finding is in accordance with a recent review in which, decrease in appetite, gastrointestinal pain, and headache were considered as the most frequently reported adverse reactions, with very few of them being rated as serious. However, since a large number of children drop out of studies due to serious side effects, it is believed that their actual number is probably higher. These side effects are reported in clinical studies of short duration, whereas long term safety is still a matter of research [69, 71]. Concerns about possible harm, especially, from the newly developed ADHD drugs have arisen, focusing on both minor adverse effects and extremely serious issues such as sudden cardiac death and suicidality [72]. Another important finding in this study was that a great percentage of the ADHD parents expressed at least moderate satisfaction from the long acting MPH. This is not surprising since previous studies had advocated overall medication satisfaction, as expressed by patients, parents/caregivers and/or physicians. Generally, satisfaction with stimulant medication as the sole therapy has been shown to be relatively high and 63–87% of patients, parents and teachers made positive assessments [11, 64, 69 -70]. In most of these studies, the researchers explored satisfaction rates for long acting MPH as compared to short acting MPH. In a study presented at the 2004 Annual Meeting of the Canadian Academy of Child and Adolescent Psychiatry, on the pharmacological evolutions concerning ADHD, Swanson and Hechtman reported significantly higher remission rates and significantly higher Clinical Global Impression and parent satisfaction scores with long acting MPH as compared to short acting MPH (results from an 8-week open-label trial) [71]. Similar results were presented in 2006, in another 8 week, multicentre, randomized, open-label study in which 147 ADHD patients (6-12 years old) received either once-daily long acting MPH or usual care with the short acting regimen. The first drug proved to be superior to the latter in terms of remission rate, severity of ADHD and

ODD symptoms, Clinical Global Impression-Improvement, Parent Satisfaction with treatment (50% of parents were 'completely satisfied' with long acting MPH given once daily, compared with 21% with the short acting MPH given two or three times daily) and other secondary outcome scores [10]. In 2005, Hoare at al, also, reported that in the case of children previously treated with the short acting regimen and then switched to the long lasting one (n=105), the parent/caregiver global assessment of satisfaction ranged from 49 to 69% after an initial 21-day trial, and 49 to 71% of investigators rated the treatment as adequate [51]. Finally, in a double-blind comparison of a long-acting MPH formulation (osmotic release oral system [OROS] MPH [Concerta, Janssen-Cilag Ltd]) given once-daily versus three-times-daily MPH-IR, 47% of parents preferred the long-acting formulation, 31% the IR formulation, and 15% their previous MPH treatment [72].

In this study, the vast majority (~81%) of the patients' subgroup previously treated with the short-acting regimen were at least moderately satisfied. From those parents who reported a good response with the short acting MPH, 26/34 were satisfied with the long acting one and only 8/34 were not. From those exhibiting an inadequate response with the short acting MPH, 12/13 subsequently report moderate to full satisfaction. This is consistent with previous results, according to which, switching from one MPH preparation to another appears to be a valid clinical approach that may contribute to treatment success. Four factors were postulated to be responsible of the observed improvement in various treatment outcomes: first, the increase (and thus optimization) of MPH dose; second, the shorter intervals between visits directly after switching, leading to more intense education and guidance of those involved; third, a positive expectation of improvement by all participants; and fourth, a possible increase in adherence in the long-term [18, 73-74]. On the other hand, dissatisfaction rate does not necessarily reflect low efficiency. In the study of Gortz-Dorten et al, approximately 30% of parents were dissatisfied with the medication, while efficacy was highly rated, making treatment individualization a very important aspect of the pharmacological treatment [18].

In our study, most parents reported satisfaction with the MPH effect especially for inattention symptoms, followed by the satisfaction rate on the hyperkinetic behavior. This high satisfaction rate on the grounds of improvement in attention had also been reported in a recent study, in the school setting and in academic situations [18]. The overall parental satisfaction with the medication exceeded the percentage of 70% (63-75.6%). The parents were also very satisfied with the effects of the drug in the children's social interactions with other children and within the family. Finally, almost 56% of parents also reported high satisfaction with how the medication helped their child feel good. These results are supported by other studies, performed in the UK and in Sweden [70, 75].

Finally, according to our results, age at treatment initiation was a significant determinant of level of parent satisfaction. We were not able though to relate parent satisfaction with type of ADHD, sex of the patient or the previous experience with short acting MPH. In 2005, Hoare et al, exploring the efficacy of long acting MPH in the long term (12 months) reported that efficacy and satisfaction were more common in patients of older age (10-16 years), those on a higher dose (36 mg or 54 mg) and those with the predominantly inattentive ADHD subtype [51], results only partly in aggreement with ours. In another study, parents expressed higher satisfaction rates if their children showed a greater reduction in ADHD symptoms and greater improvements in all QoL domains [18]. They argued that symptom severity and/or functional impairment at the end of the study, as well as QoL, were the most significant predictors for parent and patient satisfaction. They also showed that satisfaction with medication slightly but significantly increased during the treatment and as time passed (from visit 1 to visit 3).

The results of our study need to be viewed in light of several limitations.

Limitation 1: One major limitation of this study was that parents' satisfaction was assessed by asking parents how satisfied they were, using a Likert scale. At the time of study conduction, there were no standardized and validated rating scales for satisfaction in Greek, not to mention that the whole concept of using such scales was new. The method we used is clearly not consistent or uniform and prevents the conduction of immediately comparable studies [19]. In the literature on ADHD, measures of satisfaction with medication such as the medication satisfaction questionnaire (MSS) [76] or the parent consumer satisfaction questionnaire (PCSQ) [77] exist and these were not used by us. In a recent study, another measure, the satisfaction with medication scale (SAMS) has been validated [18]. This new rating scale was designed to assess the satisfaction with ADHD medication of parents and children on a per item basis. It would be very informative if a new study using these measures is conducted in our setting.

Limitation 2: Satisfaction level in our study was reported only for parents/caregivers. Patient satisfaction with medication though may be an important factor in the evaluation of overall treatment outcome [64]. In order for treatments to be considered effective, they have to be viewed favorably by patients who also have to be willing to use them [19]. Although parental satisfaction is usually in accordance with the child's feeling on treatment effect, this is not always the case. In a double-blind crossover study child and parent perceptions of treatment with stimulant medication in a sample of 102 children with ADHD was attempted; disagreement between child and parental perceptions of treatment response existed in >25%. This involved mostly parental viewing of the child's response favorably, while the child's rating was unfavorable; side-effects were the main determinant of children's perceptions of adverse outcome. Thus, parental report alone is not infallible in providing reliable information regarding effects as experienced by the child [58]. In another study consisting of 79 child-parent peers, few differences between parents and children for positive effects existed, although parents reported higher levels of negative effects. This result suggested that parents' considerations clearly have an influence on the way children perceive medication [69]. In the study of Gortz-Dorten et al, patients reported slightly but significantly higher satisfaction than parents. Overall satisfaction with the medication was high for 79.0% of patients and 66.1% of children also reported high satisfaction with how the medication helped them feel good. In conclusion, it is important to assess parental and child perspectives separately, with comparable questions, as their perceptions of medication are correlated, but only to a moderate degree [18].

Limitation 3: This was an observational study; assuch, selection of participants was based on loose criteria and treatment conditions are less controlled and standardized. This study design could be considered an advantage, from a different point of view, as it reflects routine care conditions in a pragmatic setting. This could be especially true for studies evaluating satisfaction with medication, in which ratings from clinical trials are less informative as they are influenced by the fact that the sample is likely to be biased, given that those who agree to participate in the studies tend to do so because they are not satisfied with their previous medication [18-19].

Limitation 4: Both of our samples are comprised of parents who have already contacted specialized help. They have accepted the diagnosis and they decided to be involved in a therapeutic procedure, with some of them not treatment naive; parents who have not yet sought health care for their child may have different impressions and experiences. This may be considered as an important bias affecting perceptions, acceptance of the medication used and satisfaction with it.

6. Conclusion

Despite medical advances, barriers for families with children with ADHD in accessing medical services still exist. In this study, parents' perceptions, teachers' low educational status for the disorder and low recognition rate from the pediatricians were important factors of low accessibility of the medical services for diagnosis and treatment of the disorder. Most of the families having a diagnosis of ADHD and a prescription of a stimulant medication, followed medical advices. Stimulants, both short and long acting, were beneficial in improving ADHD symptoms. Parents were satisfied with the use of long acting stimulants, with older age of their child with ADHD being the only significant prognostic factor of their satisfaction level.

Author details

Antigone Papavasiliou[1], Irene Nikaina[1], Anna Spyridonidou[2] and Eleanna Nianiou[3]

1 Neurology Department, Pendeli Childrens' Hospital, Athens, Greece

2 Child and Adolescent Psychiatry Department, Sismanogleio General Athens Hospital, Athens, Greece

3 Department of Neurology, Iaso General Hospital, Athens, Cyprus

References

[1] American Academy of Pediatrics: Clinical practice guideline: diagnosis and evaluation of the child with attention-deficit/hyperactivity disorder. Pediatrics 2000, 105(5): 1158-1170.

[2] Coghill D, Soutullo C, d'Aubuisson C, Preuss U, Lindback T, Silverberg M, et al. Impact of attention-deficit/hyperactivity disorder on the patient and family: results from a European survey. Child Adolesc Psychiatry Ment Health 2008; 2(1):31

[3] Anastopoulos AD, Guevremont DC, Shelton TL, DuPaul GJ. Parenting stress among families of children with Attention Deficit Hyperactivity Disorder. J Abnorm Child Psychol 1992;20(5):503-20.

[4] Klassen AF, Miller A, Fine S. Health-related quality of life in children and adolescents who have a diagnosis of attention deficit/hyperactivity disorder. Pediatrics 2004; 114 (5):e541–e547

[5] Rushton JL, Fant KE, Clerk SJ. Use of practice guidelines in the primary care of children with attention-deficit/hyperactivity disorder. Pediatrics 2004;114(1): e23-8.

[6] Concannon PE, Tang Yp. Management of attention deficit hyperactivity disorder: a parental perspective. J Paediatr Child health 2005;41(12):625-30.

[7] Odom SE. Effects of an educational intervention on mothers of male children with attention deficit hyperactivity disorder. J Community Health Nurs 1996;13(4):207-20.

[8] American Academy of Child and Adolescent Psychiatry. Practice parameter for the use of stimulant medications in the treatment of children, adolescents, and adults. J Am Acad Child Adolesc Psychiatry 2002;41(Suppl2):26S-49S.

[9] Biederman J, Faraone SV. Attention-deficit hyperactivity disorder. Lancet 2005; 366: (9481)237–248

[10] Steele M, Weiss M, Swanson J, Wang J, Prinzo RS, Binder CE. A randomized, controlled effectiveness trial of OROS- methylphenidate compared to usual care with immediate-release methylphenidate in attention deficit hyperactivity disorder. Can J Clin Pharmacol 2006; 13 (1):e50–e62

[11] DosReis S, Zito JM, Safer DJ, Soeken KL, Mitchell JW Jr, Ellwood LC. Parental perceptions and satisfaction with stimulant medications for attention deficit/hyperactivity disorder. J Dev Behav Pediatr 2003; 24(3):155-162.

[12] Chou WJ, Chen SJ, Chen YS, Liang HY, Lin CC, Tang CS, et al. Remission in Children and Adolescents Diagnosed with Attention-Deficit/Hyperactivity Disorder via an Effective and Tolerable Titration Scheme for Osmotic Release Oral System Methylphenidate. J Child Adolesc Phychiatr 2012; 22 (3); 215-25

[13] Dopfner M, Gerber WD, Banaschewski T, Breuer D, Freisleder FJ, Gerber-von MG, et al. Comparative efficacy of once-a-day extended-release methylphenidate, two-times-daily immediate-release methylphenidate, and placebo in a laboratory school setting. Eur Child Adolesc Psychiatry 2004; 13(Suppl 1):93–101

[14] Banaschewski T, Coghill D, Santosh P, Zuddas A, Asherson P, Buitelaar J, et al. Long-acting medications for the hyperkinetic disorders. A systematic review and European treatment guideline. Eur Child Adolesc Psychiatry 2006; 15(8):476–495

[15] Findling RL, Quinn D, Hatch SJ, Cameron SJ, DeCory HH, McDowell M. Comparison of the clinical efficacy of twice-daily Ritalin and once-daily Equasym XL with placebo in children with Attention Deficit/Hyperactivity Disorder. Eur Child Adolesc Psychiatry 2006; 15(8):450–459.

[16] Breuer D, Gortz-Dorten-Dorten A, Rothenberger A, Dopfner M. Assessment of daily profiles of ADHD and ODD symptoms, and symptomatology related to ADHD medication, by parent and teacher ratings. Eur Child Adolesc Psychiatry. 2011. Doi: 10.1007/ s00787-011-0206-0

[17] Pekarik G. Relationship of clients' reasons for dropping out of treatment to outcome and satisfaction. J Clin Psychol 1992; 48(1):91–98

[18] Gortz-Dorten A, Breuer D, Hautmann C, Rothenberger A, Dopfner M. What contributes to patient and parent satisfaction with medication in the treatment of children with ADHD? A report on the development of a new rating scale. Eur Child Adolesc Psychiatry 2011; 20 (Suppl 2):S297–S307. DOI 10.1007/s00787-011-0207-z.

[19] Bukstein OG. Satisfaction with treatment for attention deficit/hyperactivity disorder. Am J Manag Care 2004; 10 (4 Suppl):S107–S116

[20] DuPaul GJ, Power TJ, Anastopoulos AD, Reid R. ADHD -Rating Scale-IV: Checklists, Norms And Clinical Interpretation. Copyright 1998

[21] Biederman J, Spencer TJ. Attention Deficit Hyperactivity Disorder: Psychopharmacological Interventions. Child Adolesc Psychiatr Clin North America 2008; 17(2): 439-458

[22] Johnston C, Mash EJ. Families of children with attention-deficit/hyperactivity disorder: Review and recommendations for future research. Clin Child Fam Psychol Rev 2001;4(3):183-207.

[23] Swensen AR, Birnbaum HG, Secnik K, Marynchenko M, Greenberg P, Claxton A. Attention-deficit/hyperactivity disorder: Increased costs for patients and their families. J Am Acad Child Adolesc Psychiatry 2003;42(12):1415-1423.

[24] Designating September 7th, 2004, as "National Attention Deficit Disorder Day." S Res 370, 108th Cong 2nd Session 2004.

[25] Guevara J, Lozano P, Wickizer T, Mell L, Gephart H. Utilization and cost of health care services for children with attention-deficit/hyperactivity disorder. Pediatrics 2001;108(1):71-78.

[26] Leibson CL, Katusic SK, Barbaresi WJ, Ransom J, O'Brien PC. Use and costs of medical care for children and adolescents with and without attention-deficit/hyperactivity disorder. JAMA 2001 (1);285:60-66.

[27] Chan E, Zhan C, Homer C. Health care use and costs for children with attention-deficit/hyperactivity disorder. Arch Pediatr Adolesc Med 2002;156(5): 504-11.

[28] Wehmeier PM, Schacht A, Rothenberger A. Change in the direct cost of treatment for children and adolescents with hyperkinetic disorder in Germany over a period of four years.Child Adolesc Psychiatry Ment Health 2009;3(1):3

[29] Winterstein AG, Gerhard T, Shuster J, Zito J, Johnson M, Liu H, et al. Utilization of pharmacological treatment in youths with attention deficit/hyperactivity disorder in Medicaid database. Ann Pharmacother. 2008;42(1):24-31. Epub 2007 Nov 27.

[30] van den Ban E, Souverein P, Swaab H, van Engeland H, Heerdink R, Egberts T. Trends in incidence and characteristics of children, adolescents and adults initiating immediate – or extended – release methyl or atomoxetine in the Netherlands during 2001-2006. J Child Adolesc Psychopharmacol. 2010 Feb;20(1):55-61.

[31] Bussing R, Zima BT, Gary FA, Garvan CW. Barriers to detection, help-seeking, and service use for children with ADHD symptoms. J Behav Health Serv Res. 2003;30(2): 176-89.

[32] Sayal K, Goodman R, Ford T. Barriers to the identification of children with attention deficit/hyperactivity disorder. J Child Psychol Psychiatry 2006;47(7):744-50.

[33] Leslie LK, Plemmons D, Monn AR, Palinkas LA. Investigating ADHD treatment trajectories: listening to families' stories about medication use. J Dev Behav Pediatr 2007;28(3):179-88

[34] Lahey BB, Applegate B, McBurnett K, et al. DSM-IV field trials for attention deficit hyperactivity disorder in children and adolescents. Am J Psychiatry. 1994; 151: 1673-1685.

[35] Biederman J, Mick E, Faraone SV, et al. Influence of gender on attention deficit hyperactivity disorder in children referred to a psychiatric clinic. Am J Psychiatry. 2002; 159(1): 36-42.

[36] Biederman J, Faraone SV, Spencer T, Wilens T, Mick E, Lapey KA. Gender differences in a sample of adults with attention deficit hyperactivity disorder. Psychiatry Res. 1994; 53(1): 13-29.

[37] Arnold LE. Sex differences in ADHD: conference summary. J Abnorm Child Psychol. 1996; 24(5): 555-569.

[38] Gershon J. A meta-analytic review of gender differences in ADHD. J Attention Dis. 2002;5(3): 143-154.

[39] Sayal K, Taylor E, Beecham J, Byrne O. Pathways to care in children at risk of attention-deficit hyperactivity disorder. British J Psychiatry 2002; 181: 43 – 48.

[40] Eiraldi RB, Mazzuca LB, Clarke AT, Power TJ. Utilization among ethnic minority children with ADHD: a model of help-seeking behavior. Adm Policy Ment Health. 2006;33(5):607-22.

[41] Kendall J, Leo MC, Perrin N, Hatton D. Service needs of families with children with ADHD. J Fam Nurs. 2005;11(3):264-88.

[42] Kovshoff H, Williams S, Vrijens M, Danckaerts M, Thompson M, Yardley L, et al. The decisions regarding ADHD management (DRAMa) study: Uncertainties and complexities in assessment, diagnosis and treatment. Eur Child Adolesc Psychiatry. 2012 ;21(2):87-99. Epub 2011 Dec 18.

[43] Quinn P, Wiga S. Perceptions of Girls and ADHD: Results From a National Survey. MedGenMed. 2004; 6(2): 2. Published online 2004 May 5. PMCID: PMC1395774.

[44] Fernández JS, Mínguez TR, Casas MA. Teachers' knowledge, misconceptions, and lacks concerning Attention Deficit Hyperactivity Disorder. Psicothema. 2007;19(4): 585-90.

[45] Sonuga-Barke EJ, Balding J. British parents' beliefs about the causes of three forms of childhood psychological disturbance. J Abnorm Child Psychol. 1993;21(4):367-76.

[46] Olaniyan O, dosReis S, Garriett V, Mychailyszyn MP, Anixt J, Rowe PC et al. Community perspectives of childhood behavioral problems and ADHD among African American parents. Ambul Pediatr. 2007;7(3):226-31.

[47] Wilcox CE, Washburn R, Patel V. Seeking help for attention deficit hyperactivity disorder in developing countries: a study of parental explanatory models in Goa, India. Soc Sci Med. 2007;64(8):1600-10.

[48] Dennis T, Davis M, Johnson U, Brooks H, Humbi A. Attention deficit hyperactivity disorder: parents' and professionals'perceptions. Community Pract. 2008 Mar; 81(3): 24-8.

[49] Peters K, Jackson D. Mothers' experiences of parenting a child with attention deficit hyperactivity disorder. J Adv Nurs. 2009;65(1):62-71.

[50] Maniadaki K, Sonuga-Barke E, Kakouros E. Parents' causal attributions about attention deficit/hyperactivity disorder: the effect of child and parent sex. Child Care Health Dev. 2005;31(3):331-40.

[51] Hoare P, Resschmidt H, Medori R, Ettrich C, Rothenberger A, Santosh P, et al. 12-month efficacy and safety of OROS MPH in children and adolescents with attention-deficit/hyperactivity disorder switched from MPH. Eur Child Adolesc Psychiatry 2005;14(6):305-9.

[52] Chen CY, Yeh HH, Chen KH, Chang IS, Wu EC, Lin KM. Differential effects of predictors on methylphenidate initiation and discontinuation among young people with

newly diagnosed attention-deficit/hyperactivity disorder. J Child Adolesc Psychopharmacol. 2011;21(3):265-73.

[53] Miller A, Lee SK, Raina P, Klassen A, Zupancic J, Olsen L. A review of therapies for attention-deficit/hyperactivity disorder. 1998 Ottawa: Canadian Coordinating Office for Health Technology Assessment (CCOHTA). Available from: http://www.ccohta.ca/main-e.htm

[54] MTA Cooperative Group. Multimodal treatment Study of Children with ADHD. A 14-month randomized clinical trial of treatment strategies for attention-deficit/hyperactivity disorded. Archives of General Psychiatry 1999;56(12):1073-86.

[55] Schachter HM, Pham B, King J, Langford S, Moher d. How efficacious and safe is short-acting methylphenidate for the treatment of attention-deficit disorder in children and adolescents? A meta-analysis. Canadian Medical Association journal 2001; 165(11):1474-88.

[56] Liu F, Muniz R, Minami H, Silva RR. Review and comparison of the long acting methylphenidate preparations. Psychiatr Q 2005;76(3):259–269

[57] Power TJ, Hess LE, Bennett DS. The acceptability of interventions for attention-deficit hyperactivity disorder among elementary and middle school teachers. J Dev Behav Pediatr 1995;16(4):238–243

[58] Lin YF, Chung HH. Parenting stress and parents' willingness to accept treatment in relation to behavioral problems of children with attention-deficit hyperactive disorder. J Nurs Res. 2002;10(1):43-56.

[59] Pham AV, Carlson JS, Kosciulek JF. Ethnic differences in parental beliefs of attention-deficit/hyperactivity disorder and treatment. J Atten Disord. 2010;13(6):584-91. Epub 2009 May 4.

[60] Fiks AG, Gafen A, Hughes CC, Hunter KF, Barg FK. Using freelisting to understand shared decision making in ADHD: parents' and pediatricians' perspectives. Patient Educ Couns. 2011 Aug;84(2):236-44. Epub 2010 Aug 24.

[61] Martényi F, Treuer T, Gau SS, Hong SD, Palaczky M, Suba J, et al. Attention-deficit / hyperactivity disorder diagnosis, co-morbidities, treatment patterns, and quality of life in a pediatric population in central and eastern Europe and Asia. J Child Adolesc Psychopharmacol. 2009 Aug;19(4):363-76.

[62] Atzori P, Usala T, Carucci S, Danjou F, Zuddas A. preedictive factors for persistent use and compliance of immediate-release methylphenidate: a 36- month naturalistic study. J Child Adolesc Psychopharmacol. 2009 Dec;19(6):673-81.

[63] Berger-Jenkins E, McKay M, Newcorn J, Bannon W, Laraque D. Parent medication concerns predict underutilization of mental health services for minority children with ADHD. Clin Pediatr (Phila). 2012;51(1):65-76. doi: 10.1177/0009922811417286. Epub 2011 Aug 25.

[64] Efron D, Jarman FC, Barker MJ. Child and parent perceptions of stimulant medication treatment in attention deficit hyperactivity disorder. J Paediatr Child Health 1998; 34(3):288–292

[65] Aagaard L, Hansen EH. Thee ocuurence of adverse drug reactions reported for attention-deficit hyperactivity disorder (ADHD) medications in the pediatric population: a qualitative review of empirical studies. Neuropsychiatr Dis Treat. 2011;7:729-44. Epub 2011 Dec 16

[66] Barner JC, Khoza S, Oladapo A. ADHD medication use, adherence, persistence and cost among Texas medicaid children. Curr Med Res Opin. 2011;27 Suppl 2:13-22.

[67] van de Loo-Neus GH, Rommelse N, Buitelaar JK. To stop or not to stop? How long should medication treatment of attention-deficit hyperactivity disorder be extende? Eur Neuropsychopharmacol. 2011 Aug;21(8):584-99. Epub 2011 May 6. Review.

[68] Graham J, Banaschewski T, Buitelaar J, Coghill D, Danckaerts M, Dittmann RW, et al. European guidelines on managing adverse effects of medication for ADHD. European Guidelines Group. Eur Child Adolesc Psychiatry. 2011 Jan;20(1):17-37. Epub 2010 Nov 3.

[69] Wolraich ML, Greenhill LL, Pelham W, Swanson J, Wilens T, Palumbo D, et al. Randomized, controlled trial of oros methylphenidate once a day in children with attention deficit/hyperactivity disorder. Pediatrics 2001;108(4):883–892

[70] Thorell LB, Dahlstrom K. Children's self-reports on perceived effects on taking stimulant medication for ADHD. J Atten Disord 2009; 12(5):460–468

[71] Swanson JM, Hechtman L. Using log-acting stimulants: does it change ADHD treatment outcoma? Can Child Adolesc Psychiatr Rev 2005;14 (Supplement 1):2-3.

[72] Pelham WE, Gnagy EM, Burrows-Maclean L, Williams A, Fabiano GA, Morrisey SM, et al. Once-a-day Concerta methylphenidate versus three-times-daily methylphenidate in laboratory and natural settings. Pediatrics 2001; 107(6):E105

[73] Chou WJ, Chou MC, Tzang RF, Hsu YC, Gau SS, Chen SJ, et al. Better efficacy for the osmotic release oral system methylphenidate among poor adherents to immediate-release methylphenidate in the three ADHD subtypes. Psychiatry Clin Neurosci 2009; 63(2):167–175

[74] Gau SS, Chen SJ, Chou WJ, Cheng H, Tang CS, Chang HL, et al. National survey of adherence, efficacy, and side effects of methylphenidate in children with attention-deficit/hyperactivity disorder in Taiwan. J Clin Psychiatry 2008; 69(1):131–140

[75] Singh I, Kendall T, Taylor C, Mears A, Hollis C, Batty M, et al. Young people's experience of ADHD and stimulant medication: a qualitative study for the NICE guideline. Child Adolesc Ment Health 2010; 15:186–192

[76] Bukstein OG, Arnold LE, Landgraf JM, Hodgkins P. Does switching from oral extended-release methylphenidate to the methylphenidate transdermal system affect

health-related quality-of-life and medication satisfaction for children with attention-deficit/hyperactivity disorder? Child Adolesc Psychiatry Ment Health 2009; 3(1):39

[77] Johnston C, Fine S. Methods of evaluating methylphenidate in children with attention deficit hyperactivity disorder: acceptability, satisfaction, and compliance. J Pediatr Psychol 1993; 18(6):717–730

Chapter 4

Is ADHD a Stress-Related Disorder? Why Meditation Can Help

Sarina J. Grosswald

Additional information is available at the end of the chapter

http://dx.doi.org/10.5772/55127

1. Introduction

ADHD is the most common neurobehavioral disorder of childhood [1]. It is also one of the most extensively studied childhood disorders. In spite of the thousands of research articles written about ADHD, a cause has not been clearly identified. Theories include genetic abnormalities, structural differences in the brain, food additives, and more. Although these factors may be physiological correlates to the symptoms of ADHD, none has been established as a cause.

Factors that have been identified to increase the risk of ADHD include premature birth, low birth weight, poor maternal health, poverty, and maternal cigarette use. While at first glance it may be difficult to find a unifying relationship among these risk factors, at a closer look all of these situations place significant physiological, and potentially psychological, stress on the developing fetus and growing child.

This chapter will consider the effects of stress on the brain, the relationship between stress and ADHD, and the use of the Transcendental Meditation (TM) technique to reduce stress and reduce the symptoms of ADHD. It will also explore the potential of the technique as a means of lowering the risk, and possibly even preventing ADHD.

2. The developing brain

ADHD is a developmental disorder causing impaired executive function, or higher order functioning of the brain. Therefore, it is important to consider how the brain develops.

At birth, a baby has almost all the neurons, or brain cells, that individual will ever have. However, there are few strong connections. It is somewhat like a pile of electrical wires with a plug and a light bulb somewhere in the pile , but few of the wires are actually connected in order to send a functioning signal from the wall socket to the light bulb. During the first two years of life there is an explosion of brain connections, sometimes referred to as "neural exuberance." This is a critical period in brain development as the child learns from experience and the environment. By age three, the brain has formed about 1,000 trillion connections — twice as many as what is found in adulthood. A baby's brain is very dense, and will stay that way throughout the first decade of life.

Around age 7 the brain begins actively pruning unused or little used connections. Repeated experiences create strong connections, while processes that are used only once or twice, or are inhibited during this critical period, are pruned. The connections that remain are stronger and faster.

Though the brain reaches 90-95 percent of its adult size by age six, it continues to develop in waves, with different parts of the brain developing at different times. The brain grows and specializes, expanding from governing only the simple functions like appetite, sleep, and motor activities, to developing more complex functions such as emotions, and finally, reasoning and critical thinking – the "executive functions." Executive function is controlled by the cortex, particularly the frontal cortex, and is the last area of the brain to develop.

Roughly between the ages of 10 and 13, the frontal cortex experiences another growth spurt (Figure 1). This growth is followed by another period of pruning, particularly in the prefrontal cortex, beginning about age 12 and continuing into the early 20s. Consequently the part of the brain responsible for higher executive functions such as planning, working memory, organization, reasoning, judgment, and impulse control is undergoing major change during adolescence.

An important development during this period is the process called mylenation, development of a fatty layer around the brain cell fibers which takes place during the brain's growth spurts. Mylenation increases the speed of information processing. Since the cortex is the last part of the brain to mature, mylenation that connects the prefrontal cortex to the parts of the brain responsible for lower order functioning such as sensory functions, movement, and emotion does not begin to strengthen until the preteen and teen years. It is during this time that preadolescents and adolescents begin exerting independence, thinking for themselves, making their own decisions, and trying out independent reasoning.

As mentioned, this is also the time when the second period of pruning is taking place, particularly in the frontal area of the brain. Executive function is improving as the prefrontal cortex communicates more fully and effectively with other parts of the brain, including those areas that are particularly associated with planning and problem-solving, emotion, and impulses. As these connections strengthen over time, the teen may show mature, clear, lucid thinking. But as a consequence of pruning, the teen may forget these lucid thoughts the next day, and act in a more childish or impulsive way. Consequently, it is not surprising that it is

http://dx.doi.org/10.5772/55127

during the middle school years that these actions are often interpreted as signs of a deeper problem, and parents or teachers raise concern about ADHD.

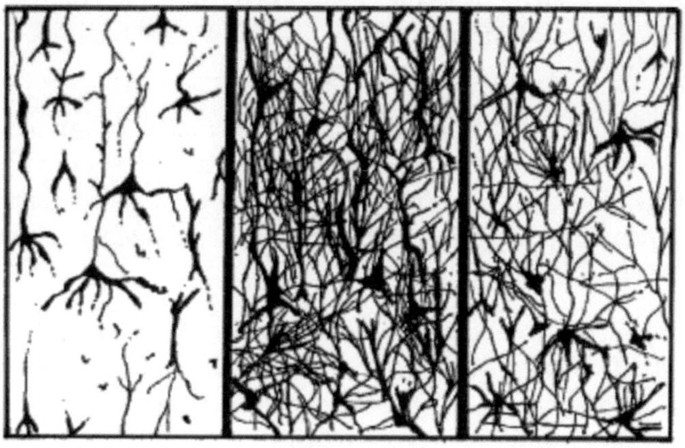

Figure 1. Density of Neuronal Connections at Different Times During Brain Development

3. Factors that negatively affect the brain

Developmental psychologists often say the "first years last forever," because this is a time of rapid development of the brain. It is a time when neurons are connecting in patterns and pathways based on the experiences to which the infant is exposed. These early experiences determine the strength and function of the brain's wiring.

Researchers have long known the importance of contact, touch and cuddling of a newborn for the child to have healthy emotional development. The "prime time" for "emotional intelligence" to develop is from birth to age 18 months. This provides the foundation for other aspects of emotional development as the child grows. The amygdala, which regulates emotion, is shaped early by experience, and forms the brain's emotional wiring. Early nurturing is important to learning empathy, happiness, hopefulness and resilience.

Traumatic events early in life, such as abuse, neglect, severe deprivation, or exposure to violence, negatively impact psychosocial development. Children who are exposed to violence and abuse at an early age tend to have both mental and physical health problems in childhood, with lasting effects in adulthood and throughout life. As they grow up, these children are more prone to aggression, conduct disorder, delinquency, antisocial behavior, anxiety, depression, and suicide [2], [3]. They are vulnerable to developing more slowly in their social and behavioral skills than their peers, or to actually getting "stuck" developmentally, perpetually acting younger than their age, consequently increasing the risk of being diagnosed with ADHD (Table 1).

Because early childhood is such a sensitive time in development, adverse influences during this time significantly increases the risk of ADHD (Table 1). For example, children whose parents divorce are almost twice as likely to be on ADHD medication after the split [2], [4]. Living with a single parent can increase the chances of a child being on ADHD medication by more than 50 percent. If a child is from a family on welfare, the likelihood of the child being on ADHD medication increases by a staggering 135 percent.

It is not only influences in the first few years that can permanently influence the growth and development of a child, but also influences during prenatal development. Studies show that when a mother drinks alcohol or takes drugs, especially early in pregnancy, it can alter the baby's brain development, reducing the number of neurons created, and affecting the way the neurotransmitters function.

Alcohol is a leading cause of the destruction of myelination in the brain. As a result of maternal alcohol abuse, the child comes into the world with neurobiological problems that include difficulties with attention, memory, problem solving, and abstract thinking – problems that will later become symptoms of ADHD.

Other aspects of the mother's health similarly influence the health of the child, and the likelihood of ADHD. Children born to mothers who have physical or mental health problems during pregnancy, including depression, anxiety, and musculoskeletal symptoms are more likely to later have ADHD [5] [6]. Similarly, if the mother experiences these problems within two years after the baby is born, the child has a higher risk of ADHD [7]. If a mother suffers from depression in the first 5 years of the child's life, the child is 2.5 times more likely to have ADHD.

Stress at birth is another factor raising the risk of ADHD. Danish researchers found that babies born prematurely have up to 70% greater risk of ADHD. Similarly, babies born of low birth weight have 50-90% greater risk of ADHD, depending on the weight at birth [8]. Babies born prematurely who are exposed to prenatal smoking can have smaller frontal and cerebellar areas of the brain, which are responsible for executive function and motor coordination, respectively. Children of mothers who smoke more than a pack of cigarettes a day are two and a half times more likely to later be taking medication for ADHD.

4. Effects of stress on the brain

Chronic physical or psychological stress can change the brain. The body's natural response to stress is to activate the sympathetic nervous system and hypothalamic-pituitary-adrenal (HPA) axis, leading to an increase in levels of catecholamines, corticotropin, and cortisol, creating the fight-or-flight response. Adrenaline and then cortisol are secreted by the adrenal glands, revving up the body, then sustaining energy flow to different systems. The lungs pump faster, and the heart begins to race. Blood pressure rises, stimulating muscles and sharpening the mind to a singular focus of attention. The release of endorphins numbs the body. Appetite, libido, and the immune system shut down. Energy normally directed to these functions is

http://dx.doi.org/10.5772/55127

Premature birth	70% increased risk
Low birth weight (3-5 lbs)	90% increased risk
Low birth weight (5-6 lbs)	50% increased risk
Mother's depression in child's first 5 years	2.5 times higher risk
Living with single parent	50% increased risk
Maternal smoking	2.5 times more likely to be on ADHD medication
Poverty	135% increased risk

Table 1. Factors that Increase the Risk of ADHD

redirected to the muscles. The response is intended to help the person react quickly and effectively to a high-pressure situation (i.e., fight or flee).

In a normal stress response, the autonomic nervous system, the HPA axis, and the cardiovascular, metabolic, and immune systems protect the body by responding to internal and external stress, then return to a balanced state.

However, chronic acute stress impairs the body's ability to return to alostasis, or baseline, leading to an out of balance biochemistry, with elevated cortisol and suppressed serotonin. Excessive levels of cortisol in the brain impair the function of the hippocampus, leading to neuronal atrophy and destruction of neurons, decreased short term and contextual memory, and poor regulation of the endocrine response to stress.

Prolonged stress hinders the body's ability to tell the hypothalamus to stop calling for more stress hormones. As a result, stress hormones flood the bloodstream, causing additional damage to the hippocampus, and additional stress. The price can be allostatic load, which is the wear and tear that results from chronic overactivity or underactivity of allostatic systems [9], [10].

The increase in cortisol inhibits utilization of blood sugar by the hippocampus, the brain's primary memory center. Reduced glucose produces an energy shortage, and the brain has no way to imprint memories. This results in the immediate short-term memory problems that are associated with stress. Further, cortisol overproduction interferes with the brain's neurotransmitters, making it hard to retrieve stored memories. Too much cortisol disrupts normal brain cell metabolism, eventually producing free radicals, which kill brain cells.

An increase in cortisol leads to a decrease in serotonin. Serotonin is a critical stress hormone, influencing body temperature, blood pressure, pain, digestion, sleep, and circadian rhythms. Deficiency in serotonin leads to behavioral concerns such as increases in irritability, aggression, impulsivity, suicide, and alcohol and drug abuse.

Chronic stress damages or kills neuronal connections. As much as 34% reduction in cells in the prefrontal cortex have been reported [11]. Significantly, chronic stress results in lower levels of expression of genes required for the function and structure of brain synapses [12]. Researchers found that a single transcription factor called GATA1, present with chronic stress, represses the expression of several genes that are necessary to form synaptic connections between brain cells in the prefrontal cortex (Figure 2).

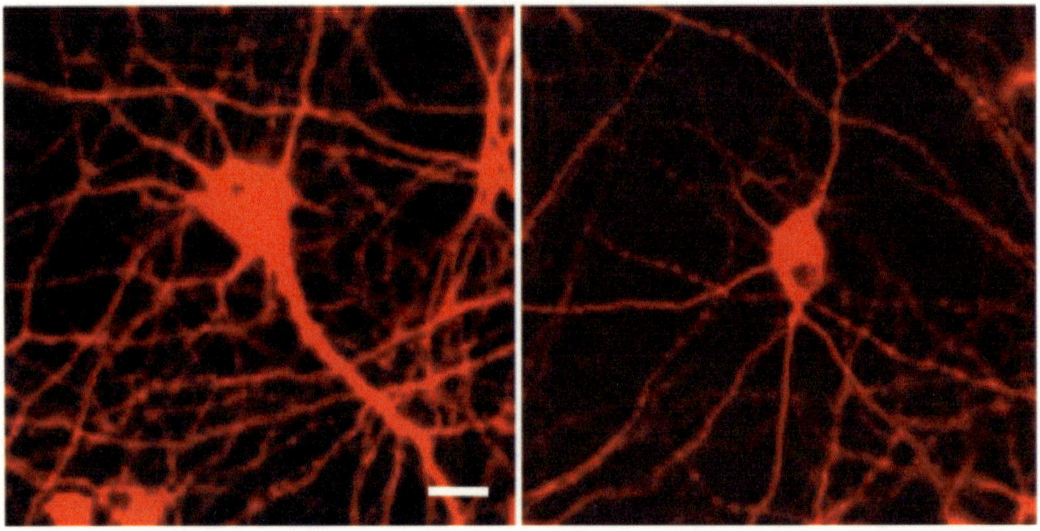

Figure 2. Tissue sample on the left from the prefrontal cortex of a Control subject. Tissue on the right, from a subject with depressive disorder shows dramatic reduction in prefrontal cortical synapses. (Figure courtesy of Kang, et al.)

5. Relationship between stress and ADHD

Disruptions of the neuronal connections in the prefrontal cortex caused by stress, interferes with executive function and behavior regulation [9]. Stress-impaired executive function is associated with impaired working memory, impaired impulse control, and lack of mental flexibility and coping strategies. Stress also dramatically compromises selective attention and the ability to sustain attention [10].

ADHD is associated with impaired executive function, specifically brain circuitry governing behavior [13], [14], [15]. Dysfunction of these circuits leads to impulsivity and lack of normal social inhibition, as well as impaired working memory, inability to focus attention, and impaired temporal organization.

In light of these similarities, the connection between stress and the symptoms of ADHD begins to emerge. Stress negatively affects brain function, resulting in the same symptoms associated with ADHD. Table 2 compares symptoms of stress identified by the US Centers for Disease Control and Prevention, and diagnostic factors for ADHD as defined by the Diagnostic and Statistical Manual of Mental Disorders (DSM-IV). The symptoms are nearly parallel. In fact it can be said that the differences are simply the difference in the way the symptom might be expressed in an adult compared to a child.

Symptoms of Stress	Symptoms of ADHD
Inability to concentrate	Difficulty sustaining attention
	Not listening when spoken to
Difficulty organizing	Difficulty organizing
Memory problems	Forgetfulness
Poor judgment	Speaks without thinking
Short temper	Impulsivity

Table 2. Symptoms of stress closely match symptoms of ADHD

Recent research sheds further light on the relationship between stress and ADHD. Vance, et al., demonstrated dysfunction of the right prefrontal regions of the brain in ADHD children [16]. This region is responsible for developing coping strategies, influencing the ability to handle stress. Early experiences of stress are believed to affect the level of responsiveness of the HPA axis and autonomic nervous system.

Young children exposed to chronic stress, can become overly accustomed to dealing with fear states, becoming conditioned to having or tolerating higher levels of adrenaline. Chronic acute stress damages the body's ability to return to non-stress levels, leading to chronically elevated levels of cortisol, a biochemical marker of stress. In children with ADHD high cortisol levels impair executive function, self-regulation, and letter knowledge [17].

Dysregulation of the central noradrenergic pathways in the brain is believed to underlie the pathophysiology of ADHD [18]. The noradrenergic system is associated with the modulation of attention, alertness, vigilance and executive function. Specifically, dopamine is associated with behavior and impulsive control, while norepinephrine is associated with focus, planning, and concept thinking including sequence and time. Disruption of the noradrenergic function seen in the presence of the "fight-or-flight" response involves the same neurochemistry associated in ADHD. In fact, the majority of ADHD medication involves increasing the presence of dopamine, norepinephrine, and serotonin.

6. The transcendental meditation technique

Given the role stress seems to play in the symptoms of ADHD, it is logical to explore stress reduction techniques, such as meditation, as a means of minimizing the effects of stress and reducing the related symptoms associated with ADHD.

There are many systems of meditation. Techniques differ widely from one another in their procedures, content, beliefs, and goals. Each technique uses a different process and thus has different effects [19], [20].

With advances in neuroscience, the study of meditation has become more specific and more evidence based. Most recently, using EEG signatures and the corresponding cognitive processes, meditation practices have been classified into three types: focused attention, open monitoring, and automatic self-transcending [21].

Techniques of focused attention are concentration techniques, and are associated with voluntary sustained control of attention on the object of meditation, such as an event, image, or sound. The brain activity during concentration meditations is characterized by EEG in the beta-2 (20-30 Hz) and gamma (30-50 Hz) frequency bands. Open monitoring or mindfulness-based techniques, involve dispassionate non-evaluative monitoring of ongoing experience. These techniques are characterized by frontal theta (5-8 Hz) EEG, and perhaps occipital gamma (30-50 Hz) EEG. Automatic self-transcending meditation is defined as effortless transcending of the meditation process itself [22], [21]. EEG activity of an automatic self-transcending technique is associated with alpha-1 (7-9 Hz), characteristic of reduced mental activity and relaxation.

The Transcendental Meditation technique falls into the category of automatic self-transcending. Concentration and open monitoring meditations both require some mental effort (i.e., holding attention on its object or maintaining attention on an ongoing experience, respectively). The Transcendental Meditation technique automatically leads to the experience of "consciousness itself," awareness without any objects of awareness, a low-stress state called transcendental or pure consciousness [23].

Practice of the technique is not based on concentrative effort, contemplation, prayer, or deliberate attempts to make the awareness more mindful or alert. Rather, the technique allows the conscious awareness, or active thinking, to spontaneously "transcend" to deeper, quieter levels of the thinking process, eventually experiencing the most settled state of awareness, where the mind is fully awake within itself, without experiencing objects of perception.

The Transcendental Meditation technique is a mental technique practiced for 10-20 minutes twice each day, sitting in a chair with eyes closed. It is easy to learn and to practice. Because it does not require concentration or controlling the mind, it is particularly well suited for children or adults with ADHD.

The technique is taught by certified Transcendental Meditation teachers in a 7-Step course. The 7-Step course of instruction involves two informational lectures (Steps 1 and 2), a brief interview with the TM instructor (Step 3), individual personal instruction (Step 4), which is followed by three days of verification of practice and additional information (Steps 5-7). The interview is about 10 minutes, while the remaining steps are approximately 1-1.5 hr each day. Each step can be conducted in a group except Steps 3 and 4, which are conducted individually, one-on-one. Periodic meetings with the student assure correct practice and reinforce regularity of the practice.

During the course of instruction, the student learns how to let the mind move from active focused levels of thinking to silent, expanded levels of wakefulness at the source of thought, without concentration or effort [24] (Figure 3).

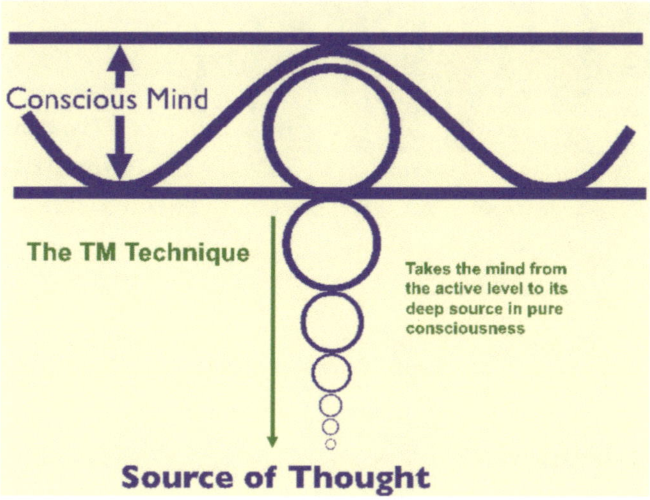

Figure 3. During the Transcendental Meditation technique the mind moves from the active, directed thinking level to the more subtle levels of thinking, to eventually go beyond the boundaries of thought to experience 'pure' consciousness.

Regular practice of the technique creates a state referred to as "restful alertness." The term reflects a combination of markedly decreased metabolism, heart rate, respiration rate, and blood flow to the limbs, similar to deep rest or sleep; while at the same time mental alertness is maintained, as demonstrated by EEG [25], [26], [27]. The TM technique produces a significantly greater degree of deep rest than sitting with eyes closed, measured by reduced respiration , reduced skin conductance (increased skin resistance), reduced plasma lactate [25], more rapid recovery from stressful stimulus, and leads to a reversal of symptomatology associated with severe and chronic stress [28].

Meta-analyses indicate that the Transcendental Meditation technique is two to four times more effective in reducing stress and anxiety than other meditation or relaxation techniques [19]. A 2012 meta-analysis found Transcendental Meditation to be the most effective technique across a broad spectrum of psychological and cognitive variables including negative emotions, neuroticism, perception, trait anxiety, behavior, and memory and learning [29] (Figure 4).

Measurements of brain function show increases in brain coherence both during the practice of the Transcendental Meditation technique, and afterwards in activity [21], [30], [31]. The primary areas of the brain that are activated are the frontal and prefrontal executive areas responsible for attention, executive function, emotional stability, and anxiety (Figure 5) [32], [31], [33], [34]. Study of college students demonstrated increased frontal coherence and reduced stress reactivity in the group practicing the Transcendental Meditation technique

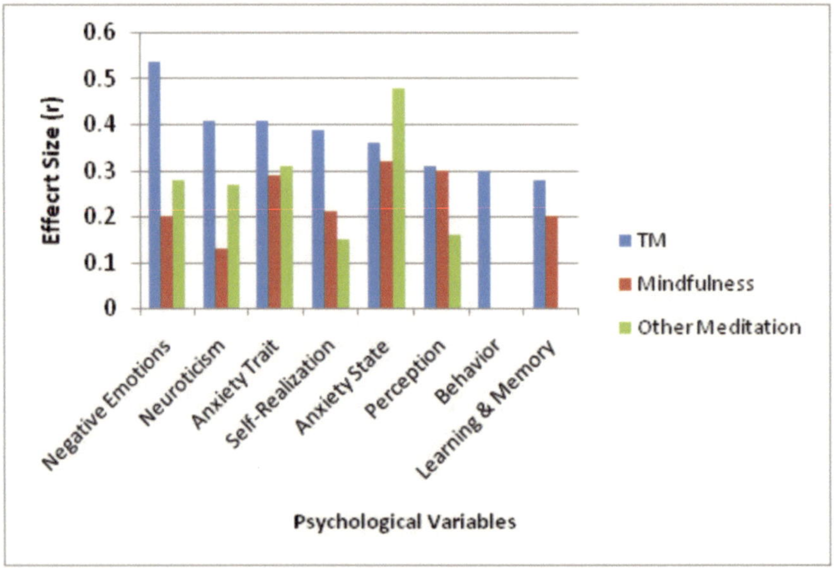

Figure 4. Meta-analysis of 163 studies of various meditation techniques, comparing the effects on psychological variables [29].

compared to controls [35], [36]. Further, students in the TM group showed that TM may lead to a foundational or 'ground' state of cerebral functioning and more focused cognitive processes [36].

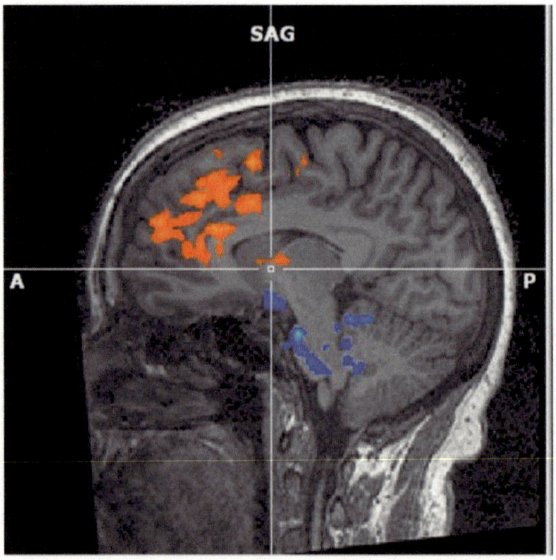

Figure 5. fMRI showing increased activation in the frontal areas of the brain during the practice of the Transcendental Meditation technique (Courtesy of M. Ludwig)

http://dx.doi.org/10.5772/55127

The effects of the Transcendental Meditation technique extend to the noradrenergic networks [26], [37], [38], resulting in a decrease in the stress hormone cortisol, both during meditation and continuing outside meditation, during activity. Practice of the technique increases serotonin availability, improving mood and reducing the activation of the brain centers for fear, anxiety, and anger.

The use of the TM technique for stress reduction in adolescents has resulted in improvement in school behavior, decreases in absenteeism and rule infractions, and reduction in suspensions due to behavior-related problems [39]. Students practicing the TM technique show higher performance on scales of self-actualization [40], increased emotional regulation, and improved well-being [41] as well as improved academic performance.

7. The Transcendental Meditation technique and ADHD

The Transcendental Meditation technique creates a neurobiological response opposite to that induced by stress. It enlivens the executive areas of the brain, and is associated with improved psychosocial behavior in normal populations.

Studies of the TM technique with students with ADHD demonstrate that the benefits of the technique also extend to this population. A 3-month pilot study was conducted with children ages 11 to 14 with the diagnosis of ADHD, and in some cases comorbidities, including general anxiety disorder, dysthymia, obsessive compulsive disorder, pervasive developmental disorder, sleep disorders, and tics [42]. These children also had language-based learning disabilities. The study measured effects of the Transcendental Meditation technique on stress, anxiety, and ADHD symptoms; and measured changes in executive function. Measures of stress and ADHD symptoms included the Achenbach Child Behavior Checklist (CBCL) completed by parents and teachers, the companion inventory the Achenbach Youth Self-Report (YSR), and the Revised Children's Manifest Anxiety Scale (RCMAS). Measures of executive function included the Behavior Rating Inventory of Executive Function (BRIEF), the Cognitive Assessment System (CAS) Expressive Attention, Delis-Kaplan Executive Function System (D-KEFS) Verbal Fluency test, and Connor's CPT II.

After three months, there were highly statistically significant reductions in anxiety and anxiousness, depression symptoms, attention problems, and total problems (Table 3).

Statistically significant improvements in executive function as measured by the BRIEF showed improved Behavioral Regulation (includes ability to Inhibit, Shift for one task to another, and Emotional Control). Similar improvements were seen in the Metacognition Index (includes ability to Initiate, Working Memory, Planning, Organize Material, and Monitoring).

A second study, a randomized control trial of a similar population as the previous study, explored improvements in brain coherence and brain development [43]. The purpose was to provide insight into the underlying mechanisms of observed changes. The study measured EEG coherence, theta/beta ratio, and executive function.

	Student					Teacher				
	Pretest		Post Test			Pretest		Post Test		
Symptom	Mean	SD	Mean	SD	ES	Mean	SD	Mean	SD	ES
Anxious/ Depressed	5.7	3.6	2.7*	3.7	.8	10.2	6.4	5.6*	3.6	.7
Withdrawn/ Depressed	4.8	2.7	3.9**	3.0	.3	4.3	3.8	3.6	4.0	.2
Affective Problems	5.8	3.4	4.1*	2.5	.5	5.0	3.7	3.6	3.6	.4
Anxiety Problems	3.2	2.0	1.6**	1.9	.8	3.7	3.5	2.1	2.4	.5
Attention Problems	7.0	4.0	5.2*	3.5	.5	23.6	10.5	22	11.0	.2
ADHD Problems	5.4	2.9	4.3	2.7	.4	12.4	5.7	11.7	5.7	.3
Total Problems	52.5	25.6	40*	27.4	.5	63.1	24.8	56*	31.2	.3

* p ≤.05. **p<.005 ES=Effect Size

Table 3. Results of Achenbach Child Behavior Checklist and Youth Self Report after three months practice of the Transcendental Meditation technique among children with ADHD.

EEG of ADHD populations show decreased activation in parietal areas of the brain that weave sensory input into concrete perception [44], higher density and amplitude of theta activity [45], [46], and lower density and amplitude of alpha and beta activity [47]. Theta is thought to block out irrelevant stimuli during memory processing. In ADHD subjects, greater theta activity may block out relevant as well as irrelevant information. Theta/beta ratios are highly correlated with severity of ADHD symptoms.

Another brain marker of ADHD is EEG coherence, a measure that reflects the number and strength of connections between different brain areas. In children diagnosed with ADHD, coherence in all frequencies is lower [48]. Alpha coherence is thought to play an important role in attention.

In the TM study, EEG of ADHD students was taken during a computer-administered paired choice reaction-time task to calculate theta/beta ratios and patterns of EEG coherence. The study also applied employed several of the same measures of executive function used in the previous study. At pretest, all students showed theta/beta ratios well above the normal range (normal average=3). Subjects were randomly assigned to the TM group and delayed-start group. The delayed-start group served as controls for the first three months, then also learned the TM technique.

Coherence maps ere calculated at pretest, 3 months, and 6 months. At 3 months, from pretest to posttests compared the TM group to the control group. At six months, changes in coherence for the control group (delayed start, who had been meditating for 3 months) were calculated from 3-month to 6-month posttests. The resulting maps showed present coherence in theta (5.0-7.5 Hz), alpha (8.0-12 Hz), beta1 (13-20 Hz), and gamma bands (20.5-50 Hz).

Results (Figure 6) indicated few sensors with higher coherence in the delayed-start group at the 3-month posttest compared to their pretest values. In contrast, in the TM group there were many frontal and parietal areas at 3-month posttest compared to pretest values. At 6-month posttest, the delayed start group (who learned TM at 3 months) also showed many frontal and parietal areas with higher coherence compared to the 3-month posttest values.

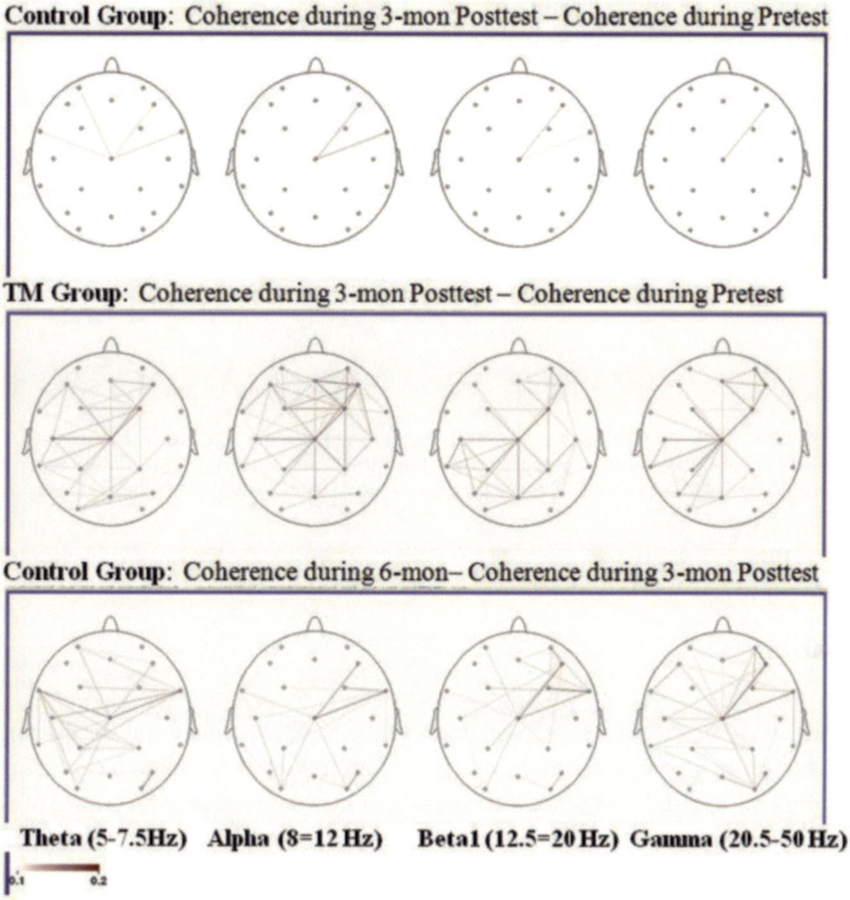

Figure 6. Coherence maps of at baseline, 3-months, and 6-months among children with ADHD. Top row is coherence during the 3-month posttest minus baseline coherence for the delayed-start subjects. Middle row is coherence during the 3-month posttest minus baseline coherence for the TM subjects. Bottom row is coherence during the 6-month posttest minus 3-month posttest for the delayed-start subjects, who had been meditating over this time.

At the 3-month posttest, theta/beta ratios increased in the delayed-start group, which is opposite to the desired effect, while the TM subjects moved closer to normal values. At the 6-month posttest, after both groups were practicing the TM technique, theta/beta ratios decreased in both groups. For the delayed start group, theta/beta ratios also significantly decreased from the 3-month to 6-month posttest after three months practice of the TM technique (Figure 7).

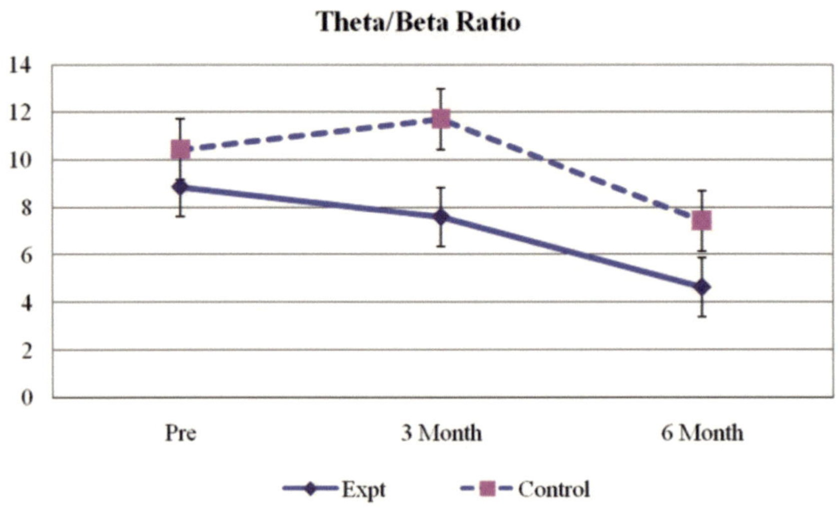

Figure 7. Theta/beta ratios compare results at pretest, 3-month and 6-month posttests. Transcendental Meditation group showed reductions at 3-months compared to delayed start controls. TM group showed continued improvements at six months. Delayed start showed significant improvements from 3-months to 6-months, after meditating for 3 months.

8. Prevention

An initial literature search of research on preventing ADHD turns up no significant contribution to the subject of effecting the underlying causes. In fact, it seems to be an area that is not actively being addressed. Most research on prevention is focused on preventing of other social problems that arise among children with ADHD, such as smoking or criminal behavior.

Without an understanding of the disorder's etiology, prevention cannot be addressed. The etiology currently gaining most attention is genetic causes. However, genetic alterations associated with ADHD may be a correlate rather than a cause. As discussed earlier, chronic stress can result in changing gene expression, resulting in structural impairment of the prefrontal cortex.

Considering the factors discussed in this chapter, a unifying underlying cause emerges. Chronic stress, whether physical or emotional, can result in structural impairment to brain, and give rise to the symptoms identified as ADHD.

http://dx.doi.org/10.5772/55127

Recognition of the role stress plays in ADHD offers an opportunity to intervene to alter the course of the disorder. Some risk factors such as maternal smoking can addressed through education and public health efforts, a child's risk of developing ADHD. Other causes of stress, however, may be more difficult to avoid or eliminate (e.g., premature birth, poverty). But many of the stress factors that raise the risk of ADHD are known (Table 1), therefore, interventions that immediately address reducing the effects of the stressors, have the potential of reducing the damaging effects on the brain, and possibly avoid development of the symptoms of ADHD.

When a child, or even an adult, begins to show signs of difficulty with attention and focus, disorganization, behavior issues, and difficulty controlling anger or impulses, a thorough approach to diagnosis should include assessment of potential causative factors. In as many as 75- 85% of cases, ADHD is complicated by the presence of other emotional or behavioral disorders [49]. Treating the underlying disorder can result in reduction of ADHD symptoms.

If the symptoms arise as a child enters school, an evaluation of learning can be useful. Approximately 20-30% of children with ADHD also have a learning disability [50]. When a child starts to show difficulty academically, he or she tends to lose interest in learning, can become easily distracted, or may engage in disruptive behaviour. This can lead to a diagnosis of ADHD since these are also clinical symptoms of the disorder. However, they may actually be caused by a learning problem, whether it is a learning disorder or simply the consequence of getting behind or confused in an academic subject and unable to catch up. An educational assessment can help distinguish the underlying problem.

If symptoms arise when a child changes schools or environments, this can be an underlying cause of stress, and consequently the appearance of ADHD related problems. Traumatic events such as conflict at home, or lose or separation from parents or close caregivers can result in ADHD symptoms.

Children who are exposed to geopolitical violence or natural disasters often display symptoms interpreted as ADHD, when they may actually be stress responses to the trauma or the chronic stress of living in fear. Each year in the US, more than five million children are exposed to some form of extreme traumatic stressor. These traumatic events include natural disasters such as tornados, floods, hurricanes; motor vehicle accidents; life threatening illness and associated painful experiences such as cancer or burns; or witnessing violence in the home or community. Over 30 percent of these traumatized children develop a clinical syndrome with emotional, behavioral, cognitive, social and physical symptoms significant enough to be diagnosed with post traumatic disorder (PTSD). Some of the symptoms of PTSD are very similar to those of ADHD. Without an exploration of the underlying causes of ADHD symptoms, other problems may go undiagnosed.

Regardless of the underlying cause of the stress, the Transcendental Meditation technique can provide an intervention that can reduce the effects of stress and related symptoms, including symptoms that might be diagnosed as ADHD.

For children as young as four or five years old, the Transcendental Meditation technique has been shown to effectively reduce stress and increase cognitive development. It can balance neurochemistry, reversing the cycle of high cortisol leading to low serotonin; thus improving mood and impulse control. (Note: for children below the age of 10 years old, the technique is slightly different, done with the eyes open, while engaged in non-focused activity.) The technique also leads to balancing dopamine and norepinephrine, the same neurotransmitters that are the target of common ADHD drugs.

For children younger than four years old, who may be too young to learn the TM technique, the Maharishi Ayurveda Mother and Baby Program provides dietary and behavioral guidelines that include foods cooked according to specific principles, and Ayurvedic massage that reduces stress and improves the baby's sleep and digestion [51]. When this approach is incorporated for the mother and the baby, along with the mother's practice of the Transcendental Meditation technique, it improves the mother's mental and physical health, and leads to a better start for the baby.

9. Case study

The following case study will illustrate how the concepts presented in this chapter can affect an individual child. At the first introduction to Jessie (not his real name), he was 7 years old and had just been diagnosed with ADHD. His mother explained, "He can't control his emotions - happy or sad emotions. He can be extreme in either direction." She described that sometimes he would be in such a rage, that he would hide under his bed or go out to his father's car to try to calm himself. "I'm afraid one day he'll be standing over me with a knife. I don't know what to do," she said. He was also having difficulty with attention and behaviour at school.

Jessie seemed like a very sweet, though rambunctious, boy. He did not seem to display any malice or meanness, but if he got frustrated or over-excited, he could not control his emotions. He was from a warm and loving family with both parents and a younger brother. They had a warm, healthy home life, and there did not seem to be cause for the level of stress that might lead to the behavior Jessie would sometimes exhibit.

Discussion with Jessie's mother, however, shed light on the situation. She had two miscarriages before Jessie was born. As a result she was very anxious during her pregnancy with Jessie. After he was born, she had another miscarriage, which led to depression and medication for her depression. When she became pregnant again, she had complications requiring bedrest for the last trimester, making it difficult to give full attention to Jessie.

During the time 2-year old Jessie's mother was in the hospital giving birth to his brother, Jessie stayed with his grandmother. While there, he got sick, requiring hospitalization, where he was temporarily put on oxygen. One can imagine how scary this would be for a young child, and though his father was with him, his mother was not.

Jessie's situation was not serious, and he was not hospitalized long. However the newborn had complications, which was finally diagnosed a year later as a digestive disease. This resulted in much attention and worry around the newborn, which to young Jessie may have seemed like a form of abandonment, creating greater stress for him. While any of these individual situations may not have caused emotional stress for Jessie, combined over an extended period of time, likely caused a significant physiological response to chronic stress. Consequently, the effect of the early adversity, several of which are known to increase the risk of ADHD, may explain Jessie's symptoms and lack of self-control, which were diagnosed as ADHD.

Jessie's parents did not want to put him on medication, so they sought another approach. At age seven, Jessie and his whole family – parents and 5-year-old brother – learned the Transcendental Meditation technique. The boys learned the young child's technique called the Word of Wisdom.

Jessie found it effective in calming himself down. It also resulted in immediate improvements in school. The next week after learning TM, he completed his weekly math test for the first time all year. He was able to maintain his attention, focus, and easily get through the task. When he turned 10 years old, Jessie learned the sitting, eyes closed technique. He does well in school, is better able to control his emotions, and gets along well with his younger brother.

Jessie eventually added a low dose of ADHD medication to augment the benefits of the meditation. He is a happy, well-adjusted child who does well in school. However, given the extreme behaviors he displayed at a younger age, his life could have quickly taken a different course. One could foresee significant behavior problems, the potential for strong life-long medication, poor success in school, and a more troubled life for him and his family. Though it is impossible to predict what would have happened over time, the value of early intervention with an effective technique for reducing stress, balancing the neurochemistry, and improving executive function can be appreciated.

10. Conclusion

A child or adult affected by trauma or severe stress looses the ability to return to a balanced state, consequently creating a cycle of chronic stress. Chronic stress alters the biochemistry and neuronal development particularly in the prefrontal cortex. The result is impaired executive function, creating lack of control of attention, focus, memory, organization, and impulses, displaying as symptoms of ADHD.

Early recognition of factors that cause severe or traumatic stress, and early intervention can help mitigate the effects. The Transcendental Meditation technique has been shown to be effective in reducing temporal and chronic stress, reducing ADHD symptoms, and improving executive function. The technique is easy to learn and easy to practice, is appropriate for people of all ages - children as young as four or five years old to adults of any age. In the presence of ADHD risk factors, the Transcendental Meditation technique offers potential for preventing full manifestation of symptoms, and provides a field for study of ADHD prevention.

Author details

Sarina J. Grosswald

Address all correspondence to: Sarina@grosswald.com

SJ Grosswald & Associates, USA

References

[1] CDC. Increasing Prevalence of Parent-Reported Attention-Deficit/Hyperactivity Disorder Among Children --- United States, 2003 and 2007. MMWR. 2010;59(44):1439–43.

[2] Repetti R., Taylor SE, Seeman TE. Risky families: Family social environments and the mental and physical health of offspring. Psychological Bulletin. 2002;128(2):330–66.

[3] Burke NJ, Hellman JL, Scott BG, Weems CF, Carrion VG. The impact of adverse childhood experiences on an urban pediatric population. Child Abuse & Neglect. 2011;35(6):408–13.

[4] Burke NJ, Hellman JL, Scott BG, Weems CF, Carrion VG. The impact of adverse childhood experiences on an urban pediatric population. Child Abuse & Neglect. 2011 Jun;35(6):408–13.

[5] Van den Bergh BRH, Marcoen A. High antenatal maternal anxiety is related to ADHD symptoms, externalizing problems, and anxiety in 8- and 9-year-olds. Child Dev. 2004 Aug;75(4):1085–97.

[6] Talge NM, Neal C, Glover V. Antenatal maternal stress and long-term effects on child neurodevelopment: how and why? J Child Psychol Psychiatry. 2007 Apr; 48(3-4):245–61.

[7] Ray GT, Croen LA, Habel LA. Mothers of children diagnosed with attention-deficit/hyperactivity disorder: health conditions and medical care utilization in periods before and after birth of the child. Med Care. 2009 Jan;47(1):105–14.

[8] Linnet KM. Gestational age, birth weight, and the risk of hyperkinetic disorder. Archives of Disease in Childhood. 2006 Aug 1;91(8):655–60.

[9] McEwen BS. Protective and damaging effects of stress mediators: central role of the brain. Dialogues Clin Neurosci. 2006;8(4):367–81.

[10] Lupien SJ, McEwen BS, Gunnar MR, Heim C. Effects of stress throughout the lifespan on the brain, behaviour and cognition. Nat Rev Neurosci. 2009 Jun;10(6):434–45.

[11] Cotter D, Mackay D, Chana G, Beasley C, Landau S, Everall IP. Reduced Neuronal Size and Glial Cell Density in Area 9 of the Dorsolateral Prefrontal Cortex in Subjects with Major Depressive Disorder. Cerebral Cortex. 2002 Apr 1;12(4):386–94.

[12] Kang HJ, Voleti B, Hajszan T, Rajkowska G, Stockmeier CA, Licznerski P, et al. Decreased expression of synapse-related genes and loss of synapses in major depressive disorder. Nat Med. 2012 Sep;18(9):1413–7.

[13] Bush G, Valera EM, Seidman LJ. Functional neuroimaging of attention-deficit/hyperactivity disorder: a review and suggested future directions. Biol. Psychiatry. 2005 Jun 1;57(11):1273–84.

[14] Durston S, Hulshoff Pol HE, Schnack HG, Buitelaar JK, Steenhuis MP, Minderaa RB, et al. Magnetic resonance imaging of boys with attention-deficit/hyperactivity disorder and their unaffected siblings. J Am Acad Child Adolesc Psychiatry. 2004 Mar; 43(3):332–40.

[15] Zametkin AJ LL. Brain metabolism in teenagers with attention-deficit hyperactivity disorder. Archives of General Psychiatry. 1993 May 1;50(5):333–40.

[16] Silk TJ, Vance A, Rinehart N, Bradshaw JL, Cunnington R. White-matter abnormalities in attention deficit hyperactivity disorder: A diffusion tensor imaging study. Human Brain Mapping. 2009 Sep 15;30(9):2757–65.

[17] Blair C, Granger D, Peters Razza R. Cortisol Reactivity Is Positively Related to Executive Function in Preschool Children Attending Head Start. Child Development. 2005 May;76(3):554–67.

[18] Biederman J, Spencer T. Attention-deficit/hyperactivity disorder (ADHD) as a noradrenergic disorder. Biol. Psychiatry. 1999 Nov 1;46(9):1234–42.

[19] Orme-Johnson DW, Walton KG. All approaches to preventing or reversing effects of stress are not the same. Am J Health Promot. 1998 Jun;12(5):297–9.

[20] Shear J, editor. Experience of Meditation: Experts Introduce the Major Traditions. Paragon House; 2006.

[21] Travis F, Shear J. Focused attention, open monitoring and automatic self-transcending: Categories to organize meditations from Vedic, Buddhist and Chinese traditions. Consciousness and Cognition. 2010 Dec;19(4):1110–8.

[22] Travis F, Arenander A, DuBois D. Psychological and physiological characteristics of a proposed object-referral/self-referral continuum of self-awareness. Consciousness and Cognition. 2004 Jun;13(2):401–20.

[23] Travis F, Pearson C. Pure Consciousness: Distinct Phenomenological and Physiological Correlates of "Consciousness Itself."Int J Neurosci. 2000 Jan 1;100(1-4):77–89.

[24] Travis F. Transcendental Meditation Technique. In: Craighead EW, Nemeroff CB, editors. Corsini Encyclopedia of Psychology and Neuroscience. New York: John Wiley and Sons; 2001. p. 1705–6.

[25] Dillbeck MC, Orme-Johnson DW. Physiological differences between transcendental meditation and rest. American Psychologist. 1987;42(9):879–81.

[26] Jevning R, Wallace RK, Beidebach M. The physiology of meditation: a review. A wakeful hypometabolic integrated response. Neurosci Biobehav Rev. 1992;16(3):415–24.

[27] Travis F, Wallace RK. Autonomic and EEG patterns during eyes-closed rest and transcendental meditation (TM) practice: the basis for a neural model of TM practice. Consciousness and Cognition. 1999;8(3):302–18.

[28] Orme-Johnson DW. Autonomic stability and Transcendental Meditation. Psychosom Med. 1973 Aug;35(4):341–9.

[29] Sedlmeier P, Eberth J, Schwarz M, Zimmermann D, Haarig F, Jaeger S, et al. The psychological effects of meditation: A meta-analysis. Psychol Bull. 2012 Nov;138(6):1139–71.

[30] Dillbeck MC, Vesely SA. Participation in the transcendental meditation program and frontal eeg coherence during concept learning. International Journal of Neuroscience. 1986 Jan;29(1-2):45–55.

[31] So KT, Orme-Johnson DW. Three randomized experiments on the longitudinal effects of the Transcendental Meditation technique on cognition. Intelligence. 2001;29:419–40.

[32] Dixon c, Dillbeck MC, Travis F, Msemaje H, Clayborne BM, Dillbeck SL, et al. Accelerating cognitive and self-development: Longitudinal studies with preschool and elementary school children. Journal of Social Behavior and Personality. 17:65–91.

[33] Fergusson LC. Field independence, transcendental mediation, and achievement in college art: a reexamination. Percept Mot Skills. 1993 Dec;77(3 Pt 2):1104–6.

[34] Travis FT, Orme-Johnson DW. Field model of consciousness: EEG coherence changes as indicators of field effects. Int. J. Neurosci. 1989 Dec;49(3-4):203–11.

[35] Travis F, Haaga DAF, Hagelin J, Tanner M, Nidich S, Gaylord-King C, et al. Effects of Transcendental Meditation practice on brain functioning and stress reactivity in college students. International Journal of Psychophysiology. 2009 Feb;71(2):170–6.

[36] Travis F, Haaga D, Hagelin J, Tanner M, Arenander A, Nidich S, et al. A self-referential default brain state: patterns of coherence, power, and eLORETA sources during eyes-closed rest and Transcendental Meditation practice. Cognitive Processing. 2010;11(1):21–30.

[37] Jevning R, Wilson AF, Davidson JM. Adrenocortical activity during meditation. Horm Behav. 1978 Feb;10(1):54–60.

[38] MacLean CR, Walton KG, Wenneberg SR, Levitsky DK, Mandarino JP, Waziri R, et al. Effects of the Transcendental Meditation program on adaptive mechanisms: changes in hormone levels and responses to stress after 4 months of practice. Psychoneuroendocrinology. 1997 May;22(4):277–95.

[39] Barnes VA, Bauza LB, Treiber FA. Impact of stress reduction on negative school behavior in adolescents. Health and Quality of Life Outcomes. 2003;1.

[40] Alexander CN, Rainforth M, Gelderloos P. Transcendental meditation, self-actualization, and psychological health: A conceptual overview and statistical meta-analysis. Journal of Social Behavior & Personality. 1991;6(5):189–248.

[41] Rosaen C, Benn R. The experience of transcendental meditation in middle school students: a qualitative report. Explore (NY). 2006 Oct;2(5):422–5.

[42] Grosswald SJ, Stixrud WR, Travis F, Bateh MA. Use of the Transcendental Meditation technique to reduce symptoms of Attention Deficit Hyperactivity Disorder (ADHD) by reducing stress and anxiety: An exploratory study. Current Issues in Education. 2008;10(2):online.

[43] Travis F, Grosswald S, Stixrud W. ADHD, Brain Functioning, and Transcendental Meditation Practice. Mind & Body, The Journal of Psychiatry. 2011;2:73–81.

[44] Silk T. Fronto-parietal activation in attention-deficit hyperactivity disorder, combined type: functional magnetic resonance imaging study. The British Journal of Psychiatry. 2005 Sep 1;187(3):282–3.

[45] di Michele F, Prichep L, John ER, Chabot RJ. The neurophysiology of attention-deficit/hyperactivity disorder. International Journal of Psychophysiology. 2005 Oct;58(1): 81–93.

[46] Janzen T, Graap K, Stephanson S, Marshall W, Fitzsimmons G. Differences in baseline EEG measures for ADD and normally achieving preadolescent males. Biofeedback Self Regul. 1995 Mar;20(1):65–82.

[47] Barry RJ, Clarke AR, Johnstone SJ. A review of electrophysiology in attention-deficit/ hyperactivity disorder: I. Qualitative and quantitative electroencephalography. Clin Neurophysiol. 2003 Feb;114(2):171–83.

[48] Clarke AR, Barry RJ, McCarthy R, Selikowitz M, Johnstone SJ, Hsu C-I, et al. Coherence in children with Attention-Deficit/Hyperactivity Disorder and excess beta activity in their EEG. Clin Neurophysiol. 2007 Jul;118(7):1472–9.

[49] Costello E MS. Prevalence and development of psychiatric disorders in childhood and adolescence. Archives of General Psychiatry. 2003 Aug 1;60(8):837–

[50] Wender PH. ADHD: attention-deficit hyperactivity disorder in children and adults. New York: Oxford University Press; 2000.

[51] Marci Freeman. Postpartum Care from Ancient India. Midwifery Today. 2002;Spring(61):23–4, 63.

Section 2

Role of Endocrine Hormones

Chapter 5

The Potential Role of Neuroendocrine in Patients with Attention-Deficit/Hyperactivity Disorder

Liang-Jen Wang and Chih-Ken Chen

Additional information is available at the end of the chapter

http://dx.doi.org/10.5772/53609

1. Introduction

Attention-Deficit/HyperactivityDisorder (**ADHD**) is one of the most prevalent neurodevelopmental **disorders** among children. It affects 3-10% of school-age children (Polanczyk et al., 2007), and a prevalence rate of 7.5% was reported in a local Taiwan study (Gau et al., 2005). The core symptoms of ADHD are inattention, hyperactivity, and impulsivity, and ADHD patients are commonly comorbid with other neuropsychiatric disorders, such as Oppositional Defiant Disorder (ODD), Conduct Disorder (CD), and tic disorders (American Psychiatric Association, 2000; Spencer et al., 2007). The most well-known neurobiological hypotheses to account for the complexity in etiology of ADHD are the dysregulation of catecholaminergic neurotransmission (Biederman & Faraone, 2002). In recent years, many researchers have raised concerns with regards to the potential roles of the neuroendocrine system in the pathogenesis of ADHD (Dubrovsky, 2005; Golubchik et al., 2007; Goodyer et al., 2001; Martel et al., 2009; Strous et al., 2006), based on observations of the epidemiological data of ADHD. ADHD is more prevalent in boys than in girls, with the ratio ranging from 4 to 1 to as much as 9 to 1, and boys generally exhibit more impaired cognitive control than girls (American Psychiatric Association, 2000). In addition, longitudinal studies have shown that there is a clear decline of symptoms with age, and a possible remission occurs after the age of 12 (Polanczyk & Rohde, 2007). The neuroendocrine system, the activation of which is closely associated with age and gender, may influence developing neural circuitry and behavioral systems; thus it has reasonably been speculated that this system plays a role in the pathogenesis of ADHD (Martel et al., 2009).

Methylphenidate (MPH), classified as a psychostimulant, is the most widely used drug for the pharmacological management of children with ADHD (Swanson et al., 2002). The effects of MPH on attention result from a combination of noradrenergic and dopaminergic mechanisms (Overtoom et al., 2003; Wilens, 2008). MPH exerts treatment effects by reducing impulsivity and disruptive behavior (Huang & Tsai, 2011), and it improves plenty of dimensions of neurocognitive function in ADHD patients (Huang et al., 2007; Pollak et al., 2010). Furthermore, some evidence has been revealed that MPH treatment possibly influences the neuroendocrine system (Hibel et al., 2007; Lurie & O'Quinn, 1991), and these influences possibly play a role as a mediator of the therapeutic effects for ADHD patients. Therefore, we herein review the related literature which investigates the relationship between ADHD, neuroendocrine, and MPH administration.

2. ADHD and neurosteroids

The term "neurosteroid" was first introduced by Baulieu (1981), which indicated steroid hormones synthesized in brain cells from cholesterol, independent of peripheral endocrine sources, acted at the central nervous system. Initially, neurosteroid referred to dehydroepiandrosterone sulfate (DHEA-S) (Baulieu & Robel, 1996). DHEA-S concentration in the brain was found to remain stable following adrenalectomy and gonadectomy. This implied that DHEA-S levels in the central neural system appeared to be independent of peripheral formation in the adrenals or gonads (Strous et al., 2006). Subsequently, progesterone, allopregnanolone, pregnenolone, dehydroepiandrosterone (DHEA) and their corresponding sulfate esters were identified as neurosteroids (Baulieu & Robel, 1998). Neurosteroids are important substrates that have been demonstrated to affect mood expression, energy level, aggression, and general activity (Wolkowitz et al., 1999).

2.1. DHEA and DHEA-S

DHEA is one of the major circulating neurosteroids in human, and it is also an ACTH-regulated steroid and a substrate for the synthesis of androstenedione and testosterone (Gurnell & Chatterjee, 2001). DHEA has been demonstrated to play several vital neurophysiological roles and to be affected by various physiological processes, including those associated with neurotrophic and neuronal excitability effects, circadian rhythms, sexual responses, immunological and stress reactions, memory, and sleep (Baulieu & Robel, 1996; Herbert, 1998). DHEA-S is a sulfated form of DHEA that is believed to be the most abundant steroid in the body (Wolf et al., 1997). DHEA-S is measured more frequently than DHEA because circulating levels of DHEA-S are approximately 500 times higher due to its lower metabolic clearance rate and minimal diurnal variation (Longcope, 1996).

Strous et al. (2001) demonstrated that DHEA and DHEA-S levels in blood are inversely related to the severity of hyperactivity/impulsivity symptoms in children with ADHD aged between 7 and 12 years. Another study found that ADHD patients treated with methylphenidate for 3 months exhibited pre- to post-treatment increases in plasma levels of DHEA and DHEA-S for 23% and 53.6%, respectively (Maayan et al., 2003). Subsequently, Lee et al. (2008) were the first research group investigating the role of neurosteroids in Asian ADHD population. They suggested that plasma DHEA-S levels in ADHD patients increased signifi-

http://dx.doi.org/10.5772/53609

cantly during a 12-week MPH treatment and under a 12-week bupropion treatment as well. These studies revealed a substantial increase in DHEA levels among pre-pubertal ADHD patients; however, there was no data with regards to age- and gender-matched healthy controls for comparison. Finally, our research team demonstrated that salivary DHEA levels were significantly lower in ADHD patients than those in healthy controls (Wang et al., 2011b). Salivary DHEA levels were not significantly correlated with ADHD clinical symptom severity, but positively correlated with performance in a neuropsychological test (Conner's Continuous Performance Test, CPT). Thus the authors suggested that lower morning DHEA levels might be a biological laboratory marker for ADHD, particularly for performance during CPT. In the longitudinal analyses, we found that morning salivary DHEA levels significantly increased under the 6-month MPH treatment course for ADHD patients. However, the salivary DHEA levels in healthy age- and gender- matched controls remain unchanged during the 6-month natural observation. Similar with the findings in the cross-sectional survey, DHEA levels exhibited a significant and independent association with overall CPT performance during the course of MPH treatment (Wang et al., 2011a). We could thus determine that the elevation of DHEA levels among ADHD patients is not derived from natural physiological change, but from MPH administration.

There is interesting coincidence in the similarity of the natural course of ADHD, brain development and age-related change in DHEA/DHEA-S levels. ADHD symptoms generally decline in severity between puberty and the early twenties (Biederman et al., 2000). Some brain imaging studies have found there to be a dysfunction of the cerebellar-striatal-prefrontal circuitry in ADHD (Gogtay et al., 2002), and that this may be the result of delayed maturation of the cerebral cortex, especially the prefrontal region (Shaw et al., 2007; McAlonan et al., 2009). Plasma DHEA/DHEA-S levels change with age, being low in the first years of life, then rapidly increasing from about eight years of age through puberty to reach their highest levels during early adulthood (de Peretti & Forest, 1978). DHEA-S has antiamnestic effects, and also anxiolytic and anti-aggressive properties (Wolf & Kirschbaum, 1999). Both DHEA and DHEA-S have been shown to regulate the motility and growth of neocortical neurons in the rodent brain (Compagnone & Mellon, 1998). This implies that DHEA/DHEA-S exert biological actions that may play crucial roles in guiding cortical projections to appropriate targets, and thus may be important for the regulation of neurodevelopment (Golubchik et al., 2007). It has been proposed that DHEA/DHEA-S exerts its positive effects in ADHD patients through stimulatory or antagonist effects at the gammaaminobutyric acid A ($GABA_A$) receptor and facilitation of the N-methyl-*D*-aspartate (NMDA) activity (Davies et al., 2009; Strous et al., 2001; Tang et al., 1999). DHEA protects hippocampal neuronal activity from glutamate toxicity. DHEA-S also protects hippocampal neuronal cells from excitatory amino acid induced neurotoxicity. Taken together, DHEA and DHEA-S may provide an important antioxidant function and may thus play a role in neurodevelopment and have neuroprotective effects (Strous et al., 2006).

Some molecular genetic studies demonstrated candidate genes contributing to ADHD. The steroid sulfatase (STS) gene, which escapes X inactivation in humans, desulfates several sulfatedsteroids, including DHEA-S to DHEA. In an animal study, it has been noticed that the

STS may modify the attentional function and motor impulsivity through administration of the substrate DHEA and DHEA-S (Davies et al., 2009). The same research team showed that the 39,X(Y*)O mice (which lack the STS gene but no other known genes as a consequence of end-to-end fusion of the X and Y chromosomes) exhibited significantly lower DHEA serum levels than 40,XY mice. They concluded that STS-deficient mice exhibit endophenotypes relevant to ADHD (Trent et al., 2012). In human studies, Kent et al. (2008) have demonstrated that boys with X-linked ichthyosis who have a deletion or point mutation of STS are at an increased risk of ADHD. In addition, Brookes et al. (2008) indicated that common variants within the STS gene may increase susceptibility to ADHD. The over transmitted risk allele of rs12861247 was also associated with reduced STS mRNA expression, and hence deficit in STS protein production is at a significantly increased risk of developing ADHD (Brookes et al., 2010). However, ethnic differences in epidemiology and genetic polymorphism of ADHD patients have been demonstrated in some studies (Nikolaidis & Gray, 2009; Pastor & Reuben, 2005). It remains unclear whether the relationships between the STS gene, ADHD and neurosteroids also exist among non-Caucasian populations.

Neurochemical findings showing MPH exerts its effects on catecholamines in areas such as the prefrontal cortex, nucleus accumbens, and striatum are consistent with the neurobiological and clinical effects of MPH on memory, attention, and movement (Wilens, 2008). The neuroendocrine effects of MPH administration might be related to its dopaminergic and adrenergic agonistic activity (Hibel et al., 2007; Lurie & O'Quinn, 1991; Weizman et al., 1987). Hibel et al. (2007) demonstrated that children taking concerta (methylphenidate extended-release tablets) had higher average levels of DHEA than those who were non-medicated. Several studies suggested that MPH increased DHEA or DHEA-S levels of ADHD patients during a 3-month treatment (Lee et al., 2008; Maayan et al., 2003; Wang et al., 2011a). One possible neurochemical explanation for this phenomenon is that MPH-induced increases in DHEA or DHEA-S may act either by decreasing levels of the $GABA_A$ antagonist-like pregnenolone sulfate, or by increasing levels of the $GABA_A$ agonist-like progesterone metabolites (Robel & Baulieu, 1995). In addition, the direct influence of medications on salivary hormones may act on the secretion and feedback control of the HPA and hypothalamic-pituitary-gonadal (HPG) axes. MPH may also indirectly influence DHEA or DHEA-S by attenuating or potentiating the impact of environmental events and subjective experience on HPA axis and HPG activity (Hibel et al., 2007). However, it is not clear whether DHEA or DHEA-S exerts effects in conjunction with or independently of MPH on neurocognitive function in ADHD. It remains to be clarified whether DHEA or DHEA-S plays a role as a mediator of the therapeutic effects of MPH, or if these associations are epiphenomena of the benefits of MPH treatment. Moreover, it would also be interesting to investigate whether DHEA or DHEA-S could directly benefit the treatment of ADHD patients.

2.2. Other neurosteroids and gonadal hormones

Neurosteroids, other than DHEA and DHEA-S, mainly contain pregnenolone (PREG) and progesterone, which is metabolized to 5a-dihydroprogesterone (5α-DH PROG) and 3α,5α-tetrahydroprogesterone (3α,5α-TH PROG), also named allopregnanolone (Vallee et al.,

http://dx.doi.org/10.5772/53609

2001). PREG is the principal precursor of DHEA. The sulfated form of **pregnenolone** (PREG-S) exerts its neurochemical action as a negative modulator of the $GABA_A$ and also as a positive modulator of the NMDA subtype of glutamate receptor (Mayo et al., 2001). PREG-S is also capable of modulating acetylcholine neurotransmission associated with paradoxical sleep modifications (Mayo et al., 2003). **In animal studies,** PREG-S in the hippocampus region plays a physiological role in preserving and enhancing cognitive abilities, possibly via an interaction with central cholinergic systems (Vallee et al., 1997; Vallee et al., 2001). Among humans, PREG appears to improve clinical symptoms in patients with mood disorders (Osuji et al., 2010), and in patients with schizophrenia as well (Marx et al., 2011). To date, there has been only one study investigating the relationship of PREG and ADHD (Strous et al., 2001), and this study revealed that PREG levels in the blood are inversely related to the severity of hyperactivity/impulsivity symptoms in children with ADHD.

Gonadal hormones may act on the prenatal development of dopaminergic neural circuitry and dopamine function in the nucleus accumbens, striatum, and prefrontal cortex via its masculinizing effects (Martel et al., 2009). Therefore, gonadal hormones may modulate corresponding deficits in cognitive control and reward processes in ADHD. In animal studies, estradiol and progesterone both appear capable of inducing increases in dendritic spine density during development. Estradiol and progesterone have been also proposed to play a role in ADHD, because they are synthesized *de novo* in the cerebellum during critical developmental periods (Dean & McCarthy, 2008). In addition, estrogen has been identified to have neuroprotective effects through protection against oxidative stress, and neurotrophic cross-talk through the signal cascade shared with neurotrophic factors (Sawada & Shimohama, 2000). However, the relationship of estradiol, progesterone and ADHD in humans has not yet been well-established in clinical studies.

Prenatal **testosterone** exposure has been implied in the etiology of **ADHD**. High levels of prenatal testosterone may moderate the relationship between prenatal risk factors, and further affect dopaminergic neural circuitry by slowing down neural development globally (Morris et al., 2004). Several studies have examined the association between the presence of **ADHD phenotype** and the ratio of the length of the second and fourth digits (2D:4D ratio), which is a marker of fetal **testosterone** exposure (de Bruin et al., 2006; Lemiere et al., 2010; Stevenson et al., 2007). However, the findings are inconsistent between these studies. Furthermore, Yu & Shi (2009) found that salivary testosterone levels are higher in children with aggressive tendencies than those without aggressive tendencies. Whereas Dorn et al., (2009) suggested that no significant difference in salivary testosterone levels between children with and without disruptive behavior disorders. Regarding the effects of MPH on testosterone, Avital et al., (2011) indicated that long-term exposure to MPH led to elevated **testosterone** levels in rodents. However, Mattison et al., (2011) reported that MPH administration in rhesus macaques, beginning before puberty, led to delay in pubertal testicular development until 5 years of age. Among humans, Hibel et al. (2007) investigated the relationship of salivary biomarker levels, diurnal variation and the effects of medications among maltreated or low-income disadvantaged children. They found that testosterone in non-medicated children decreased along with time in a day, but those in children taking psychostimulants remained unchanged. In summary, evidence about the role of gonadal hormones in the aetiology of **ADHD in humans is remains scarce, thus future clinical studies are warranted to elucidate this issue.**

3. Cortisol

Dysfunction of the hypothalamic-pituitary-adrenal (HPA) axis in ADHD children was proposed to address the complexity in the pathophysiology of ADHD (Kaneko et al., 1993; Ma et al., 2011). The HPA axis plays an important role in regulating central nervous system neurotransmitters and behavior, such as attention, emotion, memory, and learning (Talge et al., 2007). The function of the HPA axis has typically been assessed by cortisol levels, which can be measured from a number of sources (saliva, urine, and blood plasma) (Hellhammer et al., 2009). Low cortisol levels generally reflect under arousal or an elevated threshold for the detection of stressors (Freitag et al., 2009; Kaneko et al., 1993). Many clinical studies investigated cortisol levels in either a stress response or an awakening response (Freitag et al., 2009; Popma et al., 2006; Stadler et al., 2011; Yang et al., 2007). For example, Popma et al. (2006) reported that patients with disruptive behavior disorders showed a significantly decreased cortisol response after a standard public speaking task as compared with the normal controls. Yang et al. (2007) demonstrated that the magnitude of the increase in cortisol reactivity to stress was inversely correlated with aggression tendency in patients with ADHD. Freitag et al. (2009) indicated that ADHD children comorbid with ODD showed a weaker cortisol awakening response compared to ADHD children without comorbidity and control children. Stadler et al. (2011) reported that ADHD patients scoring high on callous unemotional traits showed a blunted HPA axis reactivity to the experimentally induced stress. Moreover, it has also been suggested that the cortisol reactivity to stress at baseline in ADHD patients could predict treatment effects (van de Wiel et al., 2004), and was associated with the one-year outcome (King et al., 1998).

On the other hand, some studies aimed to determine the basal level of morning cortisol in ADHD patients, and to determine the relationship between cortisol levels and ADHD related social/behavioral symptoms or cognition deficit. Among these, Schulz et al., (1997) showed that there was no significant difference in basal cortisol levels between aggressive and nonaggressive boys with ADHD. In addition, the basal level of morning cortisol was not significantly correlated with the severity of ADHD hyperactivity/impulsivity symptoms (Strous et al., 2001) and the performance in neuropsychological test (Wang et al., 2011b). However, there is one study which demonstrated gender differences in the cortisol levels among a community sample of adolescents, which showed that females carry a positive and males a negative association between cortisol and conduct symptoms (Young et al., 2012). For ADHD subtypes, Ma et al. (2011) reported that the level of cortisol in the ADHD group was significantly lower than that of the control group. There was a significant difference in cortisol levels between ADHD subtypes: The level of cortisol of the ADHD-predominantly hyperactive impulsive type was significantly lower than that of ADHD-predominantly inattention type and ADHD-combined type (Ma et al., 2011). Furthermore, a recent meta-analysis revealed that the age of the children significantly moderated the relation between basal cortisol and externalizing behavior. Externalizing behavior was associated with higher basal cortisol in preschoolers, and with lower basal cortisol in elementary school-aged children (Alink et al., 2008).

Regarding with the effects of MPH on cortisol, Weizman et al. (1987) reported that plasma cortisol levels of ADHD patients increased under acute challenge of MPH; nevertheless, the effects disappeared when subjects were re-challenged after 4 weeks. Similar effect of acute challenge MPH for increasing cortisol levels was also observed among normal adults (Joyce et al., 1986). However, Lee et al. (2008) showed that during a 12-week period, there was no significant change in cortisol levels in ADHD patients under MPH treatment. In contrast, Chen et al. (2012) reported that basal plasma cortisol levels were significant increased after treatment either with MPH or with atomoxetine. Furthermore, our research team showed that the morning levels of salivary cortisol in the patients with ADHD were significantly increased from baseline at 1 month after the MPH treatment was started (Wang et al., 2012). Subsequently, the cortisol levels dropped to an intermediary level that differed from the baseline and 1-month values. The effects of MPH on the neuroendocrine system were proposed to result from a combination of noradrenergic and dopaminergic mechanisms (Lurie & O'Quinn, 1991). The higher concentrations of dopamine and norepinephrine could promote the release of corticotropin releasing hormone (CRH) and the adrenocorticotropic hormone (ACTH) (Biondi & Picardi, 1999). It might be a possible explanation of MPH-induced cortisol elevation; however, the effect of MPH on cortisol secretion seems to be temporary. Acute tolerance to MPH has long been reported in the treatment of ADHD in children (Swanson et al., 1999). It warrants further investigation to clarify whether the transient effect on cortisol increment shares similar neurobiological mechanisms with the tolerance of MPH.

4. Conclusion

Awareness of the prominent position that the neuroendocrine system has to play in pathophysiology of ADHD is increasing. DHEA and DHEA-S are important neurosteroids substrates which demonstrate a potential correlation to symptoms severity and neurocognitive function in ADHD patients. MPH, the most therapeutically efficient drugs in

ADHD, exerts its pharmacological effects via increasing the level of the dopamine and norepinephrine. Extant studies almost identically indicate that MPH administration would lead to increases in the levels of DHEA or DHEA-S. With regards to other neurosteroids or gonadal hormones, their influence on developing neural circuitry and behavioral systems has already been established in animal models. However, many findings noted in animal studies have yet to be replicated in humans, in particular patients with ADHD. The HPA-axis dysfunction, which was measured by cortisol levels, has also been indicated to address the complexity in the pathogenesis of ADHD. Current studies revealed that ADHD patients, especially for those with higher aggression tendencies or comorbidities, might have lower levels of cortisol than healthy controls. MPH administration is able to elevate cortisol levels, but the effects seem to be temporary. To date, much remains unclear about the complex interaction between neuroendocrine system, pathophysiology of ADHD and effects of MPH. Further research at the basic scientific level as well as in the context of double-blinded placebo controlled investigation is mandated to better elucidate the role of neuroendocrine in the understanding and management of ADHD patients.

Author details

Liang-Jen Wang[1,2] and Chih-Ken Chen[2,3]

1 Department of Child and Adolescent Psychiatry, Chang Gung Memorial Hospital - Kaohsiung Medical Center, Chang Gung University College of Medicine, Kaohsiung, Taiwan

2 Chang Gung University School of Medicine, Taoyuan, Taiwan

3 Department of Psychiatry, Chang Gung Memorial Hospital, Keelung, Taiwan

References

[1] Alink, L.R., Van Ijzendoorn, M.H., Bakermans-Kranenburg, M.J., Mesman, J., Juffer, F. & Koot, H.M. (2008). Cortisol and externalizing behavior in children and adolescents: mixed meta-analytic evidence for the inverse relation of basal cortisol and cortisol reactivity with externalizing behavior. *Dev Psychobiol*, 50, 427-450.

[2] American Psychiatric Association (2000). Diagnostic and Statistical Manual of Mental disorders. *American Psychiatric Association*, Washington, DC.

[3] Avital, A., Dolev, T., Aga-Mizrachi, S. & Zubedat, S. (2011). Environmental enrichment preceding early adulthood methylphenidate treatment leads to long term increase of corticosterone and testosterone in the rat. *PLoS One*, 6, e22059.

[4] Baulieu, E.E. & Robel, P. (1996). Dehydroepiandrosterone and dehydroepiandrosterone sulfate as neuroactive neurosteroids. *J Endocrinol*, 150 Suppl, S221-239.

[5] Baulieu, E.E. & Robel, P. (1998). Dehydroepiandrosterone (DHEA) and dehydroepiandrosterone sulfate (DHEAS) as neuroactive neurosteroids. *Proc Natl Acad Sci U S A*, 95, 4089-4091.

[6] Biederman, J. & Faraone, S.V. (2002). Current concepts on the neurobiology of Attention-Deficit/Hyperactivity Disorder. *J Atten Disord*, 6 Suppl 1, S7-16.

[7] Biederman, J., Mick, E. & Faraone, S.V. (2000). Age-dependent decline of symptoms of attention deficit hyperactivity disorder: impact of remission definition and symptom type. *Am J Psychiatry*, 157, 816-818.

[8] Biondi, M. & Picardi, A. (1999). Psychological stress and neuroendocrine function in humans: the last two decades of research. *Psychother Psychosom*, 68, 114-150.

[9] Brookes, K.J., Hawi, Z., Kirley, A., Barry, E., Gill, M. & Kent, L. (2008). Association of the steroid sulfatase (STS) gene with attention deficit hyperactivity disorder. *Am J Med Genet B Neuropsychiatr Genet*, 147B, 1531-1535.

[10] Brookes, K.J., Hawi, Z., Park, J., Scott, S., Gill, M. & Kent, L. (2010). Polymorphisms of the steroid sulfatase (STS) gene are associated with attention deficit hyperactivity disorder and influence brain tissue mRNA expression. *Am J Med Genet B Neuropsychiatr Genet*, 153B, 1417-1424.

[11] Chen, Y.H., Lin, X.X., Chen, H., Liu, Y.Y., Lin, G.X., Wei, L.X., et al. (2012). The change of the cortisol levels in children with ADHD treated by methylphenidate or atomoxetine. *J Psychiatr Res*, 46, 415-416.

[12] Compagnone, N.A. & Mellon, S.H. (1998). Dehydroepiandrosterone: a potential signalling molecule for neocortical organization during development. *Proc Natl Acad Sci U S A*, 95, 4678-4683.

[13] Davies, W., Humby, T., Kong, W., Otter, T., Burgoyne, P.S. & Wilkinson, L.S. (2009). Converging pharmacological and genetic evidence indicates a role for steroid sulfatase in attention. *Biol Psychiatry*, 66, 360-367.

[14] De Bruin, E.I., Verheij, F., Wiegman, T. & Ferdinand, R.F. (2006). Differences in finger length ratio between males with autism, pervasive developmental disorder-not otherwise specified, ADHD, and anxiety disorders. *Dev Med Child Neurol*, 48, 962-965.

[15] De Peretti, E. & Forest, M.G. (1978). Pattern of plasma dehydroepiandrosterone sulfate levels in humans from birth to adulthood: evidence for testicular production. *J Clin Endocrinol Metab*, 47, 572-577.

[16] Dean, S.L. & Mccarthy, M.M. (2008). Steroids, sex and the cerebellar cortex: implications for human disease. *Cerebellum*, 7, 38-47.

[17] Dorn, L.D., Kolko, D.J., Susman, E.J., Huang, B., Stein, H., Music, E., et al. (2009). Salivary gonadal and adrenal hormone differences in boys and girls with and without disruptive behavior disorders: Contextual variants. *Biol Psychol*, 81, 31-39.

[18] Dubrovsky, B.O. (2005). Steroids, neuroactive steroids and neurosteroids in psychopathology. *Prog Neuropsychopharmacol Biol Psychiatry*, 29, 169-192

[19] Freitag, C.M., Hanig, S., Palmason, H., Meyer, J., Wust, S. & Seitz, C. (2009). Cortisol awakening response in healthy children and children with ADHD: impact of comorbid disorders and psychosocial risk factors. *Psychoneuroendocrinology*, 34, 1019-1028.

[20] Gau, S.S., Chong, M.Y., Chen, T.H. & Cheng, A.T. (2005). A 3-year panel study of mental disorders among adolescents in Taiwan. *Am J Psychiatry*, 162, 1344-1350.

[21] Gogtay, N., Giedd, J. & Rapoport, J.L. (2002). Brain development in healthy, hyperactive, and psychotic children. *Arch Neurol*, 59, 1244-1248.

[22] Golubchik, P., Lewis, M., Maayan, R., Sever, J., Strous, R. & Weizman, A. (2007). Neurosteroids in child and adolescent psychopathology. *Eur Neuropsychopharmacol*, 17, 157-164.

[23] Goodyer, I.M., Park, R.J., Netherton, C.M. & Herbert, J. (2001). Possible role of cortisol and dehydroepiandrosterone in human development and psychopathology. *Br J Psychiatry*, 179, 243-249.

[24] Gurnell, E.M. & Chatterjee, V.K. (2001). Dehydroepiandrosterone replacement therapy. *Eur J Endocrinol*, 145, 103-106.

[25] Hellhammer, D.H., Wust, S. & Kudielka, B.M. (2009). Salivary cortisol as a biomarker in stress research. *Psychoneuroendocrinology*, 34, 163-171.

[26] Herbert, J. (1998). Neurosteroids, brain damage, and mental illness. *Exp Gerontol*, 33, 713-727.

[27] Hibel, L.C., Granger, D.A., Cicchetti, D. & Rogosch, F. (2007). Salivary biomarker levels and diurnal variation: associations with medications prescribed to control children's problem behavior. *Child Dev*, 78, 927-937.

[28] Huang, Y.S., Chao, C.C., Wu, Y.Y., Chen, Y.Y. & Chen, C.K. (2007). Acute effects of methylphenidate on performance during the Test of Variables of Attention in children with attention deficit/hyperactivity disorder. *Psychiatry Clin Neurosci*, 61, 219-225.

[29] Huang, Y.S. & Tsai, M.H. (2011). Long-term outcomes with medications for attention-deficit hyperactivity disorder: current status of knowledge. *CNS Drugs*, 25, 539-554.

[30] Joyce, P.R., Donald, R.A., Nicholls, M.G., Livesey, J.H. & Abbott, R.M. (1986). Endocrine and behavioral responses to methylphenidate in normal subjects. *Biol Psychiatry*, 21, 1015-1023.

[31] Kaneko, M., Hoshino, Y., Hashimoto, S., Okano, T. & Kumashiro, H. (1993). Hypothalamic-pituitary-adrenal axis function in children with attention-deficit hyperactivity disorder. *J Autism Dev Disord*, 23, 59-65.

[32] Kent, L., Emerton, J., Bhadravathi, V., Weisblatt, E., Pasco, G., Willatt, L.R., et al. (2008). X-linked ichthyosis (steroid sulfatase deficiency) is associated with increased risk of attention deficit hyperactivity disorder, autism and social communication deficits. *J Med Genet*, 45, 519-524.

[33] King, J.A., Barkley, R.A. & Barrett, S. (1998). Attention-deficit hyperactivity disorder and the stress response. *Biol Psychiatry*, 44, 72-74.

[34] Lee, M.S., Yang, J.W., Ko, Y.H., Han, C., Kim, S.H., Joe, S.H., et al. (2008). Effects of methylphenidate and bupropion on DHEA-S and cortisol plasma levels in attention-deficit hyperactivity disorder. *Child Psychiatry Hum Dev*, 39, 201-209.

[35] Lemiere, J., Boets, B. & Danckaerts, M. (2010). No association between the 2D:4D fetal testosterone marker and multidimensional attentional abilities in children with ADHD. *Dev Med Child Neurol*, 52, e202-208.

[36] Longcope, C. (1996). Dehydroepiandrosterone metabolism. *J Endocrinol*, 150 Suppl, S125-127.

[37] Lurie, S. & O'quinn, A. (1991). Neuroendocrine responses to methylphenidate and d-amphetamine: applications to attention-deficit disorder. *J Neuropsychiatry Clin Neurosci*, 3, 41-50.

[38] Ma, L., Chen, Y.H., Chen, H., Liu, Y.Y. & Wang, Y.X. (2011). The function of hypothalamus-pituitary-adrenal axis in children with ADHD. *Brain Res*, 1368, 159-162.

[39] Maayan, R., Yoran-Hegesh, R., Strous, R., Nechmad, A., Averbuch, E., Weizman, A., et al. (2003). Three-month treatment course of methylphenidate increases plasma levels of dehydroepiandrosterone (DHEA) and dehydroepiandrosterone-sulfate (DHEA-S) in attention deficit hyperactivity disorder. *Neuropsychobiology*, 48, 111-115.

[40] Martel, M.M., Klump, K., Nigg, J.T., Breedlove, S.M. & Sisk, C.L. (2009). Potential hormonal mechanisms of attention-deficit/hyperactivity disorder and major depressive disorder: a new perspective. *Horm Behav*, 55, 465-479.

[41] Marx, C.E., Bradford, D.W., Hamer, R.M., Naylor, J.C., Allen, T.B., Lieberman, J.A., et al. (2011). Pregnenolone as a novel therapeutic candidate in schizophrenia: emerging preclinical and clinical evidence. *Neuroscience*, 191, 78-90.

[42] Mattison, D.R., Plant, T.M., Lin, H.M., Chen, H.C., Chen, J.J., Twaddle, N.C., et al. (2011). Pubertal delay in male nonhuman primates (Macaca mulatta) treated with methylphenidate. *Proc Natl Acad Sci U S A*, 108, 16301-16306.

[43] Mayo, W., George, O., Darbra, S., Bouyer, J.J., Vallee, M., Darnaudery, M., et al. (2003). Individual differences in cognitive aging: implication of pregnenolone sulfate. *Prog Neurobiol*, 71, 43-48.

[44] Mayo, W., Le Moal, M. & Abrous, D.N. (2001). Pregnenolone sulfate and aging of cognitive functions: behavioral, neurochemical, and morphological investigations. *Horm Behav*, 40, 215-217.

[45] Mcalonan, G.M., Cheung, V., Chua, S.E., Oosterlaan, J., Hung, S.F., Tang, C.P., et al. (2009). Age-related grey matter volume correlates of response inhibition and shifting in attention-deficit hyperactivity disorder. *Br J Psychiatry*, 194, 123-129.

[46] Morris, J.A., Jordan, C.L. & Breedlove, S.M. (2004). Sexual differentiation of the vertebrate nervous system. *Nat Neurosci*, 7, 1034-1039.

[47] Nikolaidis, A. & Gray, J.R. (2009). ADHD and the DRD4 exon III 7-repeat polymorphism: an international meta-analysis. *Soc Cogn Affect Neurosci.*

[48] Osuji, I.J., Vera-Bolanos, E., Carmody, T.J. & Brown, E.S. (2010). Pregnenolone for cognition and mood in dual diagnosis patients. *Psychiatry Res*, 178, 309-312.

[49] Overtoom, C.C., Verbaten, M.N., Kemner, C., Kenemans, J.L., Van Engeland, H., Buitelaar, J.K., et al. (2003). Effects of methylphenidate, desipramine, and L-dopa on attention and inhibition in children with Attention Deficit Hyperactivity Disorder. *Behav Brain Res*, 145, 7-15.

[50] Pastor, P.N. & Reuben, C.A. (2005). Racial and ethnic differences in ADHD and LD in young school-age children: parental reports in the National Health Interview Survey. *Public Health Rep*, 120, 383-392.

[51] Polanczyk, G., De Lima, M.S., Horta, B.L., Biederman, J. & Rohde, L.A. (2007). The worldwide prevalence of ADHD: a systematic review and metaregression analysis. *Am J Psychiatry*, 164, 942-948.

[52] Polanczyk, G. & Rohde, L.A. (2007). Epidemiology of attention-deficit/hyperactivity disorder across the lifespan. *Curr Opin Psychiatry*, 20, 386-392.

[53] Pollak, Y., Shomaly, H.B., Weiss, P.L., Rizzo, A.A. & Gross-Tsur, V. (2010). Methylphenidate effect in children with ADHD can be measured by an ecologically valid continuous performance test embedded in virtual reality. *CNS Spectr*, 15, 125-130.

[54] Popma, A., Jansen, L.M., Vermeiren, R., Steiner, H., Raine, A., Van Goozen, S.H., et al. (2006). Hypothalamus pituitary adrenal axis and autonomic activity during stress in delinquent male adolescents and controls. *Psychoneuroendocrinology*, 31, 948-957.

[55] Robel, P. & Baulieu, E.E. (1995). Neurosteroids: biosynthesis and function. *Crit Rev Neurobiol*, 9, 383-394.

[56] Sawada, H. & Shimohama, S. (2000). Neuroprotective effects of estradiol in mesencephalic dopaminergic neurons. *Neurosci Biobehav Rev*, 24, 143-147.

[57] Schulz, K.P., Halperin, J.M., Newcorn, J.H., Sharma, V. & Gabriel, S. (1997). Plasma cortisol and aggression in boys with ADHD. *J Am Acad Child Adolesc Psychiatry*, 36, 605-609.

[58] Shaw, P., Eckstrand, K., Sharp, W., Blumenthal, J., Lerch, J.P., Greenstein, D., et al. (2007). Attention-deficit/hyperactivity disorder is characterized by a delay in cortical maturation. *Proc Natl Acad Sci U S A*, 104, 19649-19654.

[59] Spencer, T.J., Biederman, J. & Mick, E. (2007). Attention-deficit/hyperactivity disorder: diagnosis, lifespan, comorbidities, and neurobiology. *J Pediatr Psychol*, 32, 631-642.

[60] Stadler, C., Kroeger, A., Weyers, P., Grasmann, D., Horschinek, M., Freitag, C., et al. (2011). Cortisol reactivity in boys with attention-deficit/hyperactivity disorder and

disruptive behavior problems: The impact of callous unemotional traits. *Psychiatry Res*, 187, 204-209.

[61] Stevenson, J.C., Everson, P.M., Williams, D.C., Hipskind, G., Grimes, M. & Mahoney, E.R. (2007). Attention deficit/hyperactivity disorder (ADHD) symptoms and digit ratios in a college sample. *Am J Hum Biol*, 19, 41-50.

[62] Strous, R.D., Maayan, R. & Weizman, A. (2006). The relevance of neurosteroids to clinical psychiatry: from the laboratory to the bedside. *Eur Neuropsychopharmacol*, 16, 155-169.

[63] Strous, R.D., Spivak, B., Yoran-Hegesh, R., Maayan, R., Averbuch, E., Kotler, M., et al. (2001). Analysis of neurosteroid levels in attention deficit hyperactivity disorder. *Int J Neuropsychopharmacol*, 4, 259-264.

[64] Swanson, J., Gupta, S., Guinta, D., Flynn, D., Agler, D., Lerner, M., et al. (1999). Acute tolerance to methylphenidate in the treatment of attention deficit hyperactivity disorder in children. *Clin Pharmacol Ther*, 66, 295-305.

[65] Swanson, J.M., Gupta, S., Williams, L., Agler, D., Lerner, M. & Wigal, S. (2002). Efficacy of a new pattern of delivery of methylphenidate for the treatment of ADHD: effects on activity level in the classroom and on the playground. *J Am Acad Child Adolesc Psychiatry*, 41, 1306-1314.

[66] Talge, N.M., Neal, C. & Glover, V. (2007). Antenatal maternal stress and long-term effects on child neurodevelopment: how and why? *J Child Psychol Psychiatry*, 48, 245-261.

[67] Tang, Y.P., Shimizu, E., Dube, G.R., Rampon, C., Kerchner, G.A., Zhuo, M., et al. (1999). Genetic enhancement of learning and memory in mice. *Nature*, 401, 63-69.

[68] Trent, S., Dennehy, A., Richardson, H., Ojarikre, O.A., Burgoyne, P.S., Humby, T., et al. (2012). Steroid sulfatase-deficient mice exhibit endophenotypes relevant to attention deficit hyperactivity disorder. *Psychoneuroendocrinology*, 37, 221-229.

[69] Vallee, M., Mayo, W., Darnaudery, M., Corpechot, C., Young, J., Koehl, M., et al. (1997). Neurosteroids: deficient cognitive performance in aged rats depends on low pregnenolone sulfate levels in the hippocampus. *Proc Natl Acad Sci U S A*, 94, 14865-14870.

[70] Vallee, M., Mayo, W. & Le Moal, M. (2001). Role of pregnenolone, dehydroepiandrosterone and their sulfate esters on learning and memory in cognitive aging. *Brain Res Brain Res Rev*, 37, 301-312.

[71] Van De Wiel, N.M., Van Goozen, S.H., Matthys, W., Snoek, H. & Van Engeland, H. (2004). Cortisol and treatment effect in children with disruptive behavior disorders: a preliminary study. *J Am Acad Child Adolesc Psychiatry*, 43, 1011-1018.

[72] Wang, L.J., Hsiao, C.C., Huang, Y.S., Chiang, Y.L., Ree, S.C., Chen, Y.C., et al. (2011a). Association of salivary dehydroepiandrosterone levels and symptoms in patients

with attention deficit hyperactivity disorder during six months of treatment with methylphenidate. *Psychoneuroendocrinology*, 36, 1209-1216.

[73] Wang, L.J., Huang, Y.S., Hsiao, C.C., Chiang, Y.L., Wu, C.C., Shang, Z.Y., et al. (2011b). Salivary dehydroepiandrosterone, but not cortisol, is associated with attention deficit hyperactivity disorder. *World J Biol Psychiatry*, 12, 99-109.

[74] Wang, L.J., Huang, Y.S., Hsiao, C.C., Chen, C.K. (2012). The Trend in Morning Levels of Salivary Cortisol in Children with ADHD during 6 Months of Methylphenidate Treatment. J Attention Disorders, (In press)

[75] Weizman, R., Dick, J., Gil-Ad, I., Weitz, R., Tyano, S. & Laron, Z. (1987). Effects of acute and chronic methylphenidate administration on beta-endorphin, growth hormone, prolactin and cortisol in children with attention deficit disorder and hyperactivity. *Life Sci*, 40, 2247-2252.

[76] Wilens, T.E. (2008). Effects of methylphenidate on the catecholaminergic system in attention-deficit/hyperactivity disorder. *J Clin Psychopharmacol*, 28, S46-53.

[77] Wolf, O.T. & Kirschbaum, C. (1999). Actions of dehydroepiandrosterone and its sulfate in the central nervous system: effects on cognition and emotion in animals and humans. *Brain Res Brain Res Rev*, 30, 264-288.

[78] Wolf, O.T., Neumann, O., Hellhammer, D.H., Geiben, A.C., Strasburger, C.J., Dressendorfer, R.A., et al. (1997). Effects of a two-week physiological dehydroepiandrosterone substitution on cognitive performance and well-being in healthy elderly women and men. *J Clin Endocrinol Metab*, 82, 2363-2367.

[79] Wolkowitz, O.M., Reus, V.I., Keebler, A., Nelson, N., Friedland, M., Brizendine, L., et al. (1999). Double-blind treatment of major depression with dehydroepiandrosterone. *Am J Psychiatry*, 156, 646-649.

[80] Yang, S.J., Shin, D.W., Noh, K.S. & Stein, M.A. (2007). Cortisol is inversely correlated with aggression for those boys with attention deficit hyperactivity disorder who retain their reactivity to stress. *Psychiatry Res*, 153, 55-60.

[81] Young, R., Sweeting, H. & West, P. (2012). Associations between DSM-IV diagnosis, psychiatric symptoms and morning cortisol levels in a community sample of adolescents. *Soc Psychiatry Psychiatr Epidemiol*, 47, 723-733.

[82] Yu, Y.Z. & Shi, J.X. (2009). Relationship between levels of testosterone and cortisol in saliva and aggressive behaviors of adolescents. *Biomed Environ Sci*, 22, 44-49.

Chapter 6

Dopamine and Glutamate Interactions in ADHD: Implications for the Future Neuropharmacology of ADHD

Erin M. Miller, Theresa C. Thomas,
Greg A. Gerhardt and Paul E. A. Glaser

Additional information is available at the end of the chapter

http://dx.doi.org/10.5772/54207

1. Introduction

In this chapter, we will discuss the interactions between a neurotransmitter that has been heavily implicated in ADHD, dopamine, and a neurotransmitter just beginning to be investigated, glutamate. We will examine the literature to reveal how current treatments for ADHD affect these neurotransmitter levels in specific areas of the brain that are thought to be dysfunctional in ADHD. Additionally, we will detail new data on dopamine and glutamate dysfunction utilizing approaches that are capable of accurately measuring levels of these neurotransmitters in two separate rodent models of ADHD. Finally, we will speculate on the role that the dopamine-glutamate interaction will play in the future neuropharmacology of ADHD and how measuring these neurotransmitter levels in rodent models of ADHD may aid in furthering the future pharmacotherapy of ADHD.

Throughout the text, we will use ADHD (Attention-Deficit/Hyperactivity Disorder) without reference to the DSM-IV type, unless a specific reference pertains to combined, inattentive or hyperactive subtypes.

2. ADHD and the link to neurochemistry

When the Diagnostic and Statistical Manual of Mental Disorders (DSM-1) was first published in 1952, childhood psychiatric disorders were thought to be caused by environment and referred to as 'reactions' [1]. It wasn't until the DSM-2 was published in 1968 that ADHD began to be separated from general reactions and become its own diagnosis, referred to as the 'hyperkinetic reaction of childhood.' This reaction was characterized by a short attention span, hyperactivity, and restlessness [2], and in 1980, with the publication of the DSM-3, the ADHD diagnosis became more specific and was described as ADD (attention-deficit disorder) [3]; however, by this time, this disorder was already being treated with stimulant medications, a treatment still used to this day.

Stimulant medications were initially discovered to treat hyperactivity in the early 1900s when the psychiatrist Charles Bradley used amphetamines to treat children with headaches caused by pneumoencephalography and found it improved their school performance, social interactions and emotional responses. However, amphetamine as a treatment for ADHD was ignored until years later due to a variety of reasons [4]. In the 1950s, researchers were beginning to look for the underlying mechanisms causing behavioral problems and it was at this time that Bradley's discovery of amphetamine as a treatment for hyperactivity was uncovered and investigations into the mechanism of action of amphetamine began. The amphetamine formulation Bradley used in his patients was called Benzedrine, a racemic mixture of 50/50 d- and l-amphetamine, produced by the company Smith, Kline and French [4]. Treatment with this medication in a variety of experimental paradigms reduced hyperactivity [5]; however, of particular note is a study published in 1976 showing decreased hyperactivity when treated with amphetamine in rodents with dopamine depletion [6]. This was the first time that hyperactivity was linked to dopamine, but far from the last.

2.1. Dopamine

Dopamine, classified as a catecholamine neurotransmitter, is produced in the cells of the substantia nigra (SN, A9) and ventral tegmental area (VTA, A10) of the midbrain and project to numerous brain regions, including the prefrontal cortex (PFC), striatum and nucleus accumbens (NA, see Figure 1). Projections from the VTA to the NA are identified as the mesolimbic pathway, or the "reward pathway," because these dopamine projections are involved in rewarding behaviors, [7] firing when a reward is greater than expected or when a reward is anticipated [8-10]. Projections from the SN to the striatum are referred to as the nigrostriatal pathway and play a role in many aspects of motor control [11]. The mesocortical system consists of dopaminergic projections from the VTA to the PFC, and it is implicated in many cognitive functions including, but most certainly not limited to, attention and memory [11]. The mesocortical system will be the main focus in this chapter.

Dopamine is produced from tyrosine into 3,4-dihydroxyphenylalanine (DOPA) by the enzyme tyrosine hydroxylase. DOPA is then made into dopamine via DOPA-decarboxylase. Conversely, dopamine is broken down or converted by a number of mechanisms: 1) dopamine-β-hydroxylase converts dopamine into norepinephrine, 2) monoamine oxidase (MAO) converts dopamine into 3,4-dihydroxyphenylacetic acid (DOPAC), and 3) catechol-*o*-methyltransferase (COMT) catalyzes the formation of homovanillic acid (HVA). Dopamine-β -hydroxylase only exists in norepinephrine neurons and thus will not be a focus here; however, MAO exists on the outer mitochondrial membrane and is also thought to be in abundance extracellularly, and COMT is mostly present extracellularly and plays a major role in regu-

http://dx.doi.org/10.5772/54207

lating dopamine neurotransmission, especially in the PFC [11]. The final and most important method in which dopamine is cleared from the synapse is via the dopamine transporter (DAT). The DAT primarily exists on the presynaptic neuron and can transport dopamine either into or out of the neuron, dependent upon the concentration gradient. It has been discovered that the removal of dopamine from the synapse is predominantly performed by the DAT and not metabolism or diffusion [12].

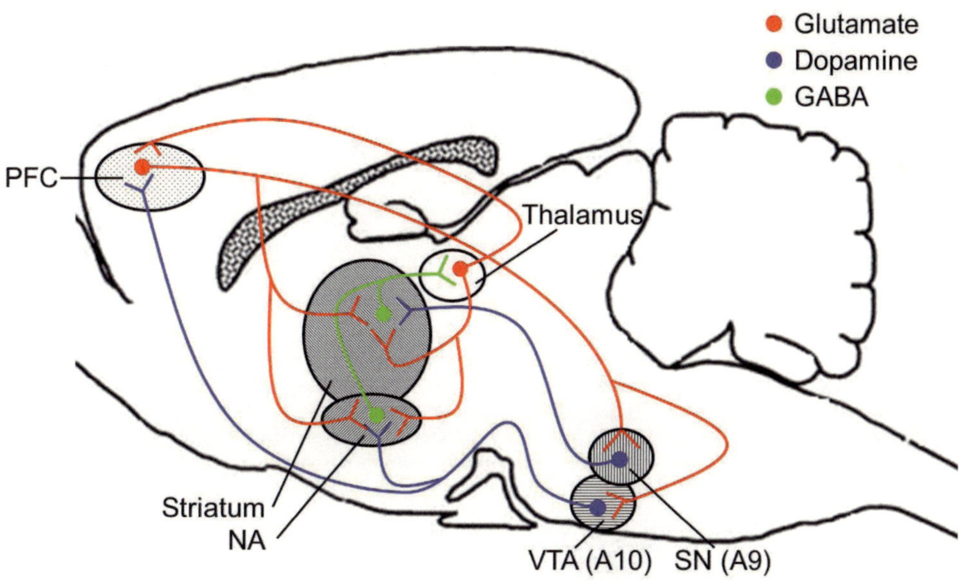

Figure 1. Modulatory dopaminergic neurons (blue) project to the dorsal striatum via the substantia nigra (SN, A9) and the ventral striatum and prefrontal cortex (PFC) via the ventral tegmental area (VTA, A10) in the rodent brain. From the striatum, inhibitory GABA neurons (green) extend to multiple regions including the thalamus, which has reciprocal excitatory glutamate connections (red) to the striatum, as well as connections to the PFC. Prefrontal cortical efferent excitatory glutamate neurons extend to the striatum, nucleus accumbens (NA), SN, as well as the VTA.

Intracellularly, dopamine is packaged into vesicles via the vesicular monoamine transporter (VMAT-2). The release of dopamine from the vesicle is Ca^{2+} and Na^{+} dependent and occurs when an action potential raises the Ca^{2+} levels in the presynaptic neuron, causing vesicles stored with dopamine to bind to the cellular membrane and release their contents. The resulting synaptic dopamine is then able to bind to dopamine receptors on both the pre- and postsynaptic neurons. These receptors are classified into two major categories: 1) D_1-type receptors, consisting of D_1 and D_5 and expressed postsynaptically, and 2) D_2-type receptors expressed both pre- and postsynaptically, consisting of D_2 (short), D_2 (long), D_3 and D_4. Stimulation of D_1-type receptors causes increased cAMP production (activating), whereas stimulation of D_2-type receptors causes inhibition of cAMP production (inhibiting). The effects of these receptors give dopamine the classification of a modulatory neurotransmitter. For a simplified PFC dopamine synapse diagram, see Figure 2.

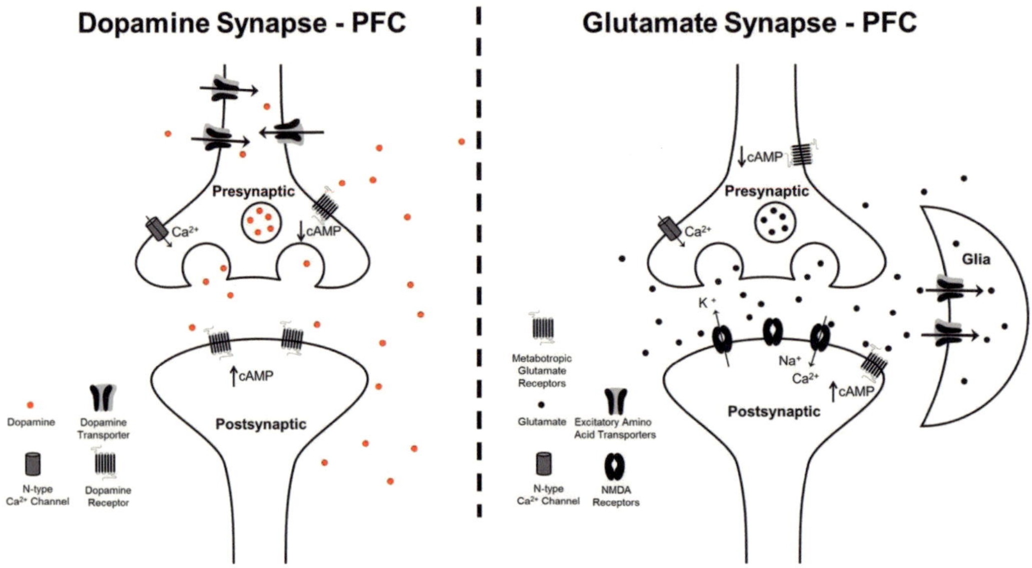

Figure 2. Dopaminergic and glutamatergic synapses in the PFC, simplified. Left: pre-synaptically, dopamine is transported into vesicles, which release their contents upon increase of the Ca^{2+} concentration. Synaptic dopamine is then able to stimulate dopamine receptors on both the pre- and postsynaptic neurons before it is cleared by the DAT or metabolism. Right: presynaptically, glutamate is stored in vesicles and then released into the extracellular space. Synaptic glutamate is then able to stimulate glutamate receptors (here represented as the NMDA and mGluR) on both the pre- and postsynaptic neurons before it is cleared by the EAAT located on nearby glial cells.

2.2. Glutamate

Recent clinical evidence has implicated glutamate in ADHD. Much of the initial evidence stems from proton magnetic resonance spectroscopy studies of children and adults with ADHD. These studies have shown increased levels of a marker for glutamate in the striatum and anterior cingulate cortex of the PFC [13-15]. Based on this evidence, new investigations into glutamatergic function in ADHD are ongoing. Glutamate is the major excitatory neurotransmitter in the central nervous system and must be tightly regulated for proper neuronal signaling to occur [16]. Unlike dopamine, glutamate is in abundance in most areas of the brain. Glutamate projections originating in the PFC extend to the striatum, NA, VTA and SN of the midbrain (see Figure 1). Glutamate is produced in the nerve terminals of these projections from two sources: 1) the Krebs cycle and 2) glutamine produced and excreted into the extracellular space via glial cells. Once produced, glutamate is transported into vesicles via the vesicular glutamate transporter (VGLUT) and when Ca^{2+} levels increase to cause an action potential, vesicles stored with glutamate bind to the cellular membrane and release their contents. Clearance of glutamate after this calcium-dependent release into the extracellular space is primarily performed by the membrane-bound glutamate transporter, called the excitatory amino acid transporter (EAAT), located on the presynaptic neuron and to the greatest extent by surrounding glial cells. The glutamate is primarily taken up by the EAATs located on the glial cells and is converted by glutamine synthetase into glutamine and transported out of the glial cell by system N transporter. The glutamine is then taken up by the system A transporter on the presynaptic neuron to help replenish glutamate levels through the mitochondrial bound glutaminase [11]. Glutamate acts on synaptic glutamate receptors in the target brain region, which are classified into two major types: 1) ionotropic, which include the NMDA, AMPA and kainate receptors and 2) metabotropic, including the excitatory mGluRs 1 and 5 (postsynaptic) and the inhibitory mGluRs 2, 3, 4, 6, 7, and 8 (presynaptic). For a simplified PFC glutamate synapse diagram, see Figure 2.

2.3. Dopamine and glutamate interactions

A dysfunctional interaction between the dopamine and glutamate systems has been implicated in numerous neuropsychiatric disorders such as drug addiction, Alzheimer's disease, schizophrenia, and ADHD. The brain regions most often linked to these disorders and the dopamine-glutamate dysfunction are the PFC and striatum, as these regions both receive heavy innervation from the dopaminergic SN/VTA and glutamate innervation from thalamic relays and other glutamate rich regions, as described in the previous section.

Studies of signaling interactions between the dopaminergic and glutamatergic systems demonstrate that the NMDA receptor is crucial in activating dopamine neurons in the VTA/SN [17, 18]. Also, it has been found that stimulation of the D_2-class dopamine receptor is involved in the downstream inhibition of the NMDA receptor, weakening the excitatory response to those neurons [19]. Likewise, it was found that activation of D_4 receptors depressed AMPA receptor-mediated excitatory synaptic transmission in PFC pyramidal neurons, which was accompanied by a D_4-induced decrease of AMPA receptors at the synapse [20]. These results provide substantial evidence that the dopamine and glutamate neuronal systems work in tandem to create a balance of neurotransmission in these regions.

The hypodopaminergic theory of ADHD asserts that the hyperactive and inattentive behaviors are caused by low levels of either tonic or phasic dopamine. If true, decreased dopamine released in the striatum and PFC would then be expected to lead to more active NMDA and AMPA receptors based on the studies mentioned above resulting in increased glutamatergic output to the striatum and SN/VTA, as well as an increased glutamate signal to the PFC. Glutamate coming into the SN/VTA would normally go on to release more dopamine [17]; however, in the ADHD brain, this feedback does not seem to occur.

2.4. Translational neuropharmacology of ADHD treatments

Investigations into the effects of stimulant action on the dopaminergic system have revealed that these medications increase extracellular dopamine levels via numerous mechanisms. First, amphetamine has been found to increase dopamine through calcium-independent mechanisms such as increased release of dopamine and blocking the reuptake of dopamine through the DAT [21, 22]. Methylphenidate (MPH), another stimulant medication commonly used to treat ADHD, increases dopamine levels by inhibiting dopamine reuptake via the DAT [23-29].

The non-stimulant medication atomoxetine (ATX) is becoming increasingly popular as a treatment for ADHD compared to the stimulant medications because it has lower abuse liability. ATX has been found to increase levels of the catecholamines by selectively blocking the norepinephrine transporter (NET), which is also able to clear dopamine [30-32] and, like stimulants, is effective at lessoning the intensity of ADHD symptoms [33-36]. *In vitro* work has shown that ATX acts as an NMDA receptor antagonist [37], providing preliminary evidence that current treatments for ADHD may have a direct effect on the glutamatergic system.

Using magnetic resonance spectroscopy, it was found that children treated with ATX, but not MPH, had decreased levels of a marker for glutamate/glutamine in the PFC, though MPH was able to decrease glutamate in the anterior cingulate cortex [38]. In the striatum, both ATX and MPH decreased the glutamate/glutamine marker levels compared to controls [13]. These results suggest that ATX may be regulating and activating prefrontal cortex neurons. However, another clinical study using a similar technique found that chronic long-acting MPH decreased glutamate levels in the PFC of children with ADHD [39]. Wiguna et al. (2012) also discovered that MPH treatment resulted in an increase in the amount of and functional state of the neurons in the PFC, supporting that the current ADHD stimulant treatment MPH can activate PFC neurons as well. Further evidence of PFC activation comes from a study of brain-derived neurotropic factor (BDNF), a marker for neuronal plasticity. ATX was found to increase BDNF expression in the PFC; however, MPH had the opposite effect and reduced BDNF expression in the PFC [40], though it must be noted that this study was completed in naïve rodents and may explain why these results do not match those seen in ADHD patients.

Many second-line and experimental treatments for ADHD are now targeting both the dopamine and glutamate systems. Memantine is an uncompetitive NMDA receptor antagonist [41] and has also been found to act as a D_2 receptor agonist [42]. It has been approved and used as a treatment for Alzheimer's disease; however, in an 8 week open-label pilot study in children with ADHD, memantine was found to improve ADHD symptoms (Findling et al, 2007). Surman et al. (2011) extended these findings to adults with ADHD in a separate open-label study lasting 12 weeks and found similar results, with memantine improving ADHD symptoms and neuropsychological performance [43]. The MAO-B inhibitor (deprenyl), which stops the degradation of dopamine and is used as a treatment in Parkinson's disease, was found to alleviate ADHD symptoms [44, 45]. These clinical data using glutamate and dopamine altering drugs provide strong links for dysfunctional dopamine-glutamate interactions in ADHD, though the importance of this dysfunction is still unknown. Based on these data, we believe it's important to not overlook the possible role of dysfunctional dopamine-glutamate interactions, but to instead focus on this relationship. Animal models of ADHD provide a unique opportunity to investigate neurotransmitter system dysfunction as well as to develop novel ways to treat ADHD targeting these systems. We will next highlight two separate models of ADHD and how they are implicating both dopamine and glutamate dysfunction in ADHD.

2.5. Animal models of ADHD: Hypotheses

The spontaneously hypertensive rat

The spontaneously hypertensive rat (SHR) has been used as an animal model for ADHD combined type since the 1970's because of its sustained attention deficits [46], motor impulsiveness [47-49], and hyperactivity [46] with the hyperactivity absent in novel situations [50]. Currently, there exists conflicting data on dopamine release and uptake levels in the brain areas thought to be involved in the pathophysiology of ADHD, including the PFC [51]. Our lab has previously reported enhanced dopamine uptake in the ventral striatum and nucleus accumbens core of the SHR [52]; however, investigations into PFC dopamine regulation are still not clear. The PFC of the SHR has been reported to have decreased dopamine uptake [53], yet a study found no differences in the levels of DAT, tyrosine hydroxylase, D_1, D_2, D_3, D_5 receptors, and dopamine-β-hydroxylase between the SHR and its progenitor strain, the Wistar Kyoto (WKY), in the PFC. Regional differences in the D_4 receptors in the PFC were found, providing evidence that the SHR's D_4 levels are lower than those of the WKY [54]. Further, it was found that PFC AMPA receptor activity was increased in the SHR [55] and inhibitory dopaminergic activity was found to be decreased while noradrenergic activity increased in the SHR [56]. These findings all convey a message that dopamine regulation is dysfunctional in the PFC of the SHR model of ADHD; however, direct observation of in vivo dopamine dynamics in the separate PFC sub-regions (cingulate, prelimbic, and infralimbic) of the SHR have not yet been accurately defined.

The dopamine receptor D4 knockout mouse

The correlation between ADHD and the 7-repeat polymorphism in the dopamine D4 receptor (DRD4.7) is supported by neuroanatomical, neurochemical, molecular genetics and pharmacological studies [57-60]. Recently, the DRD4.7 was identified as having the most significant genetic relationship to ADHD in pooled family and case-controlled studies [61]. Clinical studies in adolescents report that ADHD patients with the DRD4.7 have thinner frontal cortical structures in comparison to age matched controls [62]. The highest concentration of DRD4s is in the frontal cortex, an area implicated in the pathophysiology of ADHD using neuroimaging and neuropsychological evaluation of ADHD patients [63-66]. There is evidence that changes in DRD4 expression can affect glutamate levels in the striatum of $DRD4^{-/-}$ mice [67]. Previous studies show that $DRD4^{-/-}$ mice are supersensitive to ethanol, cocaine and methamphetamine [68]; have enhanced reactivity to unconditioned fear [69]; reduced exploration of novel stimuli [70]; and hypersensitivity to amphetamine [71]. In the cortex, hyperexcitability has been demonstrated in $DRD4^{-/-}$ mice using immunohistochemical, electrophysiological, pharmacological and ultrastructural methods, indicating that DRD4 activation has an inhibitory influence on glutamate neurons in the frontal cortex [72]. At this time, no direct studies of in vivo glutamate have been investigated in the intact PFC of the $DRD4^{-/-}$ mouse. Therefore, *in vivo* measures of glutamatergic modulation in the PFC may correlate changes in glutamate neurotransmission to the expression levels of the DRD4 and understanding the physiological role of the DRD4 may elucidate the importance of dopamine and glutamate interactions in the PFC.

Measuring neurotransmitters in these rodent models of ADHD

Recent studies point to the importance of a dysfunctional relationship between dopaminergic and glutamatergic neurotransmission in ADHD, therefore new investigations into this relationship are necessary to improve our understanding and may lead to improved therapeutics for ADHD. Based on our development of novel and revolutionary methods of measuring dopamine and glutamate in vivo, we realize we are in a unique position to test our hypotheses that dopamine and glutamate regulation play a major role in the pathophysiology of ADHD. The development of carbon fiber microelectrodes and glutamate oxidase-coated microelectrode arrays (MEAs) provide improved spatial resolution, sub-second temporal resolution, and low limits of detection (<10 nM for dopamine [52], <0.2 μM for glutamate [73]) over conventional techniques used in the past, such as microdialysis. The smaller size of these probes and decreased damage to tissue compared to microdialysis probes allows for the *in vivo* characterization of dopamine and glutamate signaling closer to the synapse. Using these technologies, we were able to explore if dysfunction in dopamine and glutamate neurotransmission occur in the PFC of the SHR and DRD4 models of ADHD. The studies described here could potentially lead to the development of novel therapies for ADHD, which will be discussed in detail later.

2.6. Neurotransmitter recording techniques: Methods

High-speed chronoamperometric recordings of dopamine release and uptake in the PFC of the SHR

Male, 8-10 weeks old, inbred spontaneously hypertensive rats (SHR, average 225 g, average PND 60), inbred Wistar Kyoto rats (WKY, average 210 g, average PND 61), and outbred Sprague Dawley rats (SD, average 289 g, average PND 69) were obtained from Charles River Laboratories (NCrl), Wilmington, Massachusetts. Animals were given access to food and water ad libitum and housed in a 12 hour light/dark cycle. Protocols for animal use were approved by the Institutional Animal Care and Use Committee, which is Association for Assessment and Accreditation of Laboratory Animal Care International approved. All procedures were carried out in accordance with the National Institutes of Health Guide for Care and Use of Laboratory Animals and all efforts were made to minimize animal suffering and to reduce the number of animals used.

High-speed chronoamperometric measurements (1 Hz sampling rate, 200 ms total) were performed using the FAST16mkII recording system (Fast Analytical Sensing Technology, Quanteon, LLC, Nicholasville, Kentucky) as previously described [52, 74]. Single carbon fiber electrodes (SF1A; 30 μm outer diameter × 150 μm length; Quanteon, LLC, Nicholasville, Kentucky) were coated with Nafion® (5% solution, 1–3 coats at 180°C, Aldrich Chemical Co., Milwaukee, Wisconsin) prior to an in vitro calibration used to determine selectivity, limit of detection, and sensitivity before use in vivo: average selectivity for all microelectrodes used in these experiments was 1877 ± 664 μM for dopamine vs. ascorbic acid; average limit of detection for the measurement of dopamine was 0.028 ± 0.008 μM (S/N of 3); average slope for the electrodes was -0.492 ± 0.111 nA/μM dopamine. After calibration, miniature Ag/AgCl reference electrodes were prepared as previously described [74]. The carbon fiber microelec-

http://dx.doi.org/10.5772/54207

trode was affixed to a micropipette (10 μm inner diameter) which was positioned approximately 200 μm from the carbon fiber electrode tip using sticky wax (Kerr USA, Romulus, Michigan).

Rats were anesthetized intraperitonealy (i.p.) using a 25% urethane solution (1.25 g/kg) and placed in a stereotaxic frame (David Kopf Instruments, Tujunga, California). A circulating heating pad (Gaymar Industries, Inc., Orchard Park, New York) was used to maintain body temperature. The skull was removed bilaterally for recordings in the PFC (AP +3.2, ML ±1.0, DV -2 to -6 in 0.5 mm increments) [75]. A small hole remote from the site of surgery was drilled for placement of the miniature Ag/AgCl reference electrode. Prior to experimentation, the micropipette was filled with filtered isotonic KCl (120 mM KCl, 29 mM NaCl, 2.5 mM $CaCl_2 \bullet 2H_2O$) solution (pH 7.2-7.4) using a 4 inch filling needle (Cadence Inc., Staunton, Virginia) and a 5 ml syringe. Experiments were then initiated with the insertion of the micropipette/microelectrode assembly into a stereotactically selected region of the left or right hemisphere's PFC. After a 30-45 minute baseline, the effect of a single local application of KCl on dopamine release was determined [52]. The KCl solution was locally applied by pressure ejection (5–25 psi for 0.5 seconds) and the single application of a set volume of KCl (75–125 nl) was delivered to each sub-region, measured by determining the amount of fluid ejected from the micropipette using a dissection microscope fitted with an eyepiece reticule that was calibrated so that 1 mm of movement was equivalent to 25 nl of fluid ejected [76, 77]. If the volume was determined to be greater or less than 75-100 nl, then that data point was excluded. After the KCl studies, the micropipette/microelectrode assembly was filled with filtered isotonic 200 μM dopamine solution containing 100 μM ascorbic acid (an antioxidant) in 0.9% saline (pH 7.2-7.4). The micropipette/microelectrode assembly was inserted stereotactically into the animal's contralateral PFC. Again, a stable baseline was achieved before the dopamine solution was locally applied by pressure ejection (10-30 psi for 0.5-10 s) to achieve a maximum amplitude between the range of 0.5 to 1 μM dopamine. The maximum concentration of the dopamine in the extracellular space was measured by subtracting the apex of the recorded peak from the baseline recorded prior to the ejection. If the peak amplitude was greater or less than 0.5 to 1 μM dopamine, then that data point was excluded. Brains were removed and processed (frozen) for histological evaluation of microelectrode recording tracks. Only data from histologically confirmed placements of microelectrodes into the PFC were used for final data analysis. Based on histological analyses, no animals were excluded due to microelectrode placement errors.

Collected data were processed using a custom Matlab®-based analysis package. For KCl-evoked DA release, maximum amplitude of the evoked dopamine peak was used. The volume of KCl applied was kept constant across depths and strains (75–125 nl). For dopamine uptake the time to 80% decay of the dopamine signal (T80) was examined. dopamine signals were amplitude matched (ranging from 0.5 to 1 μM dopamine) to ensure accurate measurement of dopamine uptake kinetics [52, 74]. Outliers were excluded via the Grubb's test before averaging if the conditions for homogeneity of variance were met. To compare dopamine dynamics in the separate PFC subregions, one-way ANOVAs followed by Bonferroni post-hoc comparisons were used. Significance was set at $p<0.05$ (GraphPad Prism 5.0).

Urethane, dopamine, ascorbic acid, sodium chloride, potassium chloride, calcium chloride and Nafion® were obtained from Sigma (St. Louis, MO). Carbon fiber microelectrodes (SF1A's) were fabricated by the Center for Microelectrode Technology.

High-speed amperometric recordings of glutamate levels in the PFC of the DRD4 knock-out mouse

Male mice (5-7 months; ~32 g) descended from the original F2 hybrid of mice with a truncated and non-expressing DRD4 gene ($DRD4^{-/-}$; 129/SvEv × C57BL/6J) were derived by back-crossing the $DRD4^{+/-}$ mouse line for 20 generations [68]. In all experiments, the $DRD4^{-/-}$ mice (n=5-8) and $DRD4^{+/-}$ (n=5-9) were compared to litter-matched $DRD4^{+/+}$ (n=5-8) animals. Mice were group-housed (2-4 per cage) with unlimited access to food and water. Mice were maintained on a twelve hour light/dark cycle. Protocols for animal use were approved by the Institutional Animal Care and Use Committee (IACUC), which is Association for Assessment and Accreditation of Laboratory Animal Care International approved, and all procedures were carried out in accordance with the National Institutes of Health Guide for Care and Use of Laboratory Animals.

Ceramic-based microelectrode arrays (MEA) that contained 4 platinum (Pt) recording surfaces (sites 1-4) in an S2 configuration (two sets of side-by-side recording sites) were prepared to selectively measure glutamate. The electrodes were fabricated for in vivo recordings using published methods [73, 78, 79]. All 4 sites were electroplated with meta-phenylene diamine (mPD) by applying a potential of +0.5 V to the Pt sites vs. a silver/silver chloride (Ag/AgCl) reference electrode (Bioanalytical Systems, RE-5) in a deoxygenated 0.05 M phosphate buffered saline (PBS; pH 7.1-7.4) with 5 mM mPD. The mPD forms a size-exclusion layer over the sites, blocking dopamine, ascorbic acid (AA), DOPAC, and other electroactive compounds. Pt sites 1 and 2 were coated with glutamate oxidase (Glu-Ox) within an inert protein matrix of bovine serum albumin (BSA) and gluteraldehyde, enabling these sites to detect glutamate levels on a sub-second timescale with low levels of detection (0.2 μM). Sites 3 and 4 were coated with only BSA and gluteraldehyde [80, 81]. In the presence of Glu-Ox, glutamate is broken down into α-ketoglutarate and peroxide (H_2O_2). The H_2O_2 is small enough to traverse the mPD layer and is readily oxidized and recorded as current using the FAST-16 equipment (Fast Analytical Sensor Technology (FAST); Quanteon L.L.C., Nicholasville, KY). For calibration details, see [73, 78]. From the calibration, average values for slope were -7.7 ± 4.8 pA/μM, selectivity 214 ± 64 to 1 and LOD 0.59 ± 0.06 μM (n=26 electrodes; 51 glutamate recording sites). After the MEA was calibrated; a single barrel glass capillary with filament (1.0 x 0.58 mm^2, 6", A-M Systems, Inc., Everett, WA) was pulled using a Kopf Pipette Puller (David Kopf Instruments, Tujunga, CA) and bumped against a glass rod so that the inner diameter of the micropipette was 10-12 μm. The tip of the micropipette was placed between the 4 Pt recording sites, approximately 50-80 μm away from the electrode surface and secured using Sticky Wax (Kerr Manufacturing Co, Detroit, Michigan).

Mice were anesthetized using i.p. injections of 10% urethane solution (1.25 g/kg) and placed in a stereotaxic frame (David Kopf Instruments, Tujunga, CA) fitted with a Cunningham™ Mouse and Neonatal Rat Adaptor (Stoelting Co., Wood Dale, IL). A circulating heating pad (Gaymar Industries, Inc., Orchard Park, NY) was used to maintain body temperature. The

http://dx.doi.org/10.5772/54207

skull overlying the PFC was removed bilaterally. The MEA–micropipette assembly was positioned in the brain according to the following stereotaxic coordinates where all anterior-posterior (AP) measures were from bregma, medial-lateral (ML) measures were from mid-line and dorsal-ventral (DV) measures were from dura: AP: +2 mm, ML: ±1 mm, DV: -1.8 to 2.6 mm at an angle of 8 degrees according to the atlas of The Mouse Brain in Stereotaxic Co-ordinates [82]. An additional hole, remote from the surgery site, was opened for a Ag/AgCl reference electrode. Prior to placement of the MEA-pipette assembly, the micropipette was filled with isotonic 125 μM glutamate (125 μM L-glutamate in 0.9% physiological saline; pH= 7.2-7.4) using a combination of a 1 ml syringe filled with glutamate solution, a 0.22 μm sterile syringe filter (Costar Corporation), and a 4" stainless steel pulled needle (30 gauge, beveled tip; Popper and Son, Inc., NY). A potential of +0.7 V was applied versus a miniature Ag/AgCl reference electrode and the data were displayed at a frequency of 2 Hz. Upon ster-eotaxic placement of the MEA-micropipette assembly, 10-20 minutes of baseline data were acquired. Extracellular levels of glutamate were measured by averaging 30 seconds of base-line recordings prior to application of glutamate or KCl. Then, a 125 μM glutamate solution was locally applied via pressure ejection using a Picospritzer II connected to the open end of the micropipette by plastic tubing (Parker Hannifin Corp., General Valve Corporation). Pressure was applied at 5-25 psi for 1 second in all of the experiments. Glutamate was ap-plied every 30-60 seconds for a total of 10 recordings. The MEA was then lowered in 350 μm increments. Baseline recordings were acquired for 5-10 minutes and the recordings were re-peated. Parameters from three of the ten signals ranging from 10-30 μM in amplitude were averaged for each Pt electrode site at each depth. Signals were analyzed for time required to rise to maximum amplitude (rise time), time for 80% of the signal to decay from maximum amplitude (T80), and the rate of uptake. The uptake rate was calculated by multiplying the first order rate constant (k^{-1}, seconds^{-1}) by the maximum amplitude (uptake rate = μM/s) [81]. All data from local applications of glutamate from a given site were pooled into a single point. Amplitude-matched signals were compared to assess genotypic differences in the rates of clearance of exogenous glutamate [83]. Brains were removed and processed for his-tological evaluation of microelectrode recording tracts. Only data from histologically con-firmed placements of microelectrodes within the PFC were used for final data analysis.

Data from the side-by-side recordings were averaged and used as a single data point. If only one microelectrode site provided usable data, then the recordings were reported as from that site. Very few data points were omitted in this study due to outlier status, with excep-tion for constraints on amplitude-matching. To determine statistical significance ($p<0.05$), processed data were analyzed using a one-way ANOVA with Tukey's post-hoc compari-sons across all genotypes (Graphpad Prism 4.0). Urethane, L-glutamate, dopamine, ascorbic acid, and 1,3-phenylenediamine dihydrochloride were obtained from Sigma-Alderich, St. Louis MO). Microelectrode arrays were provided by Quanteon L.L.C. (Nicholasville, KY).

2.7. Dopamine dysfunction in the PFC of the SHR model of ADHD: Results

High-speed chronoamperometry coupled with carbon fiber microelectrodes was used to evaluate KCl-evoked dopamine release because of its capability to record dopamine release within sub-regions of the striatum and the NA [52, 74] using a local application of 75-125 nl KCl in 500 μm increments. To examine potential differences in evoked dopamine release in the separate sub-regions of the PFC between the outbred SD, the WKY progenitor, and the SHR model of ADHD, one-way ANOVAs were used. No significant differences were found between strains (cingulate cortex, p=0.1295; prelimbic cortex, p=0.1998; infralimbic cortex, p=0.1050). These data suggests that the cingulate, prelimbic and infralimbic regions in all three strains have a similar capacity to release dopamine during an action potential event. It's important to note that in both the SD and SHR strains, dopamine peak amplitudes increased as the microelectrode was moved ventrally; however, the WKY strain displayed the opposite effect. See Figure 3. Note that all dopamine signals were indicative of the detection of dopamine and/or norepinephrine based on the reduction/oxidation rations of the signals that averaged ~0.8-1.0 for all recordings.

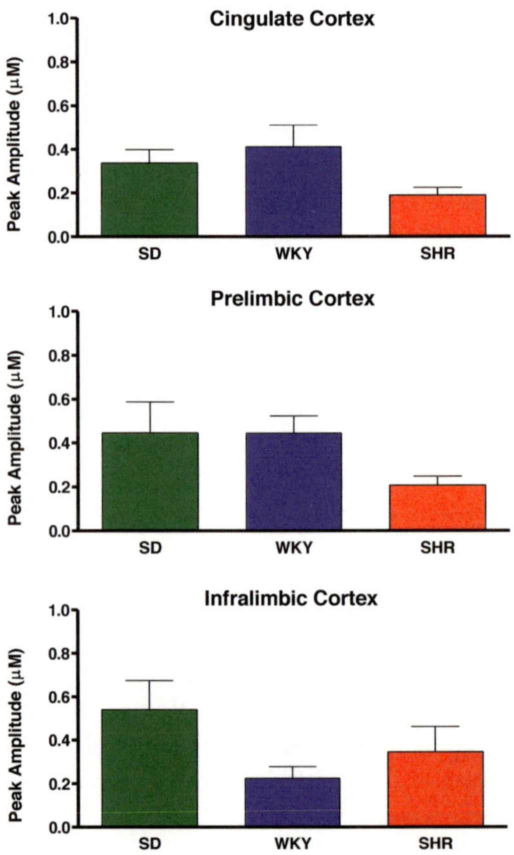

Figure 3. No differences were observed between the outbred SD control strain, the WKY progenitor strain, and the SHR model of ADHD in the KCl-evoked dopamine peak amplitudes following a local application of KCl in any of the prefrontal cortical sub-regions. Values represent the mean ± SEM.

http://dx.doi.org/10.5772/54207

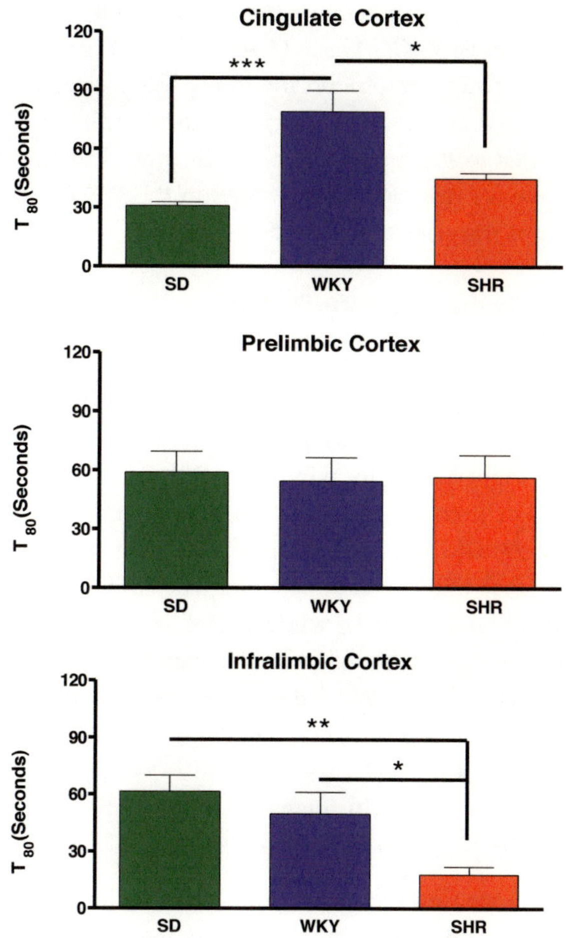

Figure 4. The SHR model of ADHD and the outbred SD control strain exhibited significantly faster dopamine uptake than the WKY strain in the cingulate cortex (*p<0.05, ***p<0.001). No dopamine uptake differences were observed in the prelimbic cortex; however, the SHR exhibited significantly faster dopamine uptake in the infralimbic cortex compared to both the SD control and WKY strain (*p<0.05, **p<0.01). Values represent the mean ± SEM.

To examine differences in dopamine uptake in the separate prefrontal cortical sub-regions, we used local applications of dopamine to directly observe the functional properties of the dopamine and norepinephrine transporters. One-way ANOVAs followed by Bonferroni post-hoc comparisons were used in each sub-region. It was discovered that the SHR model of ADHD (p<0.05) and the outbred SD control strain (p<0.001) displayed significantly faster dopamine uptake compared to the WKY strain in the cingulate cortex ($F_{(2,23)}$=11.11). The average dopamine uptake times in the cingulate cortex were: SD, 30.8 ± 2 seconds; WKY, 79.1 ± 10 seconds; and SHR, 44.8 ± 3 seconds. No dopamine uptake differences were observed in the prelimbic cortex (p=0.9605); however, the SHR exhibited significantly faster dopamine uptake compared to both the SD control ($p<0.01$) and the WKY strain ($p<0.05$) in the infralimbic cortex ($F_{(2,28)}=6.53$). The average dopamine uptake times in the infralimbic cortex were: SD, 61.6 ± 8 seconds; WKY, 49.8 ± 11 seconds; and SHR, 18 ± 4 seconds. These data reveal that the dopamine and norepinephrine transporters clear dopamine faster in the SHR in the cingulate and infralimbic cortices compared to control, but not the prelimbic cortex. It's important to note that as the microelectrode was moved ventrally in the control SD strain, the dopamine uptake became slower; however, in the WKY and SHR strains, dopamine uptake became faster as the electrode moved ventrally.

2.8. Glutamate dysfunction in the PFC of the DRD4-/- mouse model of ADHD: Results

In order to evaluate the effect of DRD4s on extracellular levels of glutamate, we compared extracellular glutamate levels across genotypes in the PFC. Extracellular resting levels of glutamate were higher by approximately 73% in the PFC of $DRD4^{-/-}$ mice in comparison to their $DRD4^{+/+}$ littermates ($DRD4^{+/+}$: 1.4 ± 0.2 μM, n=8, signals=22; $DRD4^{+/-}$: 1.9 ± 0.3 μM, n=8, signals=23; $DRD4^{-/-}$: 2.5 ± 0.3 μM, n=8, signals=24; $p<0.05$, see Figure 5). A depth analysis showed that $DRD4^{+/+}$ mice maintained similar extracellular resting glutamate levels across depths (1.4 ± 0.3 μM), while $DRD4^{-/-}$ mice tended to have higher levels throughout all areas. The most profound difference was the stepwise increase in extracellular glutamate levels in the cingulate cortex with a significant difference observed between the $DRD4^{+/+}$ and $DRD4^{-/-}$ mice ($DRD4^{+/+}$: 1.4 ± 0.3 μM, n=8; $DRD4^{+/-}$: 2.0 ± 0.6 μM, n=7 ; $DRD4^{-/-}$: 3.0 ± 0.7 μM, n=8; Student's t-test: $p<0.05$; see Figure 5) These data indicate that the loss of DRD4s results in increased extracellular resting glutamate levels in the PFC, most dramatically in the cingulate cortex.

The *in vivo* activity of glutamate uptake was examined with a high degree of temporal and spatial resolution by locally applying exogenous glutamate to the extracellular space of the brain and measuring the presence and successive clearance kinetics. Resulting data provided kinetic measures that allowed us to evaluate the efficiency of exogenous glutamate removal from the extracellular space within the 3 different brain areas of the medial PFC. Statistical comparisons were made on amplitude-matched data in order to make sure that variations in maximum amplitude would not contribute to changes in rise time, uptake rate and T80. Average maximum amplitudes were 15.39 ± 1.30 μM (n=8; signals= 21), 13.62 ± 0.78 μM (n=9; signals =25) and 13.93 ± 0.91 μM (n=8; signals = 21) in the $DRD4^{+/+}$, $DRD4^{+/-}$ and $DRD4^{-/-}$, respectively. Uptake rates within the PFC were similar across genotypes ($DRD4^{+/+}$: 4.85 ± 0.69 μM, n=8; $DRD4^{+/-}$: 4.82 ± 0.46 μM, n=9; $DRD4^{-/-}$: 5.28 ± 0.74 μM, n=8; see Figure 6). The time it took for 80% of the signal to decay (T80) was significantly longer in $DRD4^{-/-}$ mice than wildtype ($DRD4^{+/+}$: 2.50 ± 0.16 μM, n=8; $DRD4^{+/-}$: 2.84 ± 0.12 μM, n=9; $DRD4^{-/-}$: 3.00 ± 0.14 μM, n=8; $p<0.05$) with the most profound changes occurring in the prelimbic area ($p<0.05$). These kinetic measures of glutamate clearance in the PFC indicate that the DRD4 may play an important role in glutamate clearance.

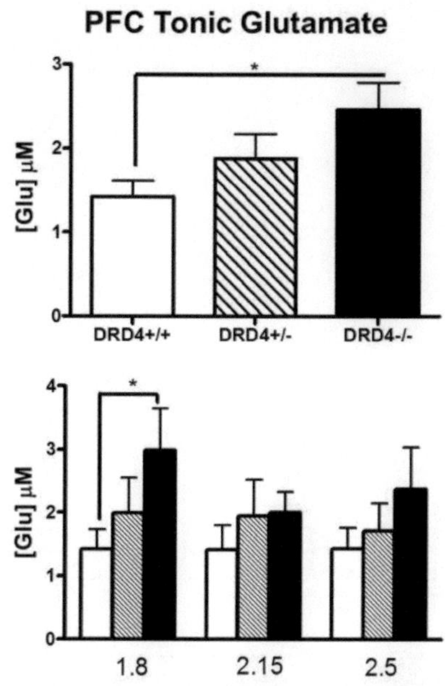

Figure 5. Extracellular resting levels of glutamate in the PFC. The top bar graph shows increased extracellular levels of glutamate in the PFC of DRD4$^{-/-}$ in comparison to DRD4$^{+/+}$ mice (*p<0.05). The bottom graph depicts extracellular resting glutamate levels broken down by depth in the PFC. The numbers on the x-axis represent the depth of the microelectrode (1.8, 2.15 and 2.5 mm) and indicate the cingulate cortex, the prelimbic area and the infralimbic area; respectively. Values represent the mean ± SEM.

2.9. Implications of dysfunctional neurotransmitter systems

The SHR and dopaminergic PFC dysfunction

Based on current stimulant treatments for ADHD that target the dopaminergic system, such as MPH, the hypofunctional catecholamine theory has evolved and states that behaviors seen with ADHD are caused by decreased levels of catecholamines in the brain regions associated with attention and reward processing [84] including the striatum and PFC. In the spontaneously hypertensive rat (SHR) model of ADHD, there have been conflicting reports of dopamine levels in the striatum and PFC; however, the techniques used varied with each study. Some studies revealed a hypodopaminergic tone [85, 86], while others found no difference in dopamine levels [87, 88]. Microdialysis measures of dopamine levels in the SHR are at most unreliable and poorly reflect concentrations of dopamine near the synapse due to the limited spatial resolution (>1 mm), slow sampling rates (1-20 min), and significant damage to the surrounding tissue [89-91]. Based on this premise, it is necessary that a technique with increased spatial and temporal resolution over microdialysis, such as carbon fiber microelectrodes coupled to high-speed chronoamperometric recordings, be used to measure dopamine dynamics in this popular animal model [92].

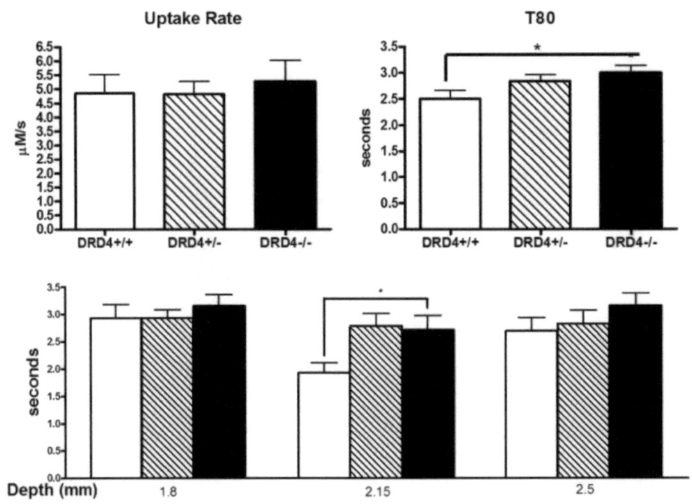

Figure 6. Glutamate clearance in the PFC. The top bar graphs represent changes in glutamate clearance in the PFC as a function of DRD4 expression for amplitude-matched signals. The T80 is significantly longer in DRD4$^{-/-}$ mice in comparison to DRD4$^{+/+}$ (*p<0.05). A depth profile of the T80 values (bottom) indicate that the most significant difference was in the prelimbic area of the PFC (2.15 mm) in the DRD4$^{-/-}$. Values represent the mean ± SEM.

Recent data from our lab using carbon fiber microelectrodes with high-speed chronoamperometry have shown decreased potassium-evoked dopamine signals in the dorsal striatum of the SHR model of ADHD compared to the WKY, as well as faster dopamine uptake in the ventral striatum and NA core in the SHR compared to both the SD and WKY controls [52]. Previous investigations have implicated the dopamine transporter (DAT) in the dopamine dysfunction of the SHR model of ADHD [93-98] and our data revealing differences in dopamine regulation in the striatum can be attributed to increased activity of the DAT in the striatum of the SHR. It is reasonable to assume that if the striatum has increased DAT activity, it's likely that similar dopamine dysfunction exists in the PFC of the SHR. It's important to clarify that the norepinephrine transporter (NET) is present in certain regions of the PFC in much greater concentrations than the DAT and dopamine uptake in the PFC is thought to be preferentially due to the NET instead of the DAT [99], so investigations into the mechanism of dopamine clearance in the PFC of the SHR should be examined in the future.

Using similar volumes of a potassium solution, evoked overflow of catecholamine nerve terminals surrounding the tip of the carbon fiber microeletrode was used to attempt to locate differences in vesicular dopamine storage in the different PFC sub-regions. Upon stimulation, no differences were observed between the inbred SHR model of ADHD, the inbred progenitor WKY and the outbred SD control strains. The lack of differences signifies to us that the separate PFC sub-regions all have the same capacity to store and release dopamine and/or norepinephrine in these strains. MAO and VMAT, both implicated in ADHD, can then be considered to be functional in the PFC of the SHR model of ADHD and drugs targeting these proteins, such as deprenyl, may not be useful in this model.

Though no differences were observed in the KCl-evoked dopamine signals, there were significant differences in the length of time required to clear exogenous dopamine applications between the SHR and control strains. Similar maximum dopamine amplitudes were achieved by applying various volumes of an exogenous dopamine solution in order to evaluate the uptake kinetics of the signals. The DAT is electrogenic and depolarization causes the DAT to change from the basal state [100-104] and in order to test the full uptake capabilities of the transporters, including both the DAT and NET, it was necessary to study the transporters in their more natural state using local applications of dopamine. Utilizing this approach, it was discovered that the SHR displayed faster uptake in the cingulate and infralimbic cortices compared to the WKY strain, but not the prelimbic cortex. The SHR model of ADHD was also discovered to have faster dopamine uptake compared to the SD strain in the infralimbic cortex. These results are significant because the cingulate cortex is involved with learning and memory, playing a vital role in the Papez circuit and the cortical control of emotions in humans [105]. These data further demonstrate that there exists a neurochemical dysfunction in a region important for linking behavioral outcomes to motivation [106, 107] in the SHR. Also, the infralimbic cortex in rodents is known to be involved with attention to stimulus features, task contingencies, and attentional set-shifting [108] – all behaviors known to be affected in individuals with ADHD [109-111].

The SHR has previously been found to have dysfunctional dopamine dynamics in the striatum and NA core [52], but here we also show evidence for faster dopamine uptake in the cingulate and infralimbic cortices of the medial PFC. These regions are heavily implicated in ADHD [66, 112, 113] and these data give further evidence for use of the SHR as a model of ADHD. Therapeutics targeting this dysfunction may prove to be useful in the SHR. However, MPH, a DAT blocker, has been investigated and found to not be useful in this model because instead of calming these animals as it does in humans, it increased locomotion in clinically relevant doses [46, 47, 114]. This signifies to us that targeting the NET instead of the DAT, such as with the use of ATX, may provide a more useful option of targeting PFC dopamine dysfunction in the SHR model of ADHD.

The DRD4 and glutamatergic PFC dysfunction

The 7-repeat polymorphism of the DRD4 has been implicated in ADHD. Little is known about the neurochemical effects of the DRD4 and thus the DRD4.7. While the DRD4$^{-/-}$ mouse is not an exact model for ADHD, it does provide insight to the neurochemistry of DRD4 signaling. In these studies we used *in vivo* amperometry coupled to a glutamate-selective MEA to measure extracellular levels of glutamate and glutamate clearance in the PFC of DRD4$^{+/+}$, DRD4$^{+/-}$ and DRD4$^{-/-}$ mice. We measured a significant increase in extracellular resting levels of glutamate, most prevalent in the cingulate cortex of the medial PFC. We also discovered increased glutamate uptake times that were seen primarily in the prelimbic area. These data support the hypothesis that DRD4 signaling is actively involved in regulating glutamate neurotransmission in the PFC.

We found that lack of DRD4 expression resulted in increased extracellular resting levels of glutamate in the PFC. We are unaware of any extracellular glutamate levels reported from the PFC of anesthetized C57BL\6 mice. Using similar technology, Hascup et al. (2007) found extracellular levels of glutamate in the PFC of awake, freely-moving C57Bl \6 mice to be 3.3 ± 0.1 μM [81]. In this study, we reported approximately 60% of the extracellular levels recorded from these prior studies in awake animals (1.42 ± 0.19 μM). Urethane anesthesia has been documented to reduce extracellular glutamate levels by 58-80% in rats and may be contributing to the lower levels of glutamate measured here [81, 115]. The relative contributions of metabolic and neuronal pools of glutamate to extracellular levels of glutamate and the role of D4 receptors in astrocytic regulation of glutamate still requires investigation. Consequences of increased extracellular levels of glutamate in the PFC would cause alterations in signaling due to increased stimulation of glutamate receptors on astrocytes and presynaptic and postsynaptic neurons. Further studies are required to test these potential changes. There is also indication that the DRD4 is localized to GABA containing interneurons in the PFC [116, 117]. Lack of inhibition resulting from loss of expression of the DRD4 could result in decreased release of GABA. This loss of inhibition could also contribute to increased tonic levels of glutamate in the PFC.

Loss of DRD4 resulted in approximately a 20% increase in clearance times in DRD4$^{-/-}$ mice. The mechanism of the increased clearance time is unknown, but the capacity of this tissue to clear similar amounts of exogenous glutamate was not significantly altered in the DRD4$^{-/-}$ mice, suggesting that transporter expression was unchanged. It is not known whether the measured effects on uptake rate were a direct or indirect effect of DRD4 signaling loss. In all areas of the brain, 80-90% of glutamate transporters are located on astrocytes [16]. Increased activation of metabotropic glutamate receptors (mGluRs) on astrocytes could potentially affect glutamate clearance in this case, depending on the affinity for glutamate by the mGluRs on astrocytes [118]. Interestingly, there have been reports of the presence of dopamine D2-receptors on the astrocytes in the PFC [119]. Prior microdialysis data suggests that extracellular dopamine content and KCl-evoked release of dopamine are lower in the striatum and NAc of DRD4$^{-/-}$ mice [120]. Alterations in dopamine neurotransmission in the PFC of these mice may elucidate a special role for the D2 receptor on astrocytes in regulation of dopa-

http://dx.doi.org/10.5772/54207

mine and glutamate interactions in DRD4$^{-/-}$ mice in PFC neurotransmission. Dopamine neurotransmission studies have not been done in these mice, but changes in whole tissue levels of dopamine and dopamine metabolites do not indicate any changes [72].

In multiple publications, the DRD4 has been indicated as having an important role in the cortico-striatal-thalamic loop. Previously, we measured increased extracellular glutamate and slower clearance of glutamate in the striatum, indicating DRD4 regulation in the corticostriatal projections [67]. In these experiments, we measured increased extracellular glutamate levels and slower glutamate clearance in the PFC, representing alterations in glutamatergic projections that primarily originate in the thalamus. Mrzljak et al. (1996) alluded that the DRD4s role in pallido-thalamic pathways may be as a regulator of GABA release [117]. By blocking these receptors, GABA release would be weakened and result in enhanced excitatory pathways beginning in the thalamus. This presents a feed forward situation in which lack of inhibitory modulation of the excitatory pathways of the cortico-striatal-thalamic loop results in increased levels of glutamate in the PFC and the striatum. Although measures of GABA in the pallido-thalamic and striatopallidal projections are necessary, our data continues to support the importance of the DRD4 in the cortico-striatal-thalamic loop, specifically in the regulation of tonic glutamate.

Region specific changes may be due to the concentration of DRD4s and cell types to which they are localized. In a study where bacterial artificial chromosomes expressed enhanced green florescent protein under the transcriptional control of the DRD4, DRD4 localization was found to be high in the orbital, prelimbic, cingulate and rostral agranular potions of the prefrontal cortex [116]. Our study found changes in the cingulate and prelimbic areas, but not the infralimbic area. Localization of DRD4s to interneurons vs. pyramidal neurons may be helpful in elucidating a relationship between altered extracellular glutamate levels in the cingulate cortex in comparison to altered clearance times in the prelimbic area. One caveat of transgenic mice is that compensatory effects may be contributing to the neurochemical effects that we measured. While compensatory effects in the PFC have not been evaluated, alterations in dopamine D1 receptor and NMDA receptor expression were reported in the striatum, nucleus accumbens and hippocampus [67, 120, 121]. Assessment of dopamine, glutamate, and GABA related receptors in the PFC would provide important information necessary for proper evaluation of receptors that could be contributing to the findings reported in this paper and need to be further investigated. Compensatory mechanisms can be indicative of developmental functions that are influenced by the absence of the DRD4 and are important to consider when evaluating glutamate function in the PFC of these knockouts.

2.10. Future directions in the neuropharmacology of ADHD

The data presented above in the SHR and DRD4$^{-/-}$ rodent models of ADHD provide evidence for dopaminergic and glutamatergic system dysfunction in the PFC. Likewise, it has previously been demonstrated that in the striatum of both models, similar neurotransmitter system dysfunction exists [52, 67]. The DRD4 knockout mouse has also been found to exhibit decreased dopamine levels in the striatum [120]. These data in the DRD4$^{-/-}$ reveal that the D_4 receptor is vital in the regulation of dopamine-glutamate interactions in the striatum and

PFC. Recent pilot data from our lab (unpublished) reveal that in the SHR model of ADHD, there exists increased resting glutamate levels in the striatum and PFC; however, further experimentation is necessary to verify these results. Glutamate dysfunction in the SHR would then create the possibility that targeting the dopamine-glutamate interaction in this model of ADHD may prove useful as well.

These animal models grant us the ability to investigate neurotransmitter system regulation *in vivo,* creating a more accurate depiction of the dysfunction in multiple subregions within the PFC. Using these animals, we plan to use common ADHD treatments, such as MPH and ATX, as well as unconventional treatments, such as memantine and deprenyl, to examine the effects of these drugs on the dopamine and glutamate neuronal systems. Our ultimate goal is to discover novel ways to treat ADHD with minimal side-effects and clear long-term safety and efficacy. Avoiding the confounding side effect of abuse potential will be especially advantageous given the difficulties this presents to prescribing stimulants. We believe that targeting the interaction between the dopamine and glutamate systems will provide a new avenue to achieve our goal.

As more and more research is beginning to implicate a dysfunctional glutamate system in ADHD, it's hard to ignore that glutamate may be playing some role in the pathophysiology of ADHD. Although it is too early to know if pharmaceuticals that modulate glutamate will be able to benefit ADHD without their own set of side-effects, it is still our hope that through modification of these interactions, we will be able to better treat individuals with ADHD and greatly improve their quality of life.

3. Conclusion

In this chapter, we have reviewed dopamine and glutamate neurotransmission, as well as dopamine-glutamate interactions, specifically relating to ADHD. We have reviewed current literature and have shown the effects of ADHD treatments on these neurotransmitters. We have discussed and detailed two rodent models of ADHD as well as the techniques used to highlight novel data revealing dopamine and glutamate dysfunction in these models of ADHD. Finally, we've examined ways these data will enable the future neuropharmacology of ADHD to move forward. Ultimately, our goal is to find novel therapies targeting dopamine-glutamate interactions to better treat ADHD in individuals of all ages.

Acknowledgements

This study was supported by USPHS grants MH070840, AG13494, and 5T32AG000242-13, NSF EEC-0310723, and DARPA N66001-09-C- 2080. In addition, the projects described were supported by the National Center for Research Resources, UL1RR033173, and the National Center for Advancing Translational Sciences, UL1TR000117. The content is solely the responsibility of the authors and does not necessarily represent the official views of the NIH.

http://dx.doi.org/10.5772/54207

Author details

Erin M. Miller[1], Theresa C. Thomas[2], Greg A. Gerhardt[1,3,5] and Paul E. A. Glaser[1,3,4]

*Address all correspondence to: pglas0@uky.edu

1 Department of Anatomy & Neurobiology, Center for Microelectrode Technology, University of Kentucky Chandler Medical Center, Lexington, KY, USA

2 Department of Child Health, University of Arizona College of Medicine-Phoenix, Phoenix, AZ, USA

3 Department of Neurology, Department of Psychiatry, University of Kentucky Chandler Medical Center, Lexington, KY, USA

4 Department of Pediatrics, University of Kentucky Chandler Medical Center, Lexington, KY, USA

5 Department of Electrical Engineering, University of Kentucky, Lexington, KY, USA

References

[1] American Psychiatric Association. Committee on Nomenclature and Statistics. and American Psychiatric Association. Committee on Statistics., *Diagnostic and statistical manual: mental disorders*. [1st ed. 1952, Washington,: American Psychiatric Assn., Mental Hospital Service. xii, 130 p.

[2] American Psychiatric Association. Committee on Nomenclature and Statistics., *Diagnostic and statistical manual of mental disorders*. 2d ed. 1968, Washington,. xv, 119 p.

[3] American Psychiatric Association. Task Force on Nomenclature and Statistics. and American Psychiatric Association. Committee on Nomenclature and Statistics., *Diagnostic and statistical manual of mental disorders*. 3d ed. 1980, Washington: American Psychiatric Assn. 494 p.

[4] Strohl, M.P., *Bradley's Benzedrine studies on children with behavioral disorders.* Yale J Biol Med, 2011. 84(1): p. 27-33.

[5] Robbins, T.W. and B.J. Sahakian, *"Paradoxical" effects of psychomotor stimulant drugs in hyperactive children from the standpoint of behavioural pharmacology.* Neuropharmacology, 1979. 18(12): p. 931-50.

[6] Shaywitz, B.A., et al., *Paradoxical response to amphetamine in developing rats treated with 6-hydroxydopamine.* Nature, 1976. 261(5556): p. 153-5.

[7] Schultz, W., *Reward signaling by dopamine neurons.* Neuroscientist, 2001. 7(4): p. 293-302.

[8] Schultz, W., *Responses of midbrain dopamine neurons to behavioral trigger stimuli in the monkey.* J Neurophysiol, 1986. 56(5): p. 1439-61.

[9] Schultz, W., *Predictive reward signal of dopamine neurons.* J Neurophysiol, 1998. 80(1): p. 1-27.

[10] Arias-Carrion, O. and E. Poppel, *Dopamine, learning, and reward-seeking behavior.* Acta Neurobiol Exp (Wars), 2007. 67(4): p. 481-8.

[11] Iversen, L.L., *Introduction to neuropsychopharmacology.* 2009, New York: Oxford University Press. x, 557 p.

[12] Cass, W.A., et al., *Clearance of exogenous dopamine in rat dorsal striatum and nucleus accumbens: role of metabolism and effects of locally applied uptake inhibitors.* J Neurochem, 1993. 61(6): p. 2269-78.

[13] Carrey, N., et al., *Glutamatergic changes with treatment in attention deficit hyperactivity disorder: a preliminary case series.* J Child Adolesc Psychopharmacol, 2002. 12(4): p. 331-6.

[14] Moore, C.M., et al., *Differences in brain chemistry in children and adolescents with attention deficit hyperactivity disorder with and without comorbid bipolar disorder: a proton magnetic resonance spectroscopy study.* Am J Psychiatry, 2006. 163(2): p. 316-8.

[15] Moore, C.M., et al., *Glutamine and glutamate levels in children and adolescents with bipolar disorder: a 4.0-T proton magnetic resonance spectroscopy study of the anterior cingulate cortex.* J Am Acad Child Adolesc Psychiatry, 2007. 46(4): p. 524-34.

[16] Danbolt, N.C., *Glutamate uptake.* Prog Neurobiol, 2001. 65(1): p. 1-105.

[17] Warton, F.L., F.M. Howells, and V.A. Russell, *Increased glutamate-stimulated release of dopamine in substantia nigra of a rat model for attention-deficit/hyperactivity disorder--lack of effect of methylphenidate.* Metab Brain Dis, 2009. 24(4): p. 599-613.

[18] Martinez-Fong, D., et al., *NMDA receptor mediates dopamine release in the striatum of unanesthetized rats as measured by brain microdialysis.* Brain Res, 1992. 595(2): p. 309-15.

[19] Kotecha, S.A., et al., *A D2 class dopamine receptor transactivates a receptor tyrosine kinase to inhibit NMDA receptor transmission.* Neuron, 2002. 35(6): p. 1111-22.

[20] Yuen, E.Y., et al., *Regulation of AMPA receptor channels and synaptic plasticity by cofilin phosphatase Slingshot in cortical neurons.* J Physiol, 2010. 588(Pt 13): p. 2361-71.

[21] Carboni, E., et al., *Amphetamine, cocaine, phencyclidine and nomifensine increase extracellular dopamine concentrations preferentially in the nucleus accumbens of freely moving rats.* Neuroscience, 1989. 28(3): p. 653-61.

[22] Kahlig, K.M. and A. Galli, *Regulation of dopamine transporter function and plasma membrane expression by dopamine, amphetamine, and cocaine.* Eur J Pharmacol, 2003. 479(1-3): p. 153-8.

[23] Kuczenski, R. and D.S. Segal, *Effects of methylphenidate on extracellular dopamine, serotonin, and norepinephrine: comparison with amphetamine.* J Neurochem, 1997. 68(5): p. 2032-7.

[24] Kuczenski, R. and D.S. Segal, *Locomotor effects of acute and repeated threshold doses of amphetamine and methylphenidate: relative roles of dopamine and norepinephrine.* J Pharmacol Exp Ther, 2001. 296(3): p. 876-83.

[25] Gerasimov, M.R., et al., *Synergistic interactions between nicotine and cocaine or methylphenidate depend on the dose of dopamine transporter inhibitor.* Synapse, 2000. 38(4): p. 432-7.

[26] Volkow, N.D., et al., *Therapeutic doses of oral methylphenidate significantly increase extracellular dopamine in the human brain.* J Neurosci, 2001. 21(2): p. RC121.

[27] Huff, J.K. and M.I. Davies, *Microdialysis monitoring of methylphenidate in blood and brain correlated with changes in dopamine and rat activity.* J Pharm Biomed Anal, 2002. 29(5): p. 767-77.

[28] Gerasimov, M.R., et al., *Comparison between intraperitoneal and oral methylphenidate administration: A microdialysis and locomotor activity study.* J Pharmacol Exp Ther, 2000. 295(1): p. 51-7.

[29] Marsteller, D.A., et al., *Acute handling stress modulates methylphenidate-induced catecholamine overflow in the medial prefrontal cortex.* Neuropsychopharmacology, 2002. 27(2): p. 163-70.

[30] Newman, L.A., J. Darling, and J. McGaughy, *Atomoxetine reverses attentional deficits produced by noradrenergic deafferentation of medial prefrontal cortex.* Psychopharmacology (Berl), 2008. 200(1): p. 39-50.

[31] Bymaster, F.P., et al., *Atomoxetine increases extracellular levels of norepinephrine and dopamine in prefrontal cortex of rat: a potential mechanism for efficacy in attention deficit/hyperactivity disorder.* Neuropsychopharmacology, 2002. 27(5): p. 699-711.

[32] Swanson, C.J., et al., *Effect of the attention deficit/hyperactivity disorder drug atomoxetine on extracellular concentrations of norepinephrine and dopamine in several brain regions of the rat.* Neuropharmacology, 2006. 50(6): p. 755-60.

[33] Michelson, D., et al., *Atomoxetine in the treatment of children and adolescents with attention-deficit/hyperactivity disorder: a randomized, placebo-controlled, dose-response study.* Pediatrics, 2001. 108(5): p. E83.

[34] Michelson, D., et al., *Atomoxetine in adults with ADHD: two randomized, placebo-controlled studies.* Biol Psychiatry, 2003. 53(2): p. 112-20.

[35] Adler, L.A., et al., *Long-term, open-label study of the safety and efficacy of atomoxetine in adults with attention-deficit/hyperactivity disorder: an interim analysis.* J Clin Psychiatry, 2005. 66(3): p. 294-9.

[36] Adler, L.A., et al., *Long-term, open-label safety and efficacy of atomoxetine in adults with ADHD: final report of a 4-year study.* J Atten Disord, 2008. 12(3): p. 248-53.

[37] Ludolph, A.G., et al., *Atomoxetine acts as an NMDA receptor blocker in clinically relevant concentrations.* Br J Pharmacol, 2010. 160(2): p. 283-91.

[38] Hammerness, P., et al., *Brain biochemical effects of methylphenidate treatment using proton magnetic spectroscopy in youth with attention-deficit hyperactivity disorder: a controlled pilot study.* CNS Neurosci Ther, 2012. 18(1): p. 34-40.

[39] Wiguna, T., et al., *Effect of 12-week administration of 20-mg long-acting methylphenidate on Glu/Cr, NAA/Cr, Cho/Cr, and mI/Cr ratios in the prefrontal cortices of school-age children in Indonesia: a study using 1H magnetic resonance spectroscopy (MRS).* Clin Neuropharmacol, 2012. 35(2): p. 81-5.

[40] Fumagalli, F., et al., *Sub-chronic exposure to atomoxetine up-regulates BDNF expression and signalling in the brain of adolescent spontaneously hypertensive rats: comparison with methylphenidate.* Pharmacol Res, 2010. 62(6): p. 523-9.

[41] Rogawski, M.A. and G.L. Wenk, *The neuropharmacological basis for the use of memantine in the treatment of Alzheimer's disease.* CNS Drug Rev, 2003. 9(3): p. 275-308.

[42] Seeman, P., C. Caruso, and M. Lasaga, *Memantine agonist action at dopamine D2High receptors.* Synapse, 2008. 62(2): p. 149-53.

[43] Surman, C.B., et al., *A pilot open label prospective study of memantine monotherapy in adults with ADHD.* World J Biol Psychiatry, 2012.

[44] Jankovic, J., *Deprenyl in attention deficit associated with Tourette's syndrome.* Arch Neurol, 1993. 50(3): p. 286-8.

[45] Feigin, A., et al., *A controlled trial of deprenyl in children with Tourette's syndrome and attention deficit hyperactivity disorder.* Neurology, 1996. 46(4): p. 965-8.

[46] Sagvolden, T., *Behavioral validation of the spontaneously hypertensive rat (SHR) as an animal model of attention-deficit/hyperactivity disorder (AD/HD).* Neurosci Biobehav Rev, 2000. 24(1): p. 31-9.

[47] Sagvolden, T., et al., *The spontaneously hypertensive rat (SHR) as an animal model of childhood hyperactivity (ADHD): changed reactivity to reinforcers and to psychomotor stimulants.* Behav Neural Biol, 1992. 58(2): p. 103-12.

[48] Sagvolden, T., E.D. Hendley, and S. Knardahl, *Behavior of hypertensive and hyperactive rat strains: hyperactivity is not unitarily determined.* Physiol Behav, 1992. 52(1): p. 49-57.

http://dx.doi.org/10.5772/54207

[49] Wultz, B. and T. Sagvolden, *The hyperactive spontaneously hypertensive rat learns to sit still, but not to stop bursts of responses with short interresponse times.* Behav Genet, 1992. 22(4): p. 415-33.

[50] Knardahl, S. and T. Sagvolden, *Open-field behavior of spontaneously hypertensive rats.* Behav Neural Biol, 1979. 27(2): p. 187-200.

[51] Russell, V., et al., *Differences between electrically-, ritalin- and D-amphetamine-stimulated release of [3H]dopamine from brain slices suggest impaired vesicular storage of dopamine in an animal model of Attention-Deficit Hyperactivity Disorder.* Behav Brain Res, 1998. 94(1): p. 163-71.

[52] Miller, E.M., et al., *The spontaneously hypertensive and Wistar Kyoto rat models of ADHD exhibit sub-regional differences in dopamine release and uptake in the striatum and nucleus accumbens.* Neuropharmacology, 2012. 63(8): p. 1327-1334.

[53] Myers, M.M., S.R. Whittemore, and E.D. Hendley, *Changes in catecholamine neuronal uptake and receptor binding in the brains of spontaneously hypertensive rats (SHR).* Brain Res, 1981. 220(2): p. 325-38.

[54] Li, Q., et al., *The usefulness of the spontaneously hypertensive rat to model attention-deficit/hyperactivity disorder (ADHD) may be explained by the differential expression of dopamine-related genes in the brain.* Neurochem Int, 2007. 50(6): p. 848-57.

[55] Russell, V.A., *Increased AMPA receptor function in slices containing the prefrontal cortex of spontaneously hypertensive rats.* Metab Brain Dis, 2001. 16(3-4): p. 143-9.

[56] Russell, V.A., *Hypodopaminergic and hypernoradrenergic activity in prefrontal cortex slices of an animal model for attention-deficit hyperactivity disorder--the spontaneously hypertensive rat.* Behav Brain Res, 2002. 130(1-2): p. 191-6.

[57] Asghari, V., et al., *Modulation of intracellular cyclic AMP levels by different human dopamine D4 receptor variants.* J Neurochem, 1995. 65(3): p. 1157-65.

[58] Faraone, S.V., et al., *Meta-analysis of the association between the 7-repeat allele of the dopamine D(4) receptor gene and attention deficit hyperactivity disorder.* Am J Psychiatry, 2001. 158(7): p. 1052-7.

[59] Sunohara, G.A., et al., *Linkage of the dopamine D4 receptor gene and attention-deficit/hyperactivity disorder.* J Am Acad Child Adolesc Psychiatry, 2000. 39(12): p. 1537-42.

[60] Swanson, J., et al., *Attention deficit/hyperactivity disorder children with a 7-repeat allele of the dopamine receptor D4 gene have extreme behavior but normal performance on critical neuropsychological tests of attention.* Proc Natl Acad Sci U S A, 2000. 97(9): p. 4754-9.

[61] Todd, R.D., et al., *Collaborative analysis of DRD4 and DAT genotypes in population-defined ADHD subtypes.* J Child Psychol Psychiatry, 2005. 46(10): p. 1067-73.

[62] Shaw, P., et al., *Polymorphisms of the dopamine D4 receptor, clinical outcome, and cortical structure in attention-deficit/hyperactivity disorder.* Arch Gen Psychiatry, 2007. 64(8): p. 921-31.

[63] Ariano, M.A., et al., *Coexpression of striatal dopamine receptor subtypes and excitatory amino acid subunits.* Synapse, 1997. 26(4): p. 400-14.

[64] Ariano, M.A., et al., *Cellular distribution of the rat D4 dopamine receptor protein in the CNS using anti-receptor antisera.* Brain Res, 1997. 752(1-2): p. 26-34.

[65] Faraone, S.V., et al., *Familial subtypes of attention deficit hyperactivity disorder: a 4-year follow-up study of children from antisocial-ADHD families.* J Child Psychol Psychiatry, 1998. 39(7): p. 1045-53.

[66] Arnsten, A.F. and B.M. Li, *Neurobiology of executive functions: catecholamine influences on prefrontal cortical functions.* Biol Psychiatry, 2005. 57(11): p. 1377-84.

[67] Thomas, T.C., et al., *Decreased dopamine D4 receptor expression increases extracellular glutamate and alters its regulation in mouse striatum.* Neuropsychopharmacology, 2009. 34(2): p. 436-45.

[68] Rubinstein, M., et al., *Mice lacking dopamine D4 receptors are supersensitive to ethanol, cocaine, and methamphetamine.* Cell, 1997. 90(6): p. 991-1001.

[69] Falzone, T.L., et al., *Absence of dopamine D4 receptors results in enhanced reactivity to unconditioned, but not conditioned, fear.* Eur J Neurosci, 2002. 15(1): p. 158-64.

[70] Dulawa, S.C., et al., *Dopamine D4 receptor-knock-out mice exhibit reduced exploration of novel stimuli.* J Neurosci, 1999. 19(21): p. 9550-6.

[71] Kruzich, P.J., K.L. Suchland, and D.K. Grandy, *Dopamine D4 receptor-deficient mice, congenic on the C57BL/6J background, are hypersensitive to amphetamine.* Synapse, 2004. 53(2): p. 131-9.

[72] Rubinstein, M., et al., *Dopamine D4 receptor-deficient mice display cortical hyperexcitability.* J Neurosci, 2001. 21(11): p. 3756-63.

[73] Hinzman, J.M., et al., *Disruptions in the regulation of extracellular glutamate by neurons and glia in the rat striatum two days after diffuse brain injury.* J Neurotrauma, 2012. 29(6): p. 1197-208.

[74] Littrell, O.M., et al., *Enhanced dopamine transporter activity in middle-aged Gdnf heterozygous mice.* Neurobiol Aging, 2012.

[75] Paxinos, G. and C. Watson, *The rat brain in stereotaxic coordinates.* 6th ed. 2009, Amsterdam ; Boston ;: Academic Press/Elsevier.

[76] Cass, W.A., et al., *Differences in dopamine clearance and diffusion in rat striatum and nucleus accumbens following systemic cocaine administration.* J Neurochem, 1992. 59(1): p. 259-66.

[77] Friedemann, M.N. and G.A. Gerhardt, *Regional effects of aging on dopaminergic function in the Fischer-344 rat.* Neurobiol Aging, 1992. 13(2): p. 325-32.

[78] Hinzman, J.M., et al., *Diffuse brain injury elevates tonic glutamate levels and potassium-evoked glutamate release in discrete brain regions at two days post-injury: an enzyme-based microelectrode array study.* J Neurotrauma, 2010. 27(5): p. 889-99.

[79] Thomas, T.C., et al., *Hypersensitive glutamate signaling correlates with the development of late-onset behavioral morbidity in diffuse brain-injured circuitry.* J Neurotrauma, 2012. 29(2): p. 187-200.

[80] Burmeister, J.J. and G.A. Gerhardt, *Self-referencing ceramic-based multisite microelectrodes for the detection and elimination of interferences from the measurement of L-glutamate and other analytes.* Anal Chem, 2001. 73(5): p. 1037-42.

[81] Hascup, K.N., et al., *Second-by-Second Measures of L-Glutamate and Other Neurotransmitters Using Enzyme-Based Microelectrode Arrays.* 2007.

[82] Franklin, K.B.J. and G. Paxinos, *The mouse brain in stereotaxic coordinates.* 1997, San Diego: Academic Press. xxii p., 186 p. of plates.

[83] Hebert, M.A., et al., *Age-related reductions in [3H]WIN 35,428 binding to the dopamine transporter in nigrostriatal and mesolimbic brain regions of the fischer 344 rat.* J Pharmacol Exp Ther, 1999. 288(3): p. 1334-9.

[84] Levy, F., *The dopamine theory of attention deficit hyperactivity disorder (ADHD).* Aust N Z J Psychiatry, 1991. 25(2): p. 277-83.

[85] Linthorst, A.C., et al., *Electrically stimulated [3H]dopamine and [14C]acetylcholine release from nucleus caudatus slices: differences between spontaneously hypertensive rats and Wistar-Kyoto rats.* Brain Res, 1990. 509(2): p. 266-72.

[86] Linthorst, A.C., et al., *Effect of the dopamine D2 receptor agonist quinpirole on the in vivo release of dopamine in the caudate nucleus of hypertensive rats.* Eur J Pharmacol, 1991. 201(2-3): p. 125-33.

[87] Versteeg, D.H., et al., *Regional concentrations of noradrenaline and dopamine in rat brain.* Brain Res, 1976. 113(3): p. 563-74.

[88] Ferguson, S.A., B.J. Gough, and A.M. Cada, *In vivo basal and amphetamine-induced striatal dopamine and metabolite levels are similar in the spontaneously hypertensive, Wistar-Kyoto and Sprague-Dawley male rats.* Physiol Behav, 2003. 80(1): p. 109-14.

[89] Obrenovitch, T.P., et al., *Excitotoxicity in neurological disorders--the glutamate paradox.* Int J Dev Neurosci, 2000. 18(2-3): p. 281-7.

[90] Borland, L.M., et al., *Voltammetric study of extracellular dopamine near microdialysis probes acutely implanted in the striatum of the anesthetized rat.* J Neurosci Methods, 2005. 146(2): p. 149-58.

[91] Wang, Y. and A.C. Michael, *Microdialysis probes alter presynaptic regulation of dopamine terminals in rat striatum.* J Neurosci Methods, 2012. 208(1): p. 34-9.

[92] Gerhardt, G.A., G.M. Rose, and B.J. Hoffer, *Release of monoamines from striatum of rat and mouse evoked by local application of potassium: evaluation of a new in vivo electrochemical technique.* J Neurochem, 1986. 46(3): p. 842-50.

[93] Leo, D., et al., *Altered midbrain dopaminergic neurotransmission during development in an animal model of ADHD.* Neurosci Biobehav Rev, 2003. 27(7): p. 661-9.

[94] Roessner, V., et al., *Methylphenidate normalizes elevated dopamine transporter densities in an animal model of the attention-deficit/hyperactivity disorder combined type, but not to the same extent in one of the attention-deficit/hyperactivity disorder inattentive type.* Neuroscience, 2010. 167(4): p. 1183-91.

[95] Simchon, Y., A. Weizman, and M. Rehavi, *The effect of chronic methylphenidate administration on presynaptic dopaminergic parameters in a rat model for ADHD.* Eur Neuropsychopharmacol, 2010. 20(10): p. 714-20.

[96] Viggiano, D., D. Vallone, and A. Sadile, *Dysfunctions in dopamine systems and ADHD: evidence from animals and modeling.* Neural Plast, 2004. 11(1-2): p. 97-114.

[97] Watanabe, Y., et al., *Brain dopamine transporter in spontaneously hypertensive rats.* J Nucl Med, 1997. 38(3): p. 470-4.

[98] Womersley, J.S., et al., *Maternal separation affects dopamine transporter function in the Spontaneously Hypertensive Rat: An in vivo electrochemical study.* Behav Brain Funct, 2011. 7: p. 49.

[99] Moron, J.A., et al., *Dopamine uptake through the norepinephrine transporter in brain regions with low levels of the dopamine transporter: evidence from knock-out mouse lines.* J Neurosci, 2002. 22(2): p. 389-95.

[100] El Ayadi, A., I. Afailal, and M. Errami, *Effects of voltage-sensitive calcium channel blockers on extracellular dopamine levels in rat striatum.* Metab Brain Dis, 2001. 16(3-4): p. 121-31.

[101] Hoffman, A.F., et al., *Voltage-dependency of the dopamine transporter in the rat substantia nigra.* Neurosci Lett, 1999. 260(2): p. 105-8.

[102] Kandasamy, S.B., *Possible involvement of L-type voltage-gated calcium channels in release of dopamine in the striatum of irradiated rats.* Radiat Res, 2000. 154(1): p. 39-43.

[103] Reith, M.E., et al., *Effect of metaphit on dopaminergic neurotransmission in rat striatal slices: involvement of the dopamine transporter and voltage-dependent sodium channel.* J Pharmacol Exp Ther, 1991. 259(3): p. 1188-96.

[104] Zahniser, N.R., et al., *Voltage-dependency of the dopamine transporter in rat brain.* Adv Pharmacol, 1998. 42: p. 195-8.

[105] Granziera, C., et al., *In-vivo magnetic resonance imaging of the structural core of the Papez circuit in humans.* Neuroreport, 2011. 22(5): p. 227-31.

[106] Adey, W.R., *An experimental study of the hippocampal connexions of the cingulate cortex in the rabbit.* Brain, 1951. 74(2): p. 233-47.

[107] Adey, W.R. and M. Meyer, *An experimental study of hippocampal afferent pathways from prefrontal and cingulate areas in the monkey.* J Anat, 1952. 86(1): p. 58-74.

[108] Dalley, J.W., R.N. Cardinal, and T.W. Robbins, *Prefrontal executive and cognitive functions in rodents: neural and neurochemical substrates.* Neurosci Biobehav Rev, 2004. 28(7): p. 771-84.

[109] Mehta, M.A., I.M. Goodyer, and B.J. Sahakian, *Methylphenidate improves working memory and set-shifting in AD/HD: relationships to baseline memory capacity.* J Child Psychol Psychiatry, 2004. 45(2): p. 293-305.

[110] Klimkeit, E.I., et al., *Motor preparation, motor execution, attention, and executive functions in attention deficit/hyperactivity disorder (ADHD).* Child Neuropsychol, 2005. 11(2): p. 153-73.

[111] Krusch, D.A., et al., *Methylphenidate slows reactions of children with attention deficit disorder during and after an error.* J Abnorm Child Psychol, 1996. 24(5): p. 633-50.

[112] Arnsten, A.F. and A.G. Dudley, *Methylphenidate improves prefrontal cortical cognitive function through alpha2 adrenoceptor and dopamine D1 receptor actions: Relevance to therapeutic effects in Attention Deficit Hyperactivity Disorder.* Behav Brain Funct, 2005. 1(1): p. 2.

[113] Arnsten, A.F., *Toward a new understanding of attention-deficit hyperactivity disorder pathophysiology: an important role for prefrontal cortex dysfunction.* CNS Drugs, 2009. 23 Suppl 1: p. 33-41.

[114] Sagvolden, T. and E.B. Johansen, *Rat Models of ADHD.* Curr Top Behav Neurosci, 2011.

[115] Day, B.K., et al., *Microelectrode array studies of basal and potassium-evoked release of L-glutamate in the anesthetized rat brain.* J Neurochem, 2006. 96(6): p. 1626-35.

[116] Noain, D., et al., *Identification of brain neurons expressing the dopamine D4 receptor gene using BAC transgenic mice.* Eur J Neurosci, 2006. 24(9): p. 2429-38.

[117] Mrzljak, L., et al., *Localization of dopamine D4 receptors in GABAergic neurons of the primate brain.* Nature, 1996. 381(6579): p. 245-8.

[118] Schoepp, D.D., *Unveiling the functions of presynaptic metabotropic glutamate receptors in the central nervous system.* J Pharmacol Exp Ther, 2001. 299(1): p. 12-20.

[119] Khan, Z.U., et al., *An astroglia-linked dopamine D2-receptor action in prefrontal cortex.* Proc Natl Acad Sci U S A, 2001. 98(4): p. 1964-9.

[120] Thomas, T.C., et al., *Dopamine D4 receptor knockout mice exhibit neurochemical changes consistent with decreased dopamine release.* J Neurosci Methods, 2007. 166(2): p. 306-14.

[121] Gan, L., et al., *Enhanced expression of dopamine D(1) and glutamate NMDA receptors in dopamine D(4) receptor knockout mice.* J Mol Neurosci, 2004. 22(3): p. 167-78.

Section 3

Assessment and Diagnosis

Chapter 7

Clinical Phenomena of ADHD

Nitin Patel

Additional information is available at the end of the chapter

http://dx.doi.org/10.5772/53789

1. Introduction

ADHD is the most common behavior diagnosis given in a approximately 5.4 million children between 4 and 17 years of age [1]. ADHD can profoundly affect the academic achievement, well being and social interactions of children. Clinically, ADHD may be confused with other medical conditions, including seizures and anxiety but not limited to behavior or paying attention only. If a child is not hyperactive, it may take a long time before it is brought to the attention of others for treatment. The American Academy of Pediatrics (AAP) recently issued new guidelines for the diagnosis and treatment of ADHD, expanding recommendations for age ranges including both early pre-school children and adolescence.

Three types of ADHD have been identified:

1. ADHD combined type; the individual displays both inattentive and hyperactive/ impulsive symptoms.

2. ADHD, predominately inattentive type; the individual has symptoms primarily related to inattention. Individuals do not display significant hyperactivity/impulsive behaviors.

3. ADHD, predominately hyperactivity/impulsive type; symptoms are primarily related to hyperactivity and impulsivity. The individual does not display significant attention problems [2]. Symptoms are typically seen early in the child's life, often when he or she enters the school setting. In order to meet the criteria for ADD/ADHD symptoms must be more excessive than would be appropriate for individual's age and developmental level. Problematic behaviors may continue through adolescence and into adulthood. The diagnosis of ADD/ADHD is a clinical diagnosis.

The individual must meet criteria requirements listed in the Diagnostic and Statistical Manual of Mental Disorders (DSM).

Six or more of the following symptoms of inattention have been present for at least 6 months to the point that it is disruptive and inappropriate for the developmental level.

Often does not give close attention to details or makes careless mistakes in school work, work or other activities.

Often has trouble keeping attention on task or play activities.

Often does not seem to listen when spoken to directly.

Often does not follow instructions and fails to finish school work, chores or duties in the workplace. Often has trouble organizing activities.

Often avoids dislikes or doesn't want to do things that take a lot of mental effort for a long period of time.

Often loses things needed for tasks and activities.

Is often easily distracted.

Is often forgetful in daily activities.

Six or more of following symptoms of hyperactivity/ impulsivity have been present for at least 6 months to an extent that it is disruptive and inappropriate for the developmental level.

2. Hyperactivity

Often fidgets with hands or feet or squirms in seat.

Often gets up from seat when remaining is seat is expected.

Often runs about or climbs where it is not appropriate.

Adolescence and adults may feel very restless.

Often has trouble playing or enjoying leisure activities quietly.

Is often "On the go" or acts as if "Driven by a motor".

Often talks excessively.

3. Impulsivity

Often blurts out answers before questions have been finished.

Often has trouble waiting when it's his turn.

Often interrupts or intrudes on others [3].

There must be clear evidence of clear impairment in social, school or work function; these symptoms do not occur only during the course of a pervasive developmental disorder,

http://dx.doi.org/10.5772/53789

schizophrenia or other psychotic disorder; and the symptoms are not better accounted for by other mental disorder, sensory disorder (hearing or visual impairment) and those who have experienced child abuse and sexual abuse [4].

The American Academy of Pediatrics (AAP) recently stated, "a primary care provider should initiate an evaluation for ADHD for any child, 4-18 years of age who presents with academic or behavior problems and symptoms of inattention, hyperactivity or impulsivity. The AAP went further in stating that the clinician should determine that the diagnostic criteria of DSM-IV have been met including documentation from parents, teachers or others school personnel and mental health clinician involved in the child's care.

There are many different rating scales available to be completed by parent, other care givers and school personnel.

The Vanderbilt ADHD diagnostic rating scale includes DSM-IV based skills with teacher and parent report forms. It screens for co-morbid conditions. It is normed for age and sex. The Vanderbilt separates inattention and hyperactivity/impulsive behaviors. It can be used free of charge [6].

The Connors rating scale has been the most utilized method of trying to diagnose ADHD and other problem childhood behavior. It follows the DSM-IV guidelines. There are forms for teachers and parents to fill that are gender specific. There is a form for the child to fill out called "a self report" [7].

Child attention profile. This is based on inattention and over reactive items from the Achenbach Child Behavior Checklist. It is normed by sex. It separates inattention and over reactive factors. This can be used free of charge [8].

The Weschsler Individual Achievement Test, 2nd edition, this provides standardized normative value academic achievement scores across a variety of subjects for individuals between the ages of 4 and 85. The reading, numerical, and spelling subtest provide brief estimates of academic achievements [9].

Changes in the definition of the diagnosis of ADHD are being considered with the next edition of the DSM that is expected to be published in May 2013. One problem with using the current DSM-IV subtypes is they are often unstable and changing over time. For example, a child may meet the criteria for one subtype at the initial evaluation and meet the criteria for another at the follow up appointment. In order for more accuracy, one proposed revision is to specify diagnosis based on current presentation of symptoms: combined presentation predominately inattentive presentation or predominately hyperactive/ impulsive presentation. In addition a fourth presentation: inattentive presentation (restrictive) may be added to be more precise in identifying individuals who display impairment only in attention not hyperactivity.

Symptoms of impulsivity are also under represented in the current DSM-IV criteria. Possible updates to the DSM-V include adding additional criteria to impulsivity.

Examples are:

tends to act without thinking, starts a task without adequate preparation or avoids listening or reading instructions.

Is often impatient, restless when waiting for others, wanting others to get to the point, speeding when driving.

Is uncomfortable doing things slowly and systematically.

Often rushes through activities or tasks.

Finds it difficult to resist temptations or opportunities, even if it means taking risks. Example: a child may play with dangerous objects; or adults may commit to a relationship after a brief acquaintance [10].

There is mounting evidence that many conditions exist with ADHD and modify the overall clinical presentation and treatment response. Co-morbid conditions should be considered simultaneously and in order to better understand and maximize therapy. These conditions may be emotional, behavioral, developmental or physical conditions. Co-morbid conditions include Oppositional Defiance Disorder (ODD), substance abuse, conduct disorder, anxiety, depression, tic disorder, Tourette's syndrome, and learning disability. Co-morbidities have their own symptoms, which may or may not overlap the symptoms of ADHD.

Oppositional Defiance Disorder (ODD). *Does the person defy you or the teacher by simply saying no or ignoring you? Does the person appear to be annoyed easily and bothered by trivial things? Does the person appear to annoy other people on purpose? Does the person appear angry, hot tempered, resentful or full of spite?*

Oppositional defiant disorder is a pattern of disobedient, hostile and defiant behavior toward authority figures. This disorder is more common in boys than girls. Children with ODD are overly stubborn, rebellious, often argue with adults and refuse to obey rules [11]. These children often blame others for their mistakes. Are in constant trouble in school. Are touchy or easily annoyed. Are spiteful and seek revenge. To fit this diagnosis, the pattern must last for at least 6 months and must be more than normal childhood misbehaviors. ODD is a less severe condition than Conduct Disorder. Frequently those who have persistent ODD later develop symptoms that qualify for diagnosis of conduct disorder [13]. Children with a diagnosis of ODD often require treatment for the ADHD as well as individual and possibly family therapy. The parents should learn how to manage the child's behavior.

Conduct Disorder. *Does the person lie a lot? Does the person get into physical fights? Does the person try of hurt people? Has the person ever stolen or damaged people's property?*

Conduct disorder is a disorder of childhood and adolescence that involves long-term (chronic) behavior problems. Conduct disorder has been associated with child abuse, drug addiction or alcoholism in the parents, genetic defects and poverty. This condition includes behaviors in which the child may lie, steal, fight, or bully others. He or she may destroy property, break into homes or play with fire. They may carry or use weapons. These children are at greater risk of using illegal substances. Children with conduct disorder are at risk of getting in trouble at school or with police [11]. The presence of negativistic, hostile

http://dx.doi.org/10.5772/53789

and defiant behaviors that include losing their temper, arguing with adults, refusing to comply with the rules of society, deliberately annoying people, consistent anger/resentment towards others. There is a history of physical aggression towards people or animals [16]. These children make no effort to hide their aggressive behaviors. They may have a hard time making friends. Children with conduct disorder require treatment for their ADHD as well as for their conduct disorder. The child's family needs to be closely involved. Parents can learn techniques to help manage their child's problem behavior. Many "behavior modification" school, "wilderness programs" or "boot camps" are sold to parents as solutions for conduct disorder. These programs use a form of "confrontation" which can actually be harmful. Treating the child at home with their family is more effective [18].

Anxiety. *Does the person appear to be nervous and anxious? Are there times when the person appears panicked, stricken, or frozen by anxiety? Does the person appear very shy compared to others his same age? Does the person repeat certain actions over and over like a ritual?*

The most common anxiety disorder with ADHD is social phobia. This condition is present in nearly 1/3 of patients with ADHD. Social phobia describes a chronic and persistent fear of being scrutinized in social situations. Many people with ADHD experience repetitive negative social encounters related to inattention which results in their misreading social cues. Disorganization causes them to be chronically tardy for social events. Impulsivity explains why they blurt out unedited and embarrassing comments. This causes them to be over whelmed and uncomfortable in social situations [12]. The treatment for this is to stabilize the ADHD [11]. Some children with anxiety did require the addition of an SSRI.

Depression. *Does the person appear sad, blue or down and how can you tell? Is the person irritable, cranky, and moody? Has the person been doing the activity once enjoyed? Does the person talk about suicide or about uselessness of life, has the person attempted suicide?*

Depression frequently occurs independently of ADHD. If depression is not identified and treated concurrently with the ADHD it can become treatment resistant depression. (12) Depression is the most common co-morbid condition in adolescents with ADHD [4]. Preliminary studies suggest that depression co-exists with the predominately inattentive and combined sub-types of ADHD [14, 15]. In many cases, ADHD related problems at school and with family and friends trigger depression by undermining a child's self esteem. This is called "secondary" depression, because it arises as the aftermath of another problem, including ADHD, it is important to taylor the treatment for the depression to the cause. If it is ADHD, treat the ADHD [19].

Bipolar disorders: *are there times where the person thinks he or she is able to do anything he or she wants? Does the person appear unusually energetic at times or almost high without drugs? Does the person miss a lot of sleep at night but still acts energetic the next day? Does the person appear to have thought that appear so fast that it is impossible to keep up with them?*

Bipolar disorder may occur with ADHD or may mimic its symptoms. Half of the boys and one-fourth of the girls with bipolar disorder also meet the criteria for ADHD. Children and adolescents with bipolar disorder often show strong emotional feelings, hyperactive behavior, overbearing manner, and difficulty waking up in the morning. Children and adolescents with sever bipolar symptoms may have excessive and lengthy temper tantrums that are destructive and often based on gross distortion of objective events. For example, when a friend wants to play a different game, bipolar children may think the friend is trying to purposefully be mean. The child gets angry at such mistreatment. This may result in a temper tantrum. Other symptoms include excessive talking, increased activity, inappropriate actions and verbal responses in social situations, lack of inhibition, chronic irritability and distractibility. The prevalence is up to 20% [21, 22]. According to an Italian study, 24% of 7-18 year old clinic attendees with bipolar disease had existing ADHD [23].

The child behavior check list score better discriminates between children with ADHD, comania in context to pediatric bipolar disorders and control subjects.

The pharmacological treatment, mood stabilizers are the first line treatment for periodic bipolar disorders. However, when ADHD symptoms are present, subjects may benefit from short-term co-concomitant treatment with a stimulant or a co-medication of a non-stimulant.

The etiology of comorbid pediatric bipolar and ADHD have distinct characteristics. Neuro imaging studies suggest general changes in prefrontal areas in both disorders. However, there are a few primary differences between the two patient groups in the areas in indifference control, working memory, planning cognitive flexibility and fluency. Several authors reported that ADHD with comorbid pediatric bipolar disorder is its own distinct form of ADHD [24]

Fifty percent of the prepubescent depressed children in one sample manifest bipolar disorder within ten year of the onset of depression [25]. Another study found 20%of depressed adolescents in another sample had revealed a bipolar disorder within 1-4 years [26]. When comparing to the children with ADHD without mania, the manic children have significantly higher rates of major depression, psychosis, multiple anxiety, conduct disorder, or oppositional defiant disorder, as well as significantly greater impairment of psychosocial functioning.

As with depression, bipolar must be treated effectively with symptoms of ADHD to resolve comorbidity affecting the individual. An atypical anti-psychotic agent appears to be effective in the elimination of juvenile mania. In an open study, Risperdal was found to be effective anti-manic but did not help ADHD symptoms, among bipolar adults comorbid for ADHD, Bupropion is effective for ADHD and depression but may lower the threshold for inducing mania.

Tic disorder and Tourette's syndrome. *Does the person have movement such as eye blinking, making an odd face, shrugging or moving an arm a lot that is not intentional? Does the person make noise without meaning to such as grunting, sniffing, or saying certain words? Do these symptoms get worse when the person is under stress or anxiety and/or are these symptoms present while the person sleeping?*

Tics are complex, stereotyped movements (motor tics) or utterances (verbal tics) that are sudden, brief and purposeless. Tics are suppressible for short periods of time, with some discomfort and never incorporated into a voluntary movement. Stress exacerbates tics and they disappear during sleep.

Tourette syndrome is any combination of verbal and motor tics. There is a strong genetic basis for Tourette syndrome and environmental factors play a role. Stimulants provoke tics in pre disposed children.

Onset is anytime from 2 to 15 years of age. The period of greatest severity is between 8 and 12 years of age and half of the children are tic free by 18 years of age. Common tics include eye blinking, grimacing, lip smacking, and shoulder shrugging. The initial verbal tics are usually throat clearing, shorting or sniffing. Symptoms wax and wane in response to stress and excitement. The decision to prescribe medication depends on whether the tics bother the child. Drug therapy is not required if the tics bother the parents but do not disturb the child's life [20].

Obsessive compulsive disorders: Obsessive –compulsive disorders are characterized by recurrent intrusive thoughts and images and repetitive behaviors that aim to reduce anxiety. Up to 30% [27] of children and adolescents with obsessive-compulsive disorders are present with ADHD symptoms. The rate of OCD among children with ADHD is 8-11% [28], but that rate is higher among children with Tourrette's disorder. Patient with comorbid ADHD and OCD were characterized by early onset of OCD symptoms. Patients with cormorbid OCD and ADHD symptoms seem to require special care and treatment because the longer those symptoms persist, the more they increase in severity. OCH can be treated with and SSRI, like Prozac, and behavior modification.

Learning disability. *Even when the person is paying attention, is learning difficult? Are there certain subjects that the person has extreme difficulty with? How does this person do in reading, writing, and mathematic? Hs the person ever been tested for a learning disability?*

Preschool children with a learning disability may have difficulty understanding certain sounds or words, or have problems expressing himself or herself in words. School age child may struggle with reading, spelling, writing, or math [11]. Poor school performance may indicate a disability in learning. Testing may be required to determine whether a discrepancy exists between the child's learning potential (intelligence quotient) and his actual academic progress (achievement test scores), indicating the presence of a learning disability [13]. If a child with ADHD also has a learning disability, neuropsychological testing can be done to help determine the best ways to help the child learn. The school can provide an Individualized education program to assist the child in learning.

Substance abuse. *Do you suspect this person smokes, uses drugs and drinks alcohol? Why do you suspect this?*

Substance abuse disorder is common in adult ADHD patients [12]. It can be seen in adolescent patients as well. These patients will demonstrate behaviors of increasing isolation from family and friends. May see the presence of drug paraphernalia. They may use alcohol or drugs to alter their mood state or to escape. There are consequences at school, in the home or authorities related to their use of alcohol or drugs [16]. Drugs may provide temporary relief from the distress caused by the anxiety, social dysfunction, stress and conflict that can result from ADHD. Parents should stay aware in child's social relationships, unexpected changes in mood, and notable declines in academic performances.

It is important to have an accurate diagnosis which involves a combination of physical examination to rule out organic causes (ear infections, elevated lead levels, seizure), behavioral observation and standard tests. Public interest in ADHD has increased along with medical debate in diagnosis and treatment. Some concerns have been emphasized over diagnosis. There is a wide variation of diagnostic criteria and treatment seen among primary care doctors. Primary care physicians should recognize ADHD as a chronic condition, therefore consider children, adolescence, and children with special health care needs. No instrument can replace clinical judgment regarding initial diagnosis and follow up of treatment assessment in children with ADHD. For treatment purposes this varies by age. The specific behavior modification in psychological counseling must be considered in addition to pharmacological treatment titrated to achieve maximum benefit with minimum side effects.

Author details

Nitin Patel*

Address all correspondence to: pateln@health.missouri.edu

University of Missouri-Columbia, Missouri, USA

References

[1] Moore, G. (2012). New guidelines for ADHD. *Chain Drug Review.*, www.findarticles.com/p/articles.141., Accessed 7/2/12.

[2] Low, K. (2012). AHDH Symptoms. Signs, and Symptoms of ADHD. http://add.about.com/od/signs and symptoms/a/sypmtoms.htm, Accessed 7/2/12.

[3] Low, K. (2009). What are the Symptoms of ADD/ADHD/ Diagnostic criteria and symptoms of ADD/ADHD. http://add.about.com/od/evaluationanddiagnosis/a/dsmcriteria.htm.

[4] Jensen, P. S. (2009). Clinical Considerations for the Diagnosis and Treatment of ADHD in the Managed Care Setting. *The AM J of Managed Care.*, 15, 5129-5140.

[5] AHDH: Clinical Practice Guideline for the Diagnosis. (2011). Evaluation and Treatment of Attention-Deficit/Hyperactivity Disorder in Children and Adolescents. Subcommittee on Attention-Deficit/Hyperactivity Disorder, Steering Committee on Quality Improvement and Management. *Pediatrics*, originally published online October 16,, DOI: 10.1542/peds 2011-2654., Accessed 9-13-12.

[6] Wolraich, M. L, Lambert, W, Doffing, M, Bickman, L, Simmons, T, & Worley, K. (2003). Pshcyometric properties of the Vanderbilt ADHD Diagnostic Parent Rating

Scale in a Referred Population. *J Pediatr, Psychol.*, 28(8), 559-568, doi/10.1093/Jpepsy/jsg046.

[7] Connors, C. K. (1969). A teacher rating scale for use in drug studies with children. *American Journal of Psychiatry,*, 126, 884-888.

[8] Barkley Clinical Interview by Barkley RA. (1991). Attention Deficit Hyperactivity Disorder: a clinical workbook.

[9] Langberg, J. M, Vaughn, A. J, Brinkman, W. B, Froehlich, T, & Epstein, J. N. (2010). Clinical Utility of the Vanderbilt ADHD Rating Scale for Ruling Out Comorbid Learning Disorders. *Pediatrics*, 1033-1038, doi: peds.2012-1267.

[10] Low, K. (2011). ADHD Diagnosis-Changes Being Considered. http://add.about.com/od/evaluationand/a/adhd-diagnosis-changes-being-considered., Accessed 7-2-12.

[11] Attention Deficit Hyperactivity Disorder. (2008). National Institute of Mental Health, US Department of Health and Human Services., http://www.nimh.nih.gov/health/topics/index.sht.ml.

[12] Young, J. L. (2010). ADHD and Psychiatric comorbities: Treatment Approaches to Improve Outcomes. Http://.medscape.org/viewarticle/704639., Accessed 6-13-12.

[13] Clinical Practice Guideline: Diagnosis and Evaluation of the child with Attention Deficit/Hyperactivity Disorder Committee on Quality Improvement, Subcommittee on Attention Deficit/Hyperactivity Disorder. Pediatrics. , 105(5), 1158-1170.

[14] Wolraich, M. L, Hannah, J. N, Pinnock, T. Y, Baumgaertel, A, & Brown, J. (1996). Comparison of diagnostic criteria for attention deficit/hyperactivity disorder in a country-wide sample. *J Am Acad Chid Adoles Psychiatry*, 35, 319-324.

[15] Wolraich, M, Hannah, J. N, Baumgaerter, A, Pinnock, T. Y, & Feurer, I. (1998). Examination of DSM-IV criteria for attention deficit/hyperactivity in a country-wide sample. *J Dev Behav Pediatr*, 19, 162-168.

[16] Dobie, C, Donald, W. B, Hanson, M, Hein, C, Huxsahl, J, Karasov, R, Kippes, C, Neumann, A, Spinner, P, Staples, T, & Steiner, L. (2013). Institute for Clinical Systems Improvement. Diagnosis and Management of Attention Deficit Hyperactivity Disorder in Primary Care for School-Age Children and Adolescents. http://bit.ly/ADHD0312., Updated March, Accessed 9-13-12.

[17] Steiner, H, & Remsing, L. (2007). Work Group on Quality Issues. Practice parameters for the assessment and treatment of children and adolescents with oppositional defiant disorder. *J Am Acad Child Adolesc Psychiatry.*, 46, 126-141.

[18] Whittinger, N. S. (2007). Clinical precursors of adolescent conduct disorder in children with attention-deficit/hyperactivity disorder. *J Am Acad Child Adolesc Psychiatry.*, 46, 179-187.

[19] Silver, L. (2006). How to treat Depression in Children with ADHD. *Attitude.*

[20] Fenichel, G. (2009). Clinical Pediatric Neurology A Signs and Symptoms Approach. 6th Ed.

[21] Singh, M. K, DelGEllo, MP, Kowatch, RA, & Strakowski, JM. Co-occurrence of bipolar and attention-deficit hyperactivity disorder in children:. *Bipolar Disorder*, 8, 710-720.

[22] Strober, M, & Carson, G. (1982). Bipolar illness in adolescents with major depression: clinical, genetic, and psycholpharmacologic predictors in three- to four year prospective follow-up investigation. *Arch Gen Psychiatry.*, 39(5), 549-55.

[23] Masi, G, Toni, C, Pergni, G, Travierson, M. C, Millipiedi, S, Mucci, M, & Akiskal, H. S. (2003). Externalizing disorders in consecutively referred children and adolescents with bipolar disorder. *Comprehensive Psychiatry*, 44, 184-189.

[24] Biederman, J, Faron, S. V, Mick, E, et al. (1999). Clinical correlates at ADHD in female: finding from large group of girls ascertained from pediatric and psychiatric referral sources. *J.AM Acad Adols C Psychiatry*, 966-75.

[25] Geller, B, Zimmerman, B, Williams, M, et al. (2002a). DSM-IV mania symptoms in a prepubertal and early onset bipolar disorder phenotype compared to attention-deficit hyperactivity and normal controls. *J Child Adolesc Psychopharmacol*, 12, 11-25.

[26] Kowatch, R. A, Fristad, M, Birmaher, B, Wagner, K. D, Findling, R. L, & Hellander, M. (2005). Child Psychiatric work group on Bipolar disorder. Treatment Guidelines for Children With Bipolar Disorder. *J. Am Acad Child Adolsc Psychiatry*, abstract.

[27] Geller, D. A, Biederman, J, Griffin, S, Jones, J, & Lefkowitz, T. R. (1996). Comorbidity of juvenile obsessive-compulsive disorder with disruptive behavior disorders. *J Am Acad Child Adolesc Psychiatry*, 35, 1637-1646.

[28] Arnold, P. D, Ickowicz, A, Chen, S, & Schachar, R. (2005). Attention-deficit hyperactivity disorder with and without obsessive-compulsive behaviours: clinical characteristics, cognitive assessment, and risk factors. *Can J Psychiatry*, 50, 59-66.

[29] Patel, N, Patel, M, & Patel, H. (2012). ADHD and Comorbid Conditions. *Attention Deficit Hyperactivity Disorder/ Book 1*,, 978-9-53307-756-7, March, 2012,, 25-46.

Chapter 8

Review of Tools Used for Assessing Teachers' Level of Knowledge with Regards Attention Deficit Hyperactivity Disorder (ADHD)

Marian Soroa, Arantxa Gorostiaga and
Nekane Balluerka

Additional information is available at the end of the chapter

http://dx.doi.org/10.5772/54277

1. Introduction

ADHD is currently one of most widely studied neuro-developmental disorders in children and adolescents. It is a severe disorder that can cause grave problems for sufferers and those around them. The interest in the study of ADHD in the scientific community is undeniable, as proved by the multitude of articles and books on the subject published annually. As indicated by Lavigne and Romero [1], interest in this condition is such that it has breached the boundaries of academic research and study and has become a social phenomenon in itself, to such an extent that any child who shows a certain degree of activity, who does not remain seated and quiet for hours and does not instantly obey each and every instruction he or she receives is immediately suspected of having ADHD. The readiness with which children are labeled as having ADHD is surely due, in part, to the lack of information about the various factors apart from ADHD, that cause lack of attention, hyperactivity and/or impulsiveness.

Neither are teachers free from the tendency to attribute ADHD to too many children in spite of having greater possibilities of obtaining more reliable information about ADHD either through professional articles and books, training courses or other professionals at their schools that work with pupils with ADHD, etc. Despite this greater ease of access to information, various studies have shown that teachers' knowledge of ADHD could be improved [2-7]. Furthermore the knowledge teachers have about ADHD is also the source of ever greater interest among scientists as they are actors with a key role in the development of the condition. The training of educators in this area is of direct benefit to students with ADHD and their families. For this reason, in order to find out exactly what level of knowledge teachers have about this problem it is crucial to have assessment tools with appropriate psychometric properties, that are reliable and valid and that provide accurate data about teachers' knowledge of ADHD.

In this chapter, the fundamental reasons for which teachers have to have a basic level of knowledge of ADHD are examined, an exhaustive analysis is carried out of the main instruments which have been developed to assess teachers' knowledge of ADHD, and the chapter ends with the main conclusions drawn from this study.

2. ADHD and teachers

ADHD is currently one of the disorders that has generated the largest number of research studies among the scientific community but despite this, in the words of Barkley [8], a lot remains unknown or misunderstood about it. Teachers, along with the family, are one of the most important agents of socialization during infancy, so they are one of the most suitable groups to receive information and training with regard to ADHD. A significant percentage of teachers have false ideas or gaps in their knowledge of ADHD, which causes them to behave inappropriately in the classroom. In this regard, it has been observed that specific training of teachers in the field and positive attitudes on their part have positive consequences for children with ADHD.

Soroa, Balluerka and Gorostiaga [9] hold that infant and primary school teachers should have general and specific knowledge about ADHD for six fundamental reasons. Firstly, because ADHD is one of the most common psychological disorders among children. The American Psychiatric Association [10] indicates that between 3% and 5% of school children suffer from ADHD, that is to say that on average there is one pupil with ADHD in every classroom of 25 [11-13].

Secondly, teachers are in a uniquely advantageous position for detecting possible cases of ADHD. They can pretty accurately distinguish normal development from what is not. Therefore, increasing teachers' knowledge about ADHD can facilitate, among other factors, early detection of the disorder and the application of the appropriate treatment [4, 14].

Thirdly, it should be noted that the role of the teacher is also essential in establishing the diagnosis. The assessments made of the behavior of the students, along with those of the parents and the results of other tests to which children are subjected, are part of the data that allow the diagnosis to be established [4-6].

Fourthly, it should be noted that teachers play a very important role in the implementation, evaluation and support of the treatment received by children with ADHD [14]. Their cooperation is necessary for the results of the treatment received by the child to be successful, and their evaluation of and opinions about the treatment of ADHD have a profound effect on its efficacy [15].

A fifth reason for teachers to be trained about ADHD lies in direct contact they have with the parents of the children. Several authors have argued that teachers make recommendations, appropriate or inappropriate, about ADHD to the parents, who tend to follow such recommendations [14, 16].

The sixth and final reason is that the knowledge that teachers have about ADHD affects their behavior and attitudes towards children with this condition [17]. Teachers with more knowledge about ADHD have a more favorable conduct and attitudes towards students with this disorder [3, 16, 18].

In spite of the existence of many reasons why teachers should have knowledge on ADHD, various studies have shown that, in general, teachers show only moderate knowledge of ADHD and that it is necessary to improve this level of knowledge [3-6, 19, 20]. Also it must be noted that many teachers present a general lack of knowledge and/or false ideas on the nature, course, consequences, causes and treatment of ADHD [21]. In some research programmes the average percentage of correct answers by teachers to questionnaires prepared in order to measure their knowledge on ADHD was around 80% [14, 18, 22-24], while in other studies the average percentage of correct answers did not exceed 53% [4-6, 20, 25]. At world level there is much research in progress on the knowledge that teachers have on ADHD; however, there is a scarcity of instruments to measure this knowledge precisely [9].

It has been found that teachers who consider that their level of knowledge about ADHD is optimum do not seek additional information; in contrast, those who consider that they do not understand many aspects referring to this topic, do look for it. For this reason, it is important that the teachers should be aware of their actual knowledge about ADHD and the possible repercussions of a lack of knowledge or erroneous knowledge. For this purpose, it is essential to use evaluation instruments which have appropriate psychometric properties for measuring such knowledge.

3. Instruments for assessing the level of knowledge of teachers regarding ADHD

Over recent decades, many instruments have been developed in order to assess the level of knowledge of teachers regarding ADHD. Given that the school setting is probably the place where children and young people spend most of the day, it is important to have a range of instruments to measure teacher knowledge about ADHD throughout the different stages of child development. These instruments, in addition to identifying gaps that teachers may have in their knowledge of the disorder, can be useful to educate the teachers about the need for more training in this area.

In this section a review is carried out of each of the main instruments developed for the evaluation of teachers' knowledge about ADHD. In the course of the description of each instrument their general characteristics are set out (the construct evaluated, items, response format, dimensionality, etc.), as well as their scoring rules and psychometric properties. Their strengths and weaknesses are also evaluated. The instruments are presented in chronological order.

3.1. ADHD Knowledge Scale (Jerome, Gordon & Hustler, 1994) [23]

3.1.1. Description and development

This instrument was developed by American and Canadian researchers, in the English language, in order to assess the general knowledge of teachers regarding ADHD. It consists of two sections, the first includes 20 items that are socio-demographic in nature (age, sex, training about ADHD, etc.) in a multiple choice format, and a second section with 20 items, 13 positive and 7 negative, with a dichotomous (True/False) response format.

In the preparation of the questionnaire, the authors contacted several teachers and directors of special education to review the instrument. The authors do not provide more information about the process.

The instrument was applied to a sample of 1289 elementary school teachers, 439 in the United States and 850 in Canada. No information is given about the sampling procedure. 46% of the sample in the United States was made up of teachers from the state of New York school district, and 54% by teachers from Broward County in Florida. The majority were women (86%), aged between 31 and 50 (67%) and had been teachers for 9 or more years. 79% taught the general school population in ordinary classes while 21% were special education teachers. The Canadian sample consisted of teachers from a wide area of south west Ontario and no further information is given by the authors about it.

3.1.2. Scoring rules

Correct answers receive 1 point and incorrect ones 0 points. So the range of possible scores goes from 0, the lowest level of knowledge, to 20, for the highest.

3.1.3. Psychometric properties

No publications have been found which provide validity evidences or reliability indices.

3.1.4. Strengths and weaknesses

This is believed to be the first study designed to test the knowledge of elementary school teachers about ADHD. A great number of subsequent studies have used this questionnaire or been inspired by it due to its simplicity and that the fact that it was a pioneer in the field that concerns us here. Furthermore, the sample used is very broad and heterogeneous. However, the response format is dichotomous, so does not provide detailed information about the real knowledge the teachers have about ADHD. Furthermore, the psychometric properties of the questionnaire are not provided.

3.2. Knowledge of Attention Deficit Disorder Questionnaire (Riley, 1994) [26]

3.2.1. Description and development

This is an instrument drawn up in the United States and in the English language to investigate teachers', counselors' and principals' knowledge of ADHD in school age children. The instrument has two sections. The first is made up of six items that gather information of a socio-demographic character (sex, training, education experience, etc.) and a second made up of 35 items which evaluates participants' knowledge of ADHD. The 35 items were taken from the DSM-III: 15 related to Attention Deficit Disorder (ADD), 11 related to diagnostic criteria for Conduct Disorder (CD) and 9 that deal with Oppositional Defiant Disorder (ODD). Participants are asked to identify the 15 statements that best characterize children with ADHD with an X marking the space before each statement.

The instrument was applied to a stratified sample of 303 participants in the Kansas School district: 160 teachers, 61 principals and 82 counselors. 91 were male and 212 female. Hardly any other information is given about the sample.

3.2.2. Scoring standards

Correct answers to the items received 1 point, while the rest of the answers received 0 points. Thus, the possible scores ranged from 0, for the lowest level of knowledge, to 15, for the highest.

3.2.3. Psychometric properties

No publications have been found which provide validity evidences or reliability indices.

3.2.4. Strengths and weaknesses

This is a simple and easy instrument to apply. The problem is that the response format is similar to the dichotomous one and respondents can try to guess the right answer. Furthermore, the psychometric properties of the instrument are not known.

3.3. ADHD Knowledge Questionnaire (Barbaresi & Olsen, 1998) [21]

3.3.1. Description and development

This is an instrument developed in the United States and in the English language in order to examine the effectiveness of a training program on ADHD given to infant and primary school teachers. The questionnaire is based on the items produced by Jerome et al. [23] and consists of two sections: A first socio-demographic section and a second section consisting of 27 items that assess teachers' knowledge regarding ADHD. The response format of the instrument is dichotomous (True, False), and includes positive and negative items (the authors do not specify the number of positive and negative items).

The questionnaire was administered to 44 teachers, of whom 33 were women and 11 men. The mean age of participants was 42 years, and they had an average of 15 years of teaching experience. 66% were ordinary classroom teachers while the remaining 34% were specialists (art, music, physical education, etc.). They had an average of 24 students per teacher. 77% had not received any training on ADHD while being trained as teachers and 27% had received no training in the subject after completion of their studies.

3.3.2. Scoring standards

Correct answers received a score of 1 and incorrect ones 0. Thus, the possible scores ranged from 0, for the lowest level of knowledge, to 27, for the highest.

3.3.3. Psychometric properties

No publications have been found which provide validity evidences or reliability indices.

3.3.4. Strengths and weaknesses

This is a simple and easy instrument to apply. However, the sample is very small and the dichotomous response format (True/False) places limits on the possibility of assessing the real level of knowledge of the teachers as the absence of a third (Don't Know) option invites respondents to guess the right answer. Furthermore, the psychometric properties of the instrument are not known.

3.4. The Knowledge of Attention Deficit Disorders Scale (KADDS)

3.4.1. Original version of The Knowledge of Attention Deficit Disorders Scale (KADDS) (Sciutto, Terjesen & Bender, 2000) [5]

3.4.1.1. Description and development

It was developed in the United States and in the English language. This is one of the most widely used instruments to assess the level of knowledge of teachers regarding ADHD, and is the first instrument whose indices of reliability and validity were published in this field. It consists of 36 items, 18 positive and 18 negative, and measures three areas of knowledge related to ADHD: 1) Symptoms/Diagnosis of ADHD (9 items), 2) General information on the nature, causes and impact of ADHD (15 items), and 3) Treatment of ADHD (12 items). It has a three option response format (True, False, Don't Know), which allows it to overcome the limits of previously used dichotomous formats (True, False) and collect more detailed information about the knowledge of teachers with respect to ADHD. The use of the three option response format allows the authors to discern those areas in which teachers have more knowledge, areas where they have the least knowledge and the areas in which they commit the greatest number of errors.

In the drawing up of the items the authors strove to include only those with the support of the scientific literature, citing references for each item in the manual accompanying the instrument. They also sought to include positive and negative aspects relating to ADHD, and positive and negative statements in nature.

Once they had drawn up the items the authors contacted a group of 40 students working for doctorates in clinical and child psychology. The participants, based on the three sub-scales provided by the authors, had to assign each item to one of the sub-scales provided. An item was considered as belonging to a particular sub-scale if at least 75% of the group was in agreement with the decision.

The authors then conducted a series of preliminary investigations to explore the reliability coefficients of the instrument. They administered an instrument of 27 items with a dichotomous response format (True, False) to 73 teachers of kindergartens and elementary schools [27] and obtained a *Cronbach's alpha* of 0.38 for the total scale. In a subsequent study they modified the items that had an inadequate item-total correlation and incorporated the three option (True, False, Don't Know) response format. The resulting scale was administered to 46 undergraduate and graduate education students and the overall *alpha* coefficient obtained for this version was 0.71 [27]. Several items were reformulated and 9 new items were included in the final version of the instrument which now had 36 items and which Bender [28] administered to 63 prospective elementary teachers, obtaining a coefficient *alpha* of 0.81.

Finally, Sciutto et al. [5] administered the resulting 36 item scale along with a socio-demographic questionnaire (age, sex, teaching experience, teaching speciality, etc.) and a scale of seven points dealing with respondents' self-perception of their effectiveness as teachers of children with ADHD to a broader sample. 149 primary school teachers from six public schools participated in the validation of the instrument. The sampling procedure is not explained. There were 134 female and 9 male participants; the sex of six participants was not given. Their average age was 41 years (*SD*=11.43) and they had an average of 12.57 years of experience as teachers (*SD*=8.06). 19% of the sample were special needs teachers and 37% said they had done special needs teaching at some point. 79% of participants had a Master's degree, whereas the other 21% reported having a Bachelor's degree. With regard to ADHD, 52% of the teachers said that had taught at least one pupil who had been diagnosed with this condition.

It is worth pointing out that Sciutto and Terjesen [29] carried out an additional study on primary school teachers and university students in the state of Ohio to expand the reliability and the evidence of validity of KADDS. This study has not been published and no more data is available about the sample. However, the authors refer to this study along with the study Sciutto, Nolfi & Bluhm [30] carried out on primary school teachers with the KADDS manual.

3.4.1.2. Scoring standards

1 point was given for correct answers and 0 for incorrect ones and gaps in knowledge. Thus, the possible scores ranged from 0, for the lowest level of knowledge, to 36, for the highest.

3.4.1.3. *Psychometric properties*

For reliability analysis, internal consistency was first calculated, producing a *Cronbach's alpha* of 0.71 for each sub-scale and 0.86 for the scale as a whole. Furthermore, it was also seen that each KADDS sub-scale had a high correlation with the total KADDS score (range r=0.85 to r=0.91) and that there was a correlation between the three sub-scales (range r=0.63 to r=0.69). In order to analyze the stability of the scale, Sciutto and Terjesen [29] administered the KADDS in two occasions to a group of 185 university students (what they were students of is not stated) leaving an interval of two weeks between one application and the other. The test-retest correlations for the KADDS scores range between r=0.59 and r=0.70 for the three sub-scales and were r=0.76 for the scale as a whole.

No test was carried out on the factorial structure of the instrument. In order to find evidence of validity, the correlations between the scale scores and a series of variable related to the construct to be measured were examined. With regard to the previous exposure of teachers in their classrooms to pupils diagnosed with ADHD, statistically significant differences were found in the KADDS scores obtained (p<0.01), as well as in various sub-scales (p<0.01 for the General information and Symptoms/Diagnosis sub-scales). The same occurred with the university students who knew a person with ADHD. In the KADDS and the Treatment sub-scale they achieved significantly higher scores (p<0.01) than those that had no contact whatever with people with ADHD [29]. Furthermore the authors of the KADDS have pointed out that the scores obtained by the teachers on the scale correlated in a statistically significant and positive way with the number of ADHD students that had in their classes (r=0.23, p<0.01 for the New York sample and r=0.31, p<0.01 for the Ohio sample in the KADDS total) [5, 30]. In this case, the same phenomenon also occurred with the university students that had some kind of contact with people with ADHD (r=0.18, p<0.01 for the KADDS total) [29]. Finally, they found that people with more information about ADHD had higher KADDS scores, both in the case of teachers (r=0.40, p<0.001 for the KADDS total) [30] and in the case of university students (r=0.36, p<0.001 for the total KADDS score) [29].

3.4.1.4. *Strengths and weaknesses*

Considering that the validation of the KADDS was carried out mainly based on the study of Sciutto et al. [5], it should be emphasized that the sample used is fairly small in size and geographically homogenous. Furthermore, the specific data from the Ohio sample are not known [29].

The reliability of the KADDS was analyzed satisfactorily. As to evidence of validity, we believe that it could be improved but this is understandable considering it was the first instrument constructed to assess knowledge of teachers regarding ADHD whose psychometric properties have been published. The authors provide information on content validity, thanks to which it is known that they tried to be careful in their selection of test items but they do not provide detailed information about the construction of the instrument (number of items initially created, etc.), and the panel of experts consulted in the process for getting content validity was fairly homogeneous (students in the same doctoral program). Furthermore, there is no factorial analysis which would justify the sub-scales defended by the authors of the KADDS.

In any case we regard the instrument developed by Sciutto et al. [5] to be a significant reference point for any researcher trying to create one with a similar purpose because it was a pioneering effort in the field with good reliability and sufficient external validity. As well as that, it is an instrument that is easy to answer due to its brief and precise instructions, its small size and its three option response format. It is also worth mentioning that it has a simple scoring system and thanks to the aforementioned response format, it provides information regarding the knowledge, false beliefs and areas of lack of knowledge of the teachers, information which the previous instruments, with their dichotomous response format, could not provide.

3.4.2. The Spanish version of The Knowledge of Attention Deficit Disorders Scale (KADDS) (Jarque, Tárraga & Miranda, 2007) [4]

3.4.2.1. Description and development

This is the Spanish adaptation of the KADDS [5]. Like the original instrument it has 36 items, 18 positive and 18 negative, and it measures three areas of knowledge related to ADHD: 1) Symptoms/Diagnosis of ADHD (9 items), 2) General information on the nature, causes and impact of ADHD (15 items), and 3) Treatment of ADHD (12 items). The three option response format (True, False, Don't Know) is the same as that of the original instrument and it has a more extensive socio-demographic section than the original instrument (age, sex, years of experience as a teacher, teaching speciality, etc.).

In the first phase of the adaptation process of the instrument, two doctoral students in developmental and educational psychology translated KADDS into Spanish making the adjustments required for the new socio-cultural context. After that, native speakers of English translated the text back into English to test the validity of the original translation. In this second phase the authors found 18 words different from the original version and agreed on a final version of the translation of those words and drew up initial version of the instrument. The initial version was sent to 15 experts in ADHD (ADHD researchers and educational psychologists) who were asked to place each of the items on one of the three sub-scales that make up the instrument. The level of agreement on the assignment of items to the sub-scales was 94%. Finally, a pilot study was conducted on a sample of 35 primary school teachers who were asked to reply to the scale and indicate errata, difficulties to understand expressions or doubts that may have arisen during completion of the questionnaire. Corrections were made and the final version was thus produced.

For the analysis of reliability and validity of the final version of the instrument, the authors contacted various public and subsidized schools in the province of Valencia. The sampling was not random. The Spanish version of the KADDS was administered to 193 teachers, 68 from infant education and 125 from primary education, of whom 130 were women and 43 men (20 teachers did not specify their sex). They had a mean age of 42 years (SD=11.40), and an average of 17 years of teaching experience (SD=12.03). 13.8% were special education teachers. 51.6% had received specific training on ADHD, with an average of 7.80 hours (*SD*=17) training. In addition, 59.1% of the teachers had had some experience teaching children with ADHD, and the average number of children with ADHD that they had in their classrooms during the previous two school years was 1.39 (*SD*=1.89).

3.4.2.2. Scoring standards

Identical to KADDS [5].

3.4.2.3. Psychometric properties

The reliability of the scale, measured by the *Cronbach's alpha* coefficient showed adequate internal consistency. The *alpha* coefficient ranged between 0.74 and 0.77 for the three sub-scales and was 0.89 for the total scale. These rates were higher than those obtained by Sciutto et al. [5] in the original instrument. In addition, each of the sub-scales showed a high correlation with the total scale score (range r=0.85 to r=0.90), and there also was correlation between the three sub-scales (range r=0.62 to r=0.69). These data are also consistent with those provided by Sciutto et al. [5]. There was no test-retest reliability check conducted.

The validity of the scale was studied using a series of *Pearson correlations* between teacher knowledge of ADHD and various socio-demographic variables, specifically, teachers' knowledge of ADHD correlated in a statistically significant way with the number of hours of training they had received, $r(152)$=0.17, p=0.036; with the number of children with ADHD they had taught, $r(180)$=0.29, p=0.001; with the number of courses during which they had children with ADHD in their classes, $r(172)$=0.23, p=0.002; and their self-perceived level of effectiveness as teachers of children with ADHD, $r(179)$=0.50, p=0.001.

3.4.2.4. Strengths and weaknesses

The sample used for the KADDS adaptation was quite small and geographically homogeneous. Also, test-retest reliability was not checked and the factorial structure of the scale was not analyzed. Apart from these weaknesses and those mentioned in the original version of KADDS, it should be noted that the instrument has adequate internal consistency and some evidence of external validity.

3.5. Attention-Deficit Hyperactivity Disorder Knowledge and Opinion Survey (AKOS-IV) – Knowledge Scale (Power & Rostain, 2003) [31]

3.5.1. Description and development

This instrument was developed in the United States in the English language and consists of 21 items, 8 positive and 13 negative with a dichotomous response format (True, False). The lead author of AKOS-IV participated in the development of different versions of the instrument. The first version was designed to analyze the level of knowledge among parents regarding ADHD [see 32]. There is a lack of published information about the second version. The third version was used to assess the level of knowledge that teachers of primary and secondary education have regarding ADHD [33], and the fourth and final version [31] has not been published, so its target population is unknown.

3.5.2. Scoring standards

1 point was given for correct answers and 0 for incorrect ones and gaps in knowledge. Thus, the possible scores ranged from 0, for the lowest level of knowledge, to 21, for the highest.

3.5.3. Psychometric properties

No publications have been found which provide validity evidences or reliability indices.

3.5.4. Strengths and weaknesses

On the positive side, it should be noted that the questionnaire is short and simple to complete, but it uses a response format with two options (True, False) which can lead to a bias in the collection of information as those subjects who did not know what to answer are required to choose one of the two alternatives provided. In addition, there is a lack of published information relating to the development of the instrument and its psychometric properties.

3.6. Attention Deficit Hyperactivity Disorder and Stimulant Medication Survey (Snider, Busch & Arrowood, 2003) [34].

3.6.1. Description and development

This is an instrument developed in the United States in the English language and it is aimed at primary school and special education teachers. Its aim is to test their knowledge of the nature of ADHD and its treatment through stimulant medication. The questionnaire is divided into six sections. The first consists of 8 socio-demographic items: The number of students the teacher has, the number of students diagnosed with ADHD, years of teaching experience, etc. The second section is made up of 47 Likert scale items with 5 options (1=Strongly Disagree, 2=Disagree; 3=Neutral/Don't know, 4=Agree, 5=Strongly Agree) divided into three blocks: A first block of 13 items to assess factual knowledge about ADHD and the use of stimulant medication, a second block of 23 items that asked participants to indicate their views about the effects of stimulant medication on classroom behavior, and a third block of 11 items assessing teachers' experience and involvement with students who have ADHD. In the third section the subjects have to state which sources they regard as most reliable for obtaining information about ADHD. In the fourth section they had to state which people usually recommend that children suspected of having ADHD be evaluated by. In the fifth section the teachers are asked about what teaching techniques they have most frequently used for dealing with children with ADHD. In the sixth and final section, there is an open question which enquires about teachers' opinions regarding the use of stimulant medication for the treatment of students with ADHD.

The pilot version was administered to 15 teachers participating in a graduate clinical experience at the University of Wisconsin. Small changes were made in the wording of the items and it was confirmed that the time required to respond to the questionnaire was about 10 to 15 minutes.

The definitive version of the questionnaire was administered to 145 teachers in Wisconsin, 29 women and 116 men. The subjects were randomly chosen from the Department of Public Instruction. Among the participants 43% were special education teachers and 30% general education teachers. The teachers had an average of 16.5 years of teaching experience (SD=9.46).

3.6.2. Scoring standards

Not provided.

3.6.3. Psychometric properties

No publications have been found which provide validity evidences or reliability indices.

3.6.4. Strengths and weaknesses

On the positive side, it should be noted that this is a questionnaire with clear instructions and is easy to fill out. However, the response format used by the authors (Likert 5 options) may complicate the interpretation of the results, since it offers the option to partially agree or disagree with the questionnaire items. Moreover, the sample used for the application of the instrument was small and geographically homogeneous, and the psychometric properties of the instrument are not known. Finally, it should be noted that one of the main objectives of the questionnaire was to analyze teachers' knowledge of stimulant medication, a very specific purpose and one distinct from the object of study of the other questionnaires that have been examined in this chapter.

3.7. Attention Deficit Hyperactivity Disorder (ADHD) Questionnaire (Kos, Richdale & Jackson, 2004) [20]

3.7.1. Description and development

This instrument was drawn up in Australia in the English language to test the perceived and real knowledge of primary teachers and trainee teachers of ADHD. Section b) of the questionnaire was drawn up to examine this main point and contains some items from Jerome et al. [23], Sciutto et al. [5] and another series of items taken from the scientific literature related to ADHD. The instrument was made up of 131 items divided into six sections. Section a) collects information on socio-demographic aspects of the sample and included an analog scale of 10 cm on which respondents had to indicate what they thought they knew about ADHD. The bottom end of this scale indicates the minimum level of knowledge (Very Little), while the upper level indicates the maximum level (A Lot). Section b) includes 27 items, 11 positive and 16 negative, with a three option response format (True, False, Don't know) drawn up to assess respondents real knowledge of ADHD. Section c) has a focus on identifying the teaching strategies which subjects might use with pupils with ADHD. For this purpose they were given a brief description of a practical case and a series of multiple choice and open questions. Section d) collects information about participants' beliefs about ADHD and the possibility of having pupils with it in their classes. For this purpose it had 31 items which required a response on an analog scale of 10 cm the bottom of which indicated complete agreement with the statement (Strongly Agree) and the top of which indicated complete disagreement (Strongly Disagree). Section e) was designed to evaluate beliefs regarding the different strategies for action possible in classes with pupils with ADHD. It has 56 items divided into various sub-sections to which respondents had to respond on 10 cm analogical scales the bottom ends of which indicated complete agreement (Strongly Agree) and the upper ends of which indicated complete disagreement (Strongly Disagree). Finally, section f) includes two multiple choice items to which subjects have to respond regarding whether or not they want more training on ADHD and to specify the way they believe most appropriate to find out more about ADHD.

The questionnaire was revised by two educational and developmental psychologists not associated with the study. It was later piloted on a sample of 9 primary school teachers from Victoria (Australia), arising from which no change was made. The questionnaire was finally administered to 120 primary school teachers in Victoria, 91 women and 29 men with an average age of 39.2 years (*SD*=10.2), and 45 students in the last year of their education degree, all women and with an average age of 23.6 years (*SD*=5.6). The sampling procedure was not explained.

3.7.2. Scoring standards

Section b) of the questionnaire had 27 items. Correct responses received a score of 1 and incorrect ones, 0. Thus, the possible scores ranged from 0, for the minimum level of knowledge, to 27, for the maximum level. The scoring standards for the other sections were not given.

3.7.3. Psychometric properties

No publications have been found which provide validity evidences or reliability indices.

3.7.4. Strengths and weaknesses

On the positive side, it should be noted that the authors have attempted to develop an instrument that collects a variety of information relating to ADHD. However, the instrument has many weaknesses: The sample used is quite small and geographically homogeneous, the information given relating to the development of the instrument is scant, the presentation of the items and response formats vary from one section to another, and there are questions with 34 possible answers and analog scales of 10 cm which make it difficult to interpret the response provided by the subject. In short, it is a long and complex questionnaire for the subject. Additionally, the psychometric properties are not known.

3.8. Knowledge of ADHD Rating Evaluation (KARE) (Vereb & DiPerna, 2004) [35]

3.8.1. Description and development

This instrument was developed in the United States and in the English language. Its purpose is to analyze the knowledge that elementary school teachers have about ADHD and assess their level of acceptance with respect to the medication and behaviorist treatments that are used with children with ADHD. The instrument is divided into three sections. The first section collects socio-demographic data. The second section consists of 43 items, positive and negative in nature (the authors do not specify the number of each), and is divided into two sub-scales: A first sub-scale assesses knowledge of the etiology, symptoms and prognosis of ADHD (31 items), and a second sub-scale assesses knowledge about treatments that are used most frequently in ADHD cases (12 items). The third and final section consists of 10 items divided into two sub-scales: The first sub-scale assesses the level of acceptance that subjects presented with respect to medication (5 items), and the second sub-scale assesses the level of acceptance of the behavioral intervention guidelines used with children with ADHD (5 items). The second section of the instrument has a response format of three options (True, False, Don't Know) and the third section, being an opinion section, has a Likert-type response format of 4 options (1=Not at all Likely, 2=Somewhat Likely, 3=Moderately Likely, 4=Very Likely).

The preliminary version of the instrument was made up of 59 items. 20 experts, members of the International Society for Research in Child and Adolescent Psychopatology who had conducted research in the area of ADHD and/or treatment acceptability were called upon to revise it. The items that received a negative evaluation from these experts were modified or removed.

Finally, the study was carried out on 47 elementary school teachers in five different districts of Pennsylvania and New Jersey. The sampling procedure was not specified. 94% of the sample was female and had an average of 13 years of teaching experience (*SD*=8.76). 85% of the teachers were general teachers, while 4.35% worked in special education and 10.6% worked in both areas.

3.8.2. Scoring standards

In the second section of the instrument 1 point was given for correct answers and 0 for incorrect ones and gaps in knowledge. Thus, the possible scores ranged from 0, for the lowest level of knowledge, to 43, for the highest. The scoring standards for the third section of the questionnaire are unknown.

3.8.3. Psychometric properties

For the reliability analysis, the internal consistency was first calculated, obtaining a *Cronbach's alpha* coefficient that ranged from 0.58 (Knowledge of treatments sub-scale) to 0.81 (Behavioral management acceptability sub-scale) for the four sub-scales in the questionnaire.

In order to analyze the stability of the instrument, the authors administered the KARE a second time to a sample of 24 subjects (without further details being given of the sample) with a time interval of four weeks between the first and the second administration. The test-retest reliability ranged from 0.76 (Behavioral management acceptability sub-scale) to 0.80 (Medication acceptability and Knowledge of treatment sub-scales).

No publications have been found which provide validity evidences.

3.8.4. Strengths and weaknesses

On the positive side, it should be noted that this is a not too long instrument with response formats that are easy to fill out. It also has an acceptable internal consistency for three of the four subs-scales that compose it, and has good test-retest stability. However, the sample used for obtaining the reliability indices is small, and no published validity evidences of the instrument have been found.

3.9. Educator ADHD knowledge (Niznik, 2004) [36]

3.9.1. Description and development

This instrument was drawn up in the United States in the English language. The main purpose of it is to assess the level of knowledge of elementary school teachers regarding ADHD before and after they received a specific training program on the subject. The instrument consists of 23 items and has a multiple choice format: Each item is followed by five possible answers, one correct and four distractors.

In the course of its development process, the instrument was administered to 10 doctors working as psychologists in the Cypress-Fairbanks school district (Texas) to receive their feedback. Adjustments have been made for a better understanding of the items and response options (the authors did not provide further details). The test authors also conducted a pilot study with 133 participants (no further description were given of the sample), as a result of which a number of items were removed.

The resulting instrument was administered to 47 elementary school teachers in the Cypress-Fairbanks school district. 91.5% of the participants were female and 8.5% male. 55.3% of them were general teachers while 44.7% were special education teachers. The age of the teachers ranged from 18 upwards, and they had an average of 11 years teaching experience. 30% of the sample had never received training about ADHD, and 95.7% had a child in their classroom with the disorder diagnosed in recent years.

3.9.2. Scoring standards

1 point was given for each correct answer so the possible scores ranged from 0, for the lowest level of knowledge, to 23, for the highest level.

3.9.3. Psychometric properties

The reliability of the instrument was calculated using the *Kuder-Richardson formula 20*, and a reliability of 0.65 was obtained. No publications have been found that provide validity evidences.

3.9.4. Strengths and weaknesses

On the positive side, it should be noted that this is a not too long instrument with a novel response format in the field that concerns us. However, the authors provide few details about the construction process of the test, the sample that has been used with the final instrument is quite small and homogeneous, and has a low reliability index. Furthermore, the validity evidences of the instrument were not provided.

3.10. The knowledge about Attention Deficit Disorder Questionnaire (KADD-Q) (West, Taylor, Houghton & Hudyma, 2005) [6]

3.10.1. Description and development

This is an instrument that was drawn up in Australia in the English language in order to assess the knowledge about ADHD of primary and secondary teachers and parents of children with the same condition. It consists of a scale of 67 items, constructed on the basis of 20 items from the KADDS [5]. It has a three option response format (True, False, Don't Know) and measures three areas of knowledge connected to ADHD: 1) Causes of ADHD, 2) Characteristics of ADHD, and 3) Treatment of ADHD. Like the KADDS scale it has positive and negative items, and for the drawing up of which the authors made efforts to use only those items with support in the scientific literature.

The KADD-Q authors obtained the sample needed for the analysis of reliability and validity of the scale by making a random selection of schools in metropolitan Perth (Western Australia) and by way of the Centre for Attention and Related Disorders of The University of Western Australia. The sample consisted of 348 participants: 256 teachers (51% primary and 43% secondary) and 92 parents. Of the teachers involved in the sample, 22% were male and 78% female. 180 teachers were recruited in their workplaces and had an average of 20.2 years (*SD*=10.3) of teaching experience, the remaining 76 teachers were recruited through the Centre for Attention and Related Disorders, and had an average amount of teaching experience of 15.8 years (*SD*=10). 96% of teachers said they had a student with ADHD in the classroom at some point and 20% were qualified in special education. As for the group of 92 parents participating in the study, it should be noted that 8% were male and 92% female. In addition, the average age at which their child had been diagnosed with ADHD was 10.3 years (*SD*=3.1). 23% of the parents were attending a support group for parents of children with ADHD and 31% had attended informational seminars about ADHD in the preceding 12 months.

3.10.2. Scoring standards

In the SPSS statistical package correct answers were coded with a 1, incorrect ones with a 0, and the gaps as a missing value. Possible answers ranged from 0, for the minimum level of knowledge, to 67, for the maximum level.

3.10.3. Psychometric properties

The reliability of the KADD-Q and its sub-scales was estimated using *Cronbach's alpha* coefficient. The results suggest that the internal consistency of the KADD-Q is high for the sample of teachers (*alpha*=0.91) and parents (*alpha*=0.93). For the sub-scales Causes, Characteristics and Treatment, *alphas* obtained were of 0.86, 0.80 and 0.79 for teachers and 0.85, 0.84 and 0.84 for the parents, respectively. In addition, each of the sub-scales of the KADD-Q had a high correlation with the total scale score (range r=0.73 to 0.92) in both the sample of teachers and parents. There were moderate correlations between the three sub-scales of teachers in the sample (range r=0.34 to 0.56), and somewhat ones higher in the sample of parents (range r=0.56 to 0.77). There was no test test-retest reliability conducted.

Convergent validity was not evaluated, nor was any test of the factorial structure of the instrument made. The scale authors present data on a series of relationships that exist between the scale scores and several variables related to the construct they purport to measure, which provide certain information concerning the external validity. The level of teachers' knowledge about ADHD was significantly higher depending on the stage of their profession they were at. Primary school teachers obtained higher scores than their secondary education colleagues (p=0.001). Teachers who had attended to professional development sessions about ADHD in the previous 12 months and those who had specific training in special education had higher scores on the scale (p<0.001 and p=0.024, respectively).

3.10.4. Strengths and weaknesses

On the positive side, it is noteworthy that the authors of KADD-Q have tried to create a single instrument to assess the knowledge of teachers in primary and secondary education and the parents of children with ADHD. This instrument has an easily completed response format and has good internal consistency. However, the teachers and parents samples used for the study were small and geographically homogeneous, the information relating to the development of the instrument is scant, the instrument lacks test-retest reliability indices, evidence of convergent validity is not provided, and nor is there any factorial analysis to confirm the presence of the three sub-scales of the instrument. To all this must be added the fact that data concerning the external validity of the instrument are scarce.

3.11. Teacher knowledge about ADHD (Jones & Chronis-Tuscano, 2008) [24]

3.11.1. Description and development

This instrument was drawn up in the United States and in the English language for the purpose of assessing teachers' knowledge of ADHD after they have receiving training related to it. It consists of 25 items with a dichotomous response format (True, False). The items were designed to cover six areas of content: 1) Causes of ADHD, 2) Assessment of ADHD, 3) ADHD sub-types, 4) Associated problems of ADHD, 5) Treatment of ADHD, and 6) Specific school-based behavioral strategies for children with ADHD.

The questionnaire was administered to a non-random sample of 142 elementary school teachers in the Washington DC metropolitan area, of whom 74 belonged to the experimental group receiving training in ADHD and the remaining 68 to a control group that did not receive such training. The average age of all participants in the sample was about 37 years (*SD*=12.45) and they had an average amount of teaching experience of 11.34 years (*SD*=10.40). 92% were women and only 17% were special education teachers. Approximately 34% of the sample had had experience of a child with ADHD in their classroom.

3.11.2. Scoring standards

1 point was given for correct answers and 0 for incorrect ones, so the range of possible scores went from 0, for the lowest possible level, to 25, for the highest possible level.

3.11.3. Psychometric properties

Internal consistency scores were 0.68 and 0.97 before and after training, respectively. No publications have been found which provide validity evidences of the instrument.

3.11.4. Strengths and weaknesses

On the positive side, it should be noted that the questionnaire is short and easy to fill out. However, it uses a dichotomous response format which prevents information being collected about the areas where the teachers' lack of knowledge is concentrated. Furthermore, information about the validity of the instrument is not available.

3.12. Questionnaire to Assess Teachers' Knowledge about ADHD

3.12.1. Basque language version of the Questionnaire to Assess Teachers' Knowledge about ADHD (Irakasleek AGHNari buruz duten ezagutza ebaluatzeko galdera-sorta – IRA-AGHN) (Soroa, Balluerka & Gorostiaga, unpublished)

3.12.1.1. Description and development

This is a newly developed questionnaire produced in Spain in the Basque language and which has yet to be published. Its purpose is to assess the knowledge of infant and primary school teachers about ADHD. It is divided into two sections. The first collects socio-demographic data (age, sex, teaching speciality, teaching experience, etc.) as well as data on the perceived knowledge of teachers of ADHD and their perceived capacity to teach children suffering from this condition. The second section assesses their real knowledge of these matters with 26 items that use a three option response format (True, False, Don't Know). The questionnaire items, 21 positive and 5 negative, assessed four areas of knowledge related to

ADHD: 1) General information about ADHD (4 items), 2) Symptoms/Diagnosis of ADHD (11 items), 3) Etiology of ADHD (4 items), and 4) Treatment of ADHD (7 items). The questionnaire items were developed from an extensive review of the literature on ADHD.

To obtain data on content validity, the authors of the instrument sought the cooperation of 8 experts in ADHD (university lecturers from different fields of knowledge and clinical or educational psychologists). Thanks to their participation the initial questionnaire of 105 items was reduced to 76 which were distributed into their corresponding sub-scales of the questionnaire when there was an agreement level of 70% among the experts. Subsequently, a pilot study was conducted on 98 infant and primary school teachers in the Autonomous Community of the Basque Country and Navarre. 83 participants were women and 15 men, with a mean age of 40 years (*SD*=9.8). They had an average of 15 years (*SD*=10) in the teaching profession, 50.5% had never received training about ADHD, and 47% said they had experience of having a child with ADHD in their classroom. 86% were infant education specialists or primary teachers and 8% were special education teachers. Thanks to the participation of these teachers, the authors of the questionnaire selected those items with high discrimination power and revised the wording of 6 statements, obtaining a preliminary instrument of 51 items.

The draft instrument was finally applied to a sample of 752 infant and primary education teachers in 84 schools in the Autonomous Community of the Basque Country and Navarre. The schools were randomly selected. 86% of participants were female and 14% male, with a mean age of 42 years (*SD*=9.68). They had an average of 17 years (*SD*=10.55) experience as teachers, 80% were infant and primary teachers and 12% special education teachers. 59% said they never received training about ADHD, and 54% stated that they had had experience of children with ADHD during their careers. The final instrument of 26 items as described earlier in this section was thus obtained.

3.12.1.2. Scoring standards

1 point was given for each correct answer and 0 for incorrect ones and gaps in knowledge. Thus, the possible scores ranged from 0, for the minimum level of knowledge, to 26, for the highest level.

3.12.1.3. Psychometric properties

With the purpose of selecting the final items for the IRA-AGHN, a factor analysis with oblique rotation was carried out. Items with a factor loading equal to or greater than .35, and which adequately reflected the underlying construct, were selected. Using the 26 selected items, the dimensionality of the instrument was examined by means of an exploratory factor analysis based on polychoric correlations. The Unweighted Least Squares (ULS) estimation method was used. Kaiser procedure was used to decide the number of factors, and the Direct Oblimin rotation method was selected in order to simplify the factor structure. The resulting structure confirmed the multi-dimensional character of the construct. Four factors were obtained which explained 53.2% of the variance: The first factor, Etiology of ADHD, explained 29.15% of the variance; the second factor, Symptoms/Diagnosis of ADHD, explained 9.8% of the variance; the third factor, General information about ADHD, explained 7.8% of the variance; and the fourth and final factor, Treatment of ADHD, explained 6.4% of the variance.

For the reliability analysis, the internal consistency was first calculated, with an *Omega* coefficient which ranged from 0.76 to 0.90 being obtained for the four sub-scales. For the purpose of analyzing the stability of the instrument the authors administered the IRA-AGHN a second time to a sample of 123 teachers with a period of four weeks between the first and second administration. The *Spearman's Rho* test-retest correlations for the IRA-AGHN scores ranged from r=0.49 to r=0.77 (p<0.01) for the four sub-scales.

Convergent validity was tested by comparing the results obtained by the subjects in the IRA-AGHN with the results obtained in the Spanish version of the KADDS [4]. The correlation between the scores obtained by the subjects in the dimensions shared by both questionnaires was r=0.54 for the General information sub-scale, r=0.45 for the Symptoms/Diagnosis sub-scale and r=0.33 for the Treatment sub-scale (p<0.01 in all cases).

Finally, to obtain evidence of external validity, the relationships between the scores obtained by the participants in the IRA-AGHN sub-scales and a series of variables related to the construct that it was sought to measure were examined. The data showed that the scores obtained by the teachers in the Symptoms/Diagnosis sub-scale had a moderate correlation with variables such as the number of children diagnosed with ADHD the teachers had taught in the course of their careers (r = .29, p = .001), the teachers' perceived knowledge of ADHD (r = .37, p = .001), and the teachers' perceived capacity to teach effectively children with ADHD (r = 0.30, p = 0.001). Meanwhile, it was observed that the scores obtained by the teachers in the General information sub-scale showed a moderate correlation with the teachers' perceived knowledge of ADHD variable (r = .30, p = .001). In addition, using the Mann-Whitney U test a comparison was drawn between the average score ranges obtained by teachers who had taught children diagnosed with ADHD in the course of their careers and those who hadn't. Results showed that there were statistically significant differences between the groups' mean score ranges in the Symptoms/Diagnosis sub-scale (*Mann-Whitney U test* = 44503; p = .0001; r = .29).

3.12.1.4. *Strengths and weaknesses*

On the positive side, it should be noted that this is a short questionnaire and easy to complete with a three option response format (True, False, Don't Know), and that it successfully evaluates teachers' knowledge, false beliefs and areas of lack of knowledge regarding ADHD. The sample used for the validation of the instrument is geographically diverse and extensive, being representative of the target population for the questionnaire. The instrument development process was thorough and rigorous, and has appropriate psychometric properties, although evidence of external validity is not supported by high levels of correlation.

3.12.2. *Spanish version of the Questionnaire to Assess Teachers' Knowledge about ADHD (Cuestionario para evaluar el conocimiento de los maestros acerca del TDAH – MAE-TDAH) (Soroa, Balluerka & Gorostiaga, unpublished)*

3.12.2.1. *Description and development*

This is a questionnaire recently produced in Spain in the Spanish language and which has yet to be published. The description is the same as that for the above mentioned version of the instrument in the Basque language.

To obtain evidence of content validity, the authors of the instrument sought the cooperation of 8 experts in ADHD (university lecturers from different fields of knowledge, child and youth psychiatrists, pediatricians, one educational psychologist and one education expert who are members of various associations of families of children with ADHD). Thanks to their participation, the initial questionnaire of 105 items was reduced to 76 items that were distributed in the corresponding sub-scales of the questionnaire with the agreement of at least 70% of the judges. Subsequently, a pilot study was conducted on 68 infant and primary school teachers in the Autonomous Community of the Basque Country and Navarre. 53 participants were women and 15 men, with a mean age of 43 years (*SD*=10.87). They had an average of 18 years (*SD*=11.67) in the teaching profession, 47% had never received training regarding ADHD, and 73% said they had a child diagnosed with ADHD in their classroom at some point in their career. 73% were infant or primary school teachers, and 15% were special education teachers. Thanks to the participation of these teachers, the authors of the questionnaire selected those items with high discrimination power and revised the wording of two of the statements, obtaining a preliminary instrument of 51 items.

Finally, the draft instrument was applied to a sample of 526 infant and primary school teachers in 57 schools in the Autonomous Community of the Basque Country and Navarre. The schools were randomly selected. 85% of participants were female and 15% male, with a mean age of 43 years (*SD*=10.89). They had an average of 17 years (*SD*=11.31) experience as teachers, 77% were infant or primary teachers and 11% were special education teachers. 56% said they had never received training regarding ADHD, and 67% stated that they had a child diagnosed with ADHD in their classroom at some point in their career. From this study the final 26 items instrument was obtained.

3.12.2.2. *Scoring standards*

Identical to those in the Basque language version of the questionnaire.

3.12.2.3. *Psychometric properties*

With the aim of selecting the final items for the MAE-TDAH, a factor analysis with oblique rotation was carried out. Items with a factor loading equal to or greater than .35, and which adequately reflected the underlying construct, were selected. Using the 26 selected items, the dimensionality of the instrument was examined by means of an exploratory factor analysis based on polychoric correlations. The Unweighted Least Squares (ULS) estimation method was used. Kaiser procedure was used to decide the number of factors, and the Direct Oblimin rotation method was selected in order to simplify the factor structure. The resulting structure confirmed the multi-dimensional character of the construct. Four factors were obtained which explained 60.73% of the variance: Etiology of ADHD explained 34.04% of the variance, General information about ADHD explained 12.14% of the variance, Treatment of ADHD explained 8.92% of the variance, and the fourth and final factor, Symptoms/Diagnosis of ADHD, explained 5.6% of the variance.

For reliability analysis, the internal consistency was first calculated and an *Omega* coefficient which ranged from 0.83 to 0.91 for four sub-scales was obtained. In order to analyze the stability of the instrument, the authors administered the MAE-TDAH a second time to a group of 112 teachers four weeks after the first application. The *Spearman's Rho* test-retest correlations for the MAE-TDAH scores ranged from r=0.62 to r=0.79 (p<0.01) for the four sub-scales.

Convergent validity was tested by comparing the results obtained by the subjects in the MAE-TDAH with the results obtained in the Spanish version of KADDS [4]. The correlations observed between the scores obtained by the subjects in the dimensions shared by both questionnaires were r=0.58 for the General information sub-scale, r=0.43 for the Symptoms/ Diagnosis sub-scale, r=0.30 for the Etiology and r=0.39 for the Treatment sub-scale (p<0.01 in all cases).

In order to find evidence of external validity the authors of the MAE-TDAH examined the correlations between the questionnaire scores and a series of variables related to the construct it was sought to measure. Significant statistical differences were found between the teachers' perceived knowledge of ADHD and the scores they obtained for all the sub-scales of the questionnaire (r=0.38 for General information, r=0.37 for Symptoms/Diagnosis, r=0.30 for Etiology and r=0.31 for Treatment; p=0.001 for all cases), as well between the teachers perceived capacity to effectively teach children with ADHD and the scores obtained in the sub-scales General information and Symptoms/Diagnosis of ADHD (r=0.29, p=0.001 and r=0.30, p=0.001, respectively).

3.12.2.4. Strengths and weaknesses

These are similar to those set out regarding the Basque language version of the questionnaire. The main difference is that in this case the sample used for the validation of the questionnaire was quite homogenous as it was confined to two autonomous communities of the Spanish state.

4. Conclusions

In the review that has been carried out in this chapter, it has been observed that there exist a great number of tools that have been developed to assess the level of knowledge of teachers regarding ADHD. However, most of them do not have good psychometric properties. The authors of this chapter consider necessary to develop and validate instruments with psychometric properties to measure teachers' knowledge of ADHD with rigor. These instruments, in addition to identifying gaps in teachers' knowledge of the disorder, can be useful in raising the awareness of teachers about the need for more training in this area, help in the design of training tailored to the needs of teachers, and ultimately, promote the welfare of children and young people with ADHD.

This lack of methodological rigor in these measurement instruments may cause the obtaining of erratic and false results. With regard to the measurement instruments used to assess teachers' knowledge of ADHD it can be seen that this knowledge varies among the studies examined here. This variability may, in part, be due to an increase in teachers' knowledge of ADHD over recent decades but it might also be due to methodological reasons such as the following: The number and content of the items in the various instruments varies; the response formats also differ and this affects the results; the size of the samples also varies considerably, in some cases being very big and in others quite small; different studies have collected different socio-demographic data from their sample, which affects the description made of it and the interpretations which might be made of the reasons for the knowledge teachers have about ADHD. All these aspects should be taken into account when it comes to interpreting, comparing and generalizing the results obtained from these instruments.

Regarding the dimensionality of the instruments analyzed here, it should be noted that five of the twelve (KADDS [4, 5], KARE [35], KADD-Q [6], Teacher Knowledge About ADHD [24], and IRA-AGHN/MAE-TDAH) used a number of dimensions ranging from 2 to 6 for the assessment of teachers knowledge of ADHD. It can be seen that Treatment is the only common to all the instruments. In general, the various dimensions proposed by the authors deal with the symptoms, sub-types, associated problems, evaluation, prognosis and etiology of ADHD. However, it should be noted that only one of the instruments reviewed, the IRA-AGHN/MAE-TDAH conducted a factor analysis to confirm the multidimensional nature of the construct.

Furthermore, the external validity of the instruments analyzed provides information about the variables that can influence the knowledge that teachers have regarding ADHD. Three of the twelve instruments reviewed (KADDS [4, 5], KADD-Q [6], and IRA-AGHN/MAE-TDAH) provide evidence of external validity. If we focus on those variables that have relationships with knowledge about ADHD with effect size equal to or greater than 0.30 in any of the instruments, it can be concluded that the variables that correlated with teachers' knowledge about ADHD are: Prior exposure of teachers to children diagnosed with ADHD in the classroom, the number of children with ADHD teachers have had in their classrooms, having had specific training about ADHD, the degree of teachers' self-perceived efficacy in teaching children with ADHD and teachers' self-perceived knowledge of ADHD.

Finally, it should be pointed out that we consider the present chapter to be of interest because it provides an exhaustive review of the main instruments identified in the scientific literature to assess teachers' knowledge of ADHD. The identification of instruments with optimal psychometric properties is fundamental because it allows for the obtaining of valid and reliable data about the construct being studied. With regard to teachers' knowledge of ADHD it has been shown that there exist a significant percentage of teachers with gaps in this area [3-7, 19, 20]. For this reason, we believe that the use of instruments which measure this knowledge with rigor could contribute to devising of training materials and courses appropriate for the needs of teachers. And this would, of course, result in benefits for the children who suffer from this condition.

Acknowledgements

The authors appreciate the cooperation of all those authors who provided additional information about the assessment instruments examined in this chapter.

This work was partially funded by a grant from the Research Bureau of the University of the Basque Country UPV/EHU (General Funding for Research Groups, GIU11/29).

Author details

Marian Soroa[1], Arantxa Gorostiaga[2] and Nekane Balluerka[2]

*Address all correspondence to: marian.soroa@ehu.es

1 Developmental and Educational Psychology Department, University Teacher Training College of Donostia of the UPV/EHU, Donostia-San Sebastián, Spain

2 Social Psychology and Methodology of the Behavioral Sciences Department, Psychology Faculty of the UPV/EHU, Donostia-San Sebastián, Spain

References

[1] Lavigne, R. & Romero, J. F. (2010). El TDAH: ¿Qué es?, ¿qué lo causa?, ¿cómo evaluarlo y tratarlo?. Madrid: Pirámide.

[2] Canu, W. H. & Mancil, E. B. (2012). An Examination of Teacher Trainees' Knowledge of Attention-Deficit/Hyperactivity Disorder. School Mental Health, 4, 105-114.

[3] Ghanizadeh, A., Bahredar, M. J., & Moeini, S. R. (2006). Knowledge and attitudes towards attention deficit hyperactivity disorder among elementary school teachers. Patient Education and Counselling, 63, 84-88.

[4] Jarque, S., Tárraga, R., & Miranda, A. (2007). Conocimientos, concepciones erróneas y lagunas de los maestros sobre el trastorno por déficit de atención con hiperactividad. Psicothema, 19(4), 585-590.

[5] Sciutto, M. J., Terjesen, M. D., & Bender, A. S. (2000). Teachers' knowledge and misperceptions of Attention-Deficit/Hyperactivity Disorder. Psychology in the Schools, 37, 115-122.

[6] West, J., Taylor, M., Houghton, S., & Hudyma, S. (2005). A Comparison of Teachers' and Parents' Knowledge and Beliefs About Attention-Deficit/Hyperactivity Disorder (ADHD). School Psychology International, 26(2), 192-208.

[7] White, S. W., Sukhodolsky, D. G., Rains, A. L., Foster, D., McGuire, J. F., & Scahill, L. (2011). Elementary School Teachers' Knowledge of Tourette Syndrome, Obsessive-Compulsive Disorder, & Attention-Deficit/Hyperactivity Disorder: Effects of Teacher Training. Journal of Developmental and Physical Disabilities, 23, 5-14.

[8] Barkley, R. A. (2005). Prólogo. In I. Moreno, El niño hiperactivo (pp. 13). Madrid: Pirámide.

[9] Soroa, M., Balluerka, N., & Gorostiaga, A. (2012). Evaluation of the level of knowledge of infant and primary school teachers with respect to the Attention Deficit Hyperactivity Disorder (ADHD): Content validity of a newly created questionnaire. In J. M. Norvilitis (Ed.), Contemporary trends in ADHD research (pp. 127-152). Rijeka: InTech. (available from: http://www.intechopen.com/articles/show/title/evaluation-of-the-level-of-knowledge-of-infant-and-primary-school-teachers-with-respect-to-the-atten)

[10] American Psychiatric Association (APA, 2000). Diagnostic and statistical manual of mental disorders (4th. ed.). Washington: Author text revision.

[11] Barkley, R. A. (1999). Niños hiperactivos: Cómo comprender y atender sus necesidades especiales. Barcelona: Paidós.

[12] Moreno, I. & Servera, M. (2002). Intervención en los trastornos del comportamiento infantil. In M. Servera (Coord.), Los trastornos por déficit de atención con hiperactividad (pp. 217-253). Madrid: Pirámide.

[13] Moreno, I. (2008). Hiperactividad infantil: Guía de actuación. Madrid: Pirámide.

[14] Ohan, J. L., Cormier, N., Hepp, S. L., Visser, T. A. V., & Strain, M. C. (2008). Does Knowledge About Attention-Deficit/Hyperactivity Disorder Impact Teachers' Reported Behaviors and Perceptions?. School Psychology Quarterly, 23, 436-449.

[15] Sherman, J., Rasmussen, C., & Baydala, L. (2008). The impact of teacher factors on achievement and behavioural outcomes of children with Attention Deficit/Hyperactivity Disorder (ADHD): A review of the literature. Educational Research, 50(4), 347-360.

[16] Kos, J., Richdale, A. L., & Hay, D. A. (2006). Children with Attention deficit Hyperactivity Disorder and their Teachers: A review of the literature. International Journal of Disability, Development and Education, 53(2), 147-160.

[17] Barkley, R. A. (2006). Attention deficit hyperactivity disorder: A handbook for diagnosis and treatment. (3rd. ed.). New York: Guilford Press.

[18] Bekle, B. (2004). Knowledge and attitudes about Attention-Deficit Hyperactivity Disorder (ADHD): A comparison between practicing teachers and undergraduate education students. Journal of Attention Disorders, 7(3), 151-161.

[19] Graczyk, P. A., Atkins, M. S., Jackon, M. M., Letendre, J. A., Kim-Cohen, J., Baumann, B. L., & McCoy, J. (2005). Urban Educators' Perceptions of Interventions for Students with Attention Deficit Hyperactivity Disorder: A Preliminary Investigation. Behavioral Disorders, 30(2), 95-104.

[20] Kos, J. M., Richdale, A. L., & Jackson, M. S. (2004). Knowledge about Attention-Deficit/Hyperactivity Disorder: A comparison of in-service and preservice teachers. Psychology in the Schools, 41(5), 517-526.

[21] Pfiffner, L. J. (1999). Potenciar la educación en la escuela y en casa: métodos para el éxito desde párvulos hasta el bachillerato. In R. Barkley (Ed.), Niños hiperactivos. Cómo comprender y atender sus necesidades especiales (pp. 245-263). Barcelona: Paidós.

[22] Barbaresi, W. J. & Olsen, R. D. (1998). An ADHD Educational Intervention for Elementary Schoolteachers: A pilot Study. Developmental and Behavioral Pediatrics, 19(2), 94-100.

[23] Jerome, L., Gordon, M., & Hustler, P. (1994). A comparison of American and Canadian Teachers' Knowledge and Attitudes Towards Attention Deficit Hyperactivity Disorder (ADHD). Canadian Journal of Psychiatry, 39, 563-567.

[24] Jones, H. A. & Chronis-Tuscano, A. (2008). Efficacy of teacher in-service training for Attention-Deficit/Hyperactivity Disorder. Psychology in the Schools, 45(10), 918-929.

[25] Stacey, M. A. (2003). Attention-Deficit/Hyperactivity Disorder: General Education Elementary School Teachers' Knowledge, Training, and Ratings of Acceptability of Interventions. (Doctoral Thesis, University of South Florida, 2003). Available from: http://etd.fcla.edu/SF/SFE0000084/Thesis.pdf

[26] Riley, N. K. (1994). Educators' Knowledge of Attention Deficit Disorder. (Doctoral Thesis, Fort Hays State University, 1994). Available from: http://catalogue.nla.gov.au/Record/5576323

[27] Sciutto, M. J. & Terjesen, M. D. (1994). (Preliminary test development data). Unpublished raw data.

[28] Bender, A. S. (1996). Effects of active learning on student teachers' identifications and referrals of attention deficit hyperactivity disorder. Unpublished doctoral dissertation, Hofstra University, Hempstead, NY.

[29] Sciutto, M. J. & Terjesen, M. D. (2004). Psychometric properties of the Knowledge of Attention Deficit Disorders Scale (KADDS). Unpublished test development data.

[30] Sciutto, M. J., Nolfi, C. J., & Bluhm, C. A. (2004). Effects of child gender and symptom type on elementary school teachers' referrals for ADHD. Journal of Emotional and Behavioral Disorders, 12, 247-253.

[31] Power, T. J. & Rostain, A. L. (2003). The Attention-Deficit/Hyperactivity Disorder Knowledge and Opinion Survey (AKOS-IV) – Knowledge Scale. Unpublished manuscript.

[32] Rostain, A. L., Power, T. J., & Atkins, M. S. (1993). Assessing parents' willingness to pursue treatment for children with attention deficit hyperactivity disorder. Journal of Academical Child and Adolescent Psychiatry, 32, 175-181.

[33] Power, T. J., Hess, L. E., & Bennett, D. S. (1995). The Acceptability of Interventions for Attention Deficit Hyperactivity Disorder Among Elementary and Middle School Teachers. Developmental and Behavioral Pediatrics, 16(4), 238-243.

[34] Snider, V. E., Busch, T., & Arrowood, L. (2003). Teacher Knowledge of Stimulant Medication and ADHD. Remedial and Special Education, 24(1), 46-56.

[35] Vereb, R. L. & DiPerna, J. (2004). Teachers' Knowledge of ADHD, Treatments for ADHD, and Treatment Acceptability: An Initial Investigation. School Psychology Review, 33(3), 421-428.

[36] Niznik, M. E. (2004). An exploratory study of the implementation and teacher outcomes of a program to train elementary educators about ADHD in the schools. (Doctoral Thesis, University of Texas, 2004). Available from: http://repositories.lib.utexas.edu/bitstream/handle/2152/1282/niznikd24758.pdf?sequence=2

Section 4

Drugs in ADHD

Chapter 9

Effects of Methylphenidate in Children with Attention Deficit Hyperactivity Disorder: A Comparison of Behavioral Results and Event–Related Potentials

Ren Yan-ling and Dong Xuan

Additional information is available at the end of the chapter

http://dx.doi.org/10.5772/53782

1. Introduction

Attention Deficit Hyperactivity Disorder (ADHD) is one of the most common mental disorders in children and adolescents, with an estimated 3–5% of children diagnosed with this disorder [1,2]. ADHD is characterized by symptoms of inattention, impulsivity and hyperactivity. It has been suggested that a core deficiency in inhibitory control accounts for many deficits in executive function observed in ADHD that underlie most of the dysfunctional behaviors associated with this syndrome [3]. The apparent importance of executive dysfunction in children with ADHD has thus led to an increasing number of investigations in this area.

Executive control is engaged in situations requiring decision making, conflict resolution, error correction, and response inhibition. An important aspect of executive function is the inhibition of a prepared response, where inhibition refers to the ability to actively suppress, interrupt or delay an action [4]. Without inhibition, there is no capacity to avoid the execution of inappropriate responses, or ensure attainment of appropriate responses, thereby preventing realization of an intended result.

One commonly used paradigm in the investigation of executive function is the continuous performance test (CPT), which is a classical GO/NOGO paradigm. CPT was firstly used as a measure of sustained attention [5], and has since been widely applied in the investigation of cognitive response control and response inhibition, in both clinical groups and healthy subjects [6].

Event-related potentials (ERPs) are electroencephalogram (EEG) recorded changes that are time locked to sensory, motor, or cognitive events. Event-related potentials provide a safe, noninvasive approach to study of the psychophysiological correlates of mental processing.

GO/NOGO tasks are a particularly suitable paradigm for investigating response inhibition with ERPs. In this task, subjects are usually required to respond either overtly or covertly to a given target stimulus (a tone or a letter) (GO condition). In a second condition, however, subjects are required to withhold a response to a given stimulus (NOGO condition). The ERPs of CPT tasks are investigated by comparing ERP differences induced by the GO condition ("9" after "1") and NOGO condition (no "9" after "1"). The NOGO condition has a more significant N2 component between 200 and 300 ms over the frontocentral scalp than the Go condition, and the subsequent frontal-central region a larger P3 component; the GO stimulus has a larger P3 component in the parietal region. The NOGO-N2 and the NOGO-P3 components are related to response inhibition [7]. The GO-P3 component is related to the attention of the GO stimulus [8]. An increasing body of recent evidence suggests that the NOGO-N2 is related to conflict monitoring, while the NOGO-P3 is related to response inhibition [9, 10]. The source of response inhibition has been localized in the anterior cingulate cortex (ACC).

Stimulant medication [11,21], particularly methylphenidate (MPH), is the most common treatment for children with ADHD, and has been shown to improve attention and behavior; low doses of MPH are highly effective and widely prescribed for the treatment of ADHD [12]. ERP analysis has been employed in efforts to gain knowledge about stimulant mechanisms and their relationship to appropriate effect, and studies have suggested that ERPs may predict the clinical response of children with ADHD to MPH [13]. Low dose MPH has been associated with reduced impulsivity (fewer false alarms) and decreased P3 latencies, whereas the higher doses have been associated with reduced impulsivity and less inattention (more hits), in addition to increased P2 and N2 latencies and decreased P3 latencies [14]. The Continuous Performance Test (CPT) is an appropriate instrument for assessment of the correlates between attention-related electrical activity levels in the brain and responses to stimulant medication [15].

This study investigates the effect of Methylphenidate on the relationship between the ERP waveform and behavioral results of children with ADHD. Therefore, based on their behavioral results pre- and post-administration of MPH, the ADHD children were divided into two groups: an ADHD good performance group and an ADHD poor performance group. We are interested in whether the changes in the ERP waveform correlate with the behavioral results, and the ERP waveform differences from the control group waveforms.

2. Materials and methods

2.1. Subjects

2.1.1. ADHD group

Twenty-eight children aged from 6 to 13 years (24 males and 4 females, mean age =9.25±1.86 years) with a primary diagnosis of ADHD participated. Children with ADHD were recruited from the ADHD clinic at the Third Affiliated Hospital of Soochow University. All of the children were identified as meeting DSM-IV criteria for ADHD based on a structured clinical interview and parent rating scales. Excluded from the study were subjects with a conduct disorder, internalizing disorder (e.g. anxiety), low intelligence (IQ<85), and gross neurological and other organic disorders. All subjects had not taken any stimulant medication. ADHD children were given a low dose of 0.3mg/kg of methylphenidate (MPH). Verbal assent was provided by the subjects and written informed consent obtained from their parents.

2.1.2. The control group

The control group consisted of 28 age- and gender-matched healthy children, 6.8-13.2 years old (mean age = 9.15 ± 1.94 years), were right-handed, with Screened IQ ≥ 85, visual or corrected visual acuity greater than 1.0, without diseases of the nervous system, and no special learning difficulties or language barriers. They were tested only one time. Verbal assent was obtained from the children and their teachers, with written informed consent obtained from their parents.

2.1.3. Behavioral results–basis for group division

Children with ADHD were tested twice. They were tested once following diagnosis (pre-administration of M PH); and a second time two hours post-administration of MPH (0.3mg/kg body weight).

The ADHD good performance group: after taking MPH, behavioral results were improved, with the number of omission errors and/or commission errors reduced by a factor of five in a total of 12 patients (1 female), mean age 9.17 ± 2.19 years old. Prior to administration of MPH, the number of omission errors and commission errors (respectively 8.37 ± 3.92, 7.78 ± 5.10) were significantly higher than the results obtained of 2 hours post-administration of MPH (respectively 2.92 ± 3.61, 3.91 ± 2.62) ($P< 0.05$).

The ADHD poor performance group: post-administration of MPH, behavioral results were not significantly improved, with behavioral changes not meeting behavioral improvement standards in a total of 16 patients (3 females), mean age 9.31 ± 1.66 years old. Prior to administration of MPH, the number of omission errors and commission errors (respectively 7.95 ± 4.61, 7.46 ± 5.81) were higher than the results obtained 2 hours post-administration MPH (respectively 5.79 ± 2.71, 5.83 ± 2.91), but the differences were not statistically significant ($P> 0.05$).

2.2. Electrophysiological paradigm

The participants were investigated electrophysiologically in an electrically shielded, dimly lit room, sitting on a comfortable chair in front of a computer screen to perform the CPT tasks, with a viewing distance of 80 cm, horizontal visual angle of 0.7°, and a vertical visual angle of 1.4°. During the task, digits were presented in a random order, and subjects instructed to press a response button whenever the digit "9"appeared immediately after the digit"1". The whole stimulus set consisted of 400 digits, with 80 prime conditions (digit"1"), 40 GO ("9" after "1") and NOGO (no "9" after "1") conditions and 240 distracters (other digits, including the digit "9", without a preceding "1") (see fig.1). The digits were presented for 200 ms each, followed by an inter-stimulus interval of 1400 ms, resulting in a total duration of approximately 11 minutes. After a short training session, subjects performed this version of the CPT while an ongoing EEG was recorded.

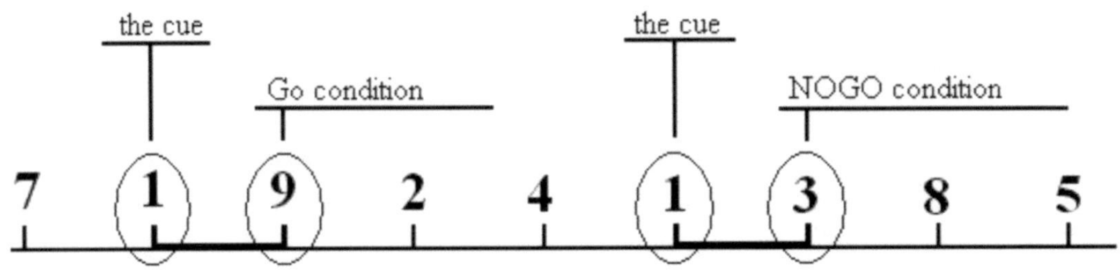

Figure 1. The sequence of stimulus presentation

2.3. EEG recording

Scalp voltages were collected with a Stellate™ System 32 channel Digital Video EEG (Stellate System Inc., CA) connected to a 32-Channel Digital Amplifier (LA MONT MEDICAL Inc., Montreal, CA). The EEG was recorded from 23 scalp electrodes which were placed according to the International 10-20 system at FP_1, FP_2, F_z, F_3, F_4, F_7, F_8, C_Z, C_3, C_4, T_3, T_4, P_Z, P_3, P_4, T_5, T_6, O_Z, O_1, O_2, M_1, M_2 and a common reference. Vertical electro-oculogram (VEOG) electrodes, located at 2 cm above and below the left eye, were used to subtract the eye movement artifact. Impedances was <5 KΩ, bandpass filtered from 0.1 to 35 Hz and digitized at 500 Hz. A midline electrode was used as the common reference for recording.

Trials were discarded from analysis if they contained eye movements (vertical EOG channel differences greater than 100μV) or more than five bad channels.

2.4. Data analysis

Grand average ERP waveforms were used to determine the individual NOGO-N2 and NOGO-P3 time window. NOGO-N2 at Fz and Cz electrodes were maximal from 250-300 ms, 280-350 ms at Pz electrode; NOGO-P3 at Fz and Cz electrodes were maximal from 400-500 ms, 420-520 ms at Pz electrode. In each time window, the amplitudes of NOGO-N2 and NOGO-P3 at Fz, Cz, Pz electrodes were measured. Latency represented the time from the stimulus onset to the wave peak; amplitude represented the vertical distance from the baseline to the wave peak.

2.5. Statistical analysis

SPSS12.0 statistical software was used for data processing, using t-test for the difference between two groups and ANOV for the differences among multiple groups. All data were expressed as Mean ± SD ($\bar{x}$± s), with the difference was considered significant if the P value was smaller than 0.05.

http://dx.doi.org/10.5772/53782

3. Results

3.1. ERP results of the ADHD good performance group

Comparing the results of this group, both pre- and post-administration of MPH, with the control group, the amplitude of the NOGO-N2 displayed no significant difference (P> 0.05). Pre-administration of MPH, the amplitude of the NOGO-P3 was significantly lower than the results obtained 2 hours post-administration of MPH and by the control group; at the Fz and Cz electrodes the differences were statistically significant (P <0.05). Comparied to the control group, the amplitude of the NOGO-P3 2 hours post-administration of MPH showed no significantly difference (P> 0.05).

See Table 1 for details.

electrode	ERP	pre- - administration of MPH	2 hours post-administration of MPH	the control group	F value	P value
Fz	N2(250-300ms)	-7.17±5.81	-5.84±4.71	-7.67±4.32	0.62	0.54
	P3(400-500ms)	20.34±11.42	30.24±10.78(1)	33.26±9.83 (2)	6.49	0.003
Cz	N2(250-300ms)	-3.01±4.68	-2.08±3.37	-4.76±6.60	1.09	0.34
	P3(400-500ms)	16.28±6.36	22.20±5.07 (1)	23.67±8.14(1)	4.52	0.02
Pz	N2(280-330ms)	-1.73±3.63	-0.28±2.71	-1.25±3.94	0.51	0.60
	P3(420-520ms)	14.34±5.72	18.20±4.41	18.88±7.69	2.00	0.15

(1) Comparing to pre- administration of MPH, P <0.05;

(2) Comparing to pre- administration of MPH, P<0.01.

Table 1. The ADHD good performance group pre- and post-administration of MPH and the control group at Fz, Cz, Pz electrodes amplitudes of the NOGO-N2 and NOGO-P3 comparison ($\bar{x}\pm$ s) (μ v)

3.2. ERP results of the ADHD poor performance group

As with the ADHD good performance group, in comparing the results pre- and post-administration of MPH with the control group, the amplitude of the NOGO-N2 also displayed no significant difference (P> 0.05). However, in this case both pre- and 2 hours post-administration of MPH, no statistically significant difference in the amplitude of the NOGP-P3 (P> 0.05) was found. Pre- and post-administration of MPH, the amplitude of the NOGO-P3 at the Fz electrode was significantly lower than that of control group (P <0.05). At the Cz electrode, the amplitude of the NOGO-P3 pre-administration of MPH was also significantly lower than that of the control group (P <0.05). However, compared to the control group, the amplitude of the NOGO-P3 post-administration of MPH showed no significant difference (P> 0.05).

See Table 2 for details.

electrode	ERP	pre-administration of MPH	2 hours post-administration of MPH	the control group	F value	P value
Fz	N2(250-300ms)	-6.88±6.59	-7.08±8.18	-7.67±4.32	0.10	0.91
	P3(400-500ms)	23.51±11.97	25.88±13.96	33.26±9.83 (1) (2)	4.23	0.02
Cz	N2(250-300ms)	-2.79±6.61	-2.22±6.33	-4.76±6.60	0.92	0.40
	P3(400-500ms)	17.28±7.56	19.94±7.09	23.67±8.14 (1)	3.68	0.03
Pz	N2(280-330ms)	0.48±6.33	-0.36±4.68	-1.25±3.94	0.66	0.52
	P3(420-520ms)	15.21±6.17	16.34±5.90	18.88±7.69	1.63	0.20

(1) Comparing to pre- administration of MPH, P <0.05;

(2) Comparing to 2 hours post-administration of MPH, P<0.05.

Table 2. The ADHD poor performance group pre- and post-administration of MPH and the control group at Fz, Cz, Pz electrodes amplitudes of the NOGO-N2 and the NOGO-P3 comparison ($\bar{x}\pm$ s) (μ v)

3.3. ERP results of the two ADHD group pre-administration of MPH

The amplitudes of the NOGO-N2 and the NOGO-P3 showed no significant differences (P> 0.05).

3.4. Grand average ERP waves

As can be seen in Figure 2, the ERP components of the ADHD good performance group, the ADHD poor performance group and the control group were consistent; all showed N1, P2, N2 and P3 components. In the ADHD good performance group, the amplitudes of the NOGO-N2 pre- and post-administration of MPH showed no significant changes; At the Fz and Cz electrodes, the amplitude of the NOGO-P3 2 hours post-administration of MPH was significantly higher than pre-administration of MPH, while the amplitude of the NOGO-P3 at the Pz electrode showed no significant changes. In the ADHD poor performance group, the amplitudes of the NOGO-N2 and NOGO-P3 at the Fz, Cz, Pz electrodes showed no significant changes both pre- and post-administration of MPH; the amplitude of the NOGO-P3 was significantly lower than that of the control group.

4. Discussion

Central stimulants are the first choice for the treatment children with ADHD, and the most widely used is Methylphenidate. MPH can improve attention deficit and interpersonal relations, lower activity levels and impulsivity, and improve academic achievement, and have a positive effect on children with ADHD. While there is a previously reported efficiency of approximately 75% [11], our clinical work indicates an efficiency rate was below this number. This study uses the continuous performance test (CPT) to s investigate the relationship

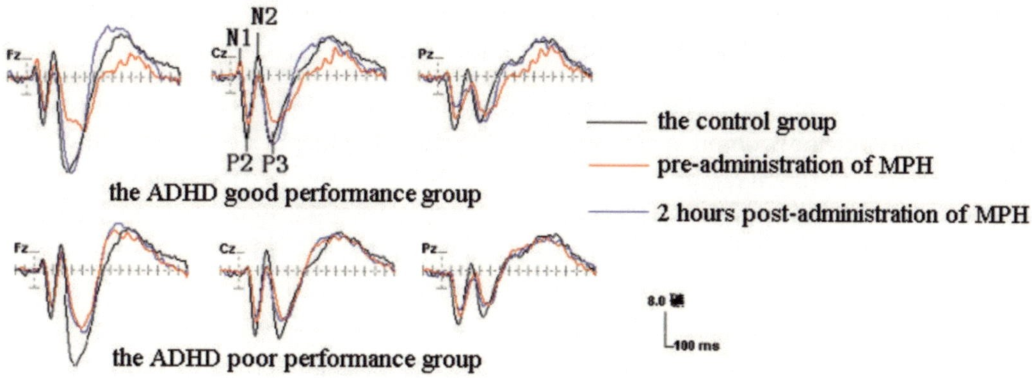

Figure 2. The grand average EPR waveforms

between behavioral results and ERP changes pre- and post-administration of MPH in children with ADHD, and compares these results to a control group.

This study found that in the ADHD group pre-administration of MPH the amplitude of the NOGO-P3 was significantly lower than that of the control group, while the amplitude of the NOGO-N2 showed no difference between the control group and the ADHD group pre-administration of MPH. This suggests the existence of frontal inhibition functional deficiencies rather than the conflict monitoring deficiencies, consistent with Fallgatter's study [16], confirming the existence of cingulate cortex dysfunction in children with ADHD.

In the ADHD good performance group, 2 hours post-administration of MPH, behavioral results were significantly improved; that is, omission errors and commission errors significantly reduced and the amplitude of the NOGO-P3 was significantly higher, although the amplitude of the NOGO-N2 showed no significant changes. Methylphenidate can improve attention deficit and the ability to inhibit impulsive reactions in children with ADHD. However, no significant changes in conflict monitoring ability were observed 2 hours post-administration of MPH. The amplitude of the NOGO-P3 was significantly increased, with no significant difference in comparison to the control group, suggesting MPH can normalize both the amplitude of the NOGO-P3 and the ability to inhibit impulsive reactions in children with ADHD.

In the ADHD poor performance group, 2 hours post-administration of MPH, behavioral results showed no significant improvement; that is, omission errors and commission errors were reduced, but the difference did not reach statistical significance. The amplitudes of the NOGO-N2 and NOGO- P3 showed no significant changes either pre- or post-administration of MPH; changes in ERP and behavioral results were consistent. This suggested that MPH had no significant impact on behavioral performance and ERP results, that it does not improve attention deficit and the ability to inhibit response, and there is no effect on the conflict monitoring and response inhibition. 2 hours post-administration of MPH, the amplitude of the NOGO-P3 was still lower than that of the control group, in which the frontal electrode had statistically significance. The result suggests that MPH failed to improve the ability of response inhibition of children with ADHD to normal levels.

Methylphenidate can be effective in improving the symptoms of children with ADHD, primarily through the promotion of dopamine (DA) and norepinephrine (NE) release to reduce reuptake. The pre-frontal region is rich with DA and NE receptors, and it is assumed that MPH acts through these receptors. ADHD is associated with a irregularity in a variety of cognitive and behavioral processes [11]. Recent studies have found that low-dose MPH in the treatment of ADHD may activate the locus coeruleus - norepinephrine (LC -NE) system, by influencing the locus coeruleus neurons in different discharge modes (phase- and tension-type) to alter behavioral and cognitive processes [17]. Neuroimaging, neuropsychological and neurochemical studies have also implicated dysfunction of fronto-striatal structures [18]. An fMRI study found that fronto-striatal activation, significantly lower in an ADHD group compared to a control group, increased post-administration of MPH [19]. The frontal lobe plays an important role in attention, executive function, working memory, regulating activities and decision-making. Most of the studies of children with ADHD consider that the frontal lobe dysfunction causes attention deficit and presents obstacles to response regulation. MPH treatment may be either effective or ineffective in children with ADHD, dependent on their age and emotional state, with treatment least effective in older age groups [20]. While this present study did not find such factors, children are nevertheless primary candidates for MPH treatment, though it should be observed that individuals respond differently

Young ES, et al [13] used an auditory oddball P300 paradigm to compare the ERP changes pre-administration and 2 hours post-administration of MPH. A prediction of the long-term benefit of medication was then made, based on the magnitude of the acute changes in P3b amplitude. The MPH challenge classification accurately predicted the outcome in 81% of cases. This present study used CPT tasks to test children with ADHD pre-administration and 2 hours post-administration of MPH. According to their behavioral results, the ADHD group was divided into an ADHD good performance group and an ADHD poor performance group. In the good performance group, the amplitude of the NOGO-P3 was significantly higher; the poor performance group, however, showed no obvious changes. The results suggested the amplitudes of the NOGO-P3 pre-administration and 2 hours post-administration of MPH were consistent with the behavioral results. Therefore, it can be posited that the amplitude of the NOGO-P3 can predict the long-term clinical efficacy of MPH treatment for ADHD. Where the amplitude of the NOGO-P3 is significantly increased post-administration of MPH, MPH may be an effective treatment; where the amplitude of the NOGO-P3 shows no significant increase post-administration of MPH, MPH is less likely to be an effective treatment. This can be primarily used to predict the efficacy of Methylphenidate for the treatment of ADHD, and assist in the selection of suitable treatment for children with ADHD. Further clinical tests will determine the accuracy of the prediction of Methylphenidate efficacy in children with ADHD. The present study can not avoid confounding medication effects with retest effects; this variable should be eliminated in future studies.

http://dx.doi.org/10.5772/53782

Acknowledgements

We wish to thank Michael Stewart for his helpful comments on this study.

This study was supported by the National Nature Science Foundation of China (NSFC Grant 30470566, 30870868), and the applied basic research Foundation of Changzhou (CJ20122016).

Author details

Ren Yan-ling and Dong Xuan*

*Address all correspondence to: dx6868@hotmail.com; ren93961981@163.com

Department of Neuroscience, The First People's Hospital of Chan Zhou (Third Affiliated Hospital of Soochow University), Chang Zhou, China

References

[1] American Psychiatric Association. Diagnostic and statistical manual of mental disorders (4th ed). Washington, 1994, DC:Author.

[2] American Psychiatric Association. Diagnostic and statistical manual of mental disorders (4th ed, text revision). Washington, 2000, DC: Author.

[3] Barkley RA. Behavioral Inhibition, Sustained Attention, and Executive FunctionsConstructing a Unifying Theory of ADHD. Psychological Bulletin 1997; 121: 65-94.

[4] Clark JM. Contributions of inhibitory mechanisms to unified theory in neuroscience and psychology. Brain Cogn 1996; 30: 127-152.

[5] Rosvold HE, Mirsky AF, Sarason I, Bransome ED, Beck LH. A continuous performance test of brain damage. J Consult Psychol 1956; 20: 343.

[6] Ehlis AC, Zielasek J, Herrmann M J, Ringel T, Jacob C, Wagener A, Fallgatter AJ. Evidence for unaltered brain electrical topography during prefrontal response control in cycloid psychoses. International Journal of Psychophysiology 2005; 55: 165– 178.

[7] Falkenstein M, Hoormann J, Hohnsbein J. ERP components in go/nogo tasks and their relation to inhibition. Acta Psychol 1999; 101: 267–291.

[8] Picton TW. The P300 wave of the human event-related potential. J. Clin. Neurophysiol 1992; 9: 456– 479.

[9] Bekker EM, Kenemans JL, Verbaten MN. Electrophysiological correlates of attention, inhibition,sensitivity and bias in a continuous performance task. Clin.Neurophysiol 2004; 115: 2001–2013.

[10] Jonkman LM. The development of preparation, conflict monitoring and inhibition from early childhood to young adulthood: a Go/Nogo ERP study. Brain research 2006; 1097: 181-193.

[11] Solanto MV. Neuropsychopharmacological mechanisms of stimulant drug action in attention-deficit hyperactivity disorder: a review and integration. Behav Brain Res 1998; 94: 127-152.

[12] Greenhill LL. Clinical effects of stimulant medication in ADHD, in Stimulant Drugs and ADHD: Basic and Clinical Neuroscience, Oxford University Press 2001, New York, 31-71.

[13] Young ES, Perros P, Price GW, Sadler T. Acute challenge ERP as a Prognostic of Stimulant therapy outcome in attention-deficit/hyperactivity disorder. Biol Psychiatry 1995; 37: 25-33.

[14] Sunohara GA, Malone MA, Rovet J. Effect of Methylphenidate on Attention in Children with Attention Deficit Hyperactivity Disorder (ADHD): ERP Evidence. Neuropsychopharmacology 1999; 21(2): 218–228.

[15] Seifert J,Scheuerpflug P,Zillessen KE,et al. Electrophysiological investigation of the effectiveness of methylphenidate in children with and without ADHD.J Neural Transm 2003; 110: 821-829.

[16] Fallgatter AJ, Ehlis AC, Seifert J, Strik WK, Scheuerpflug P, Zillessen KE, et al. Altered response control and anterior cingulated function in attention-deficit/hyperactivity disorder boys. Clinical Neurophysiolgy 2004; 115: 973-981.

[17] Devilbiss DM, Berridge CW. Low-Dose Methylphenidate Actions on Tonic and Phasic Locus Coeruleus Discharge. J Pharmacol Exp Ther 2006; 319: 1327-1335.

[18] Bush G, Valera EM, Seidman LJ. Functional Neuroimaging of Attention-Deficit/ Hyperactivity Disorder: A Review and Suggested Future Directions. BIOL PSYCHIATRY 2005; 57: 1273–1284.

[19] Vaidya CJ, Austin G, Kirkorian G, Ridlehuber HW, Desmond JE, Glover GH, Gabrieli JD. Selective effects of methylphenidate in attention deficit hyperactivity disorder: A functional magnetic resonance study. Proc Natl Acad Sci 1998; 95(24): 14494 – 14499.

[20] Sunohara GA, Voros JG, Malone MA, Taylor MJ. Effects of methylphenidate in children with attention deficit hyperactivity disorder: a comparison of event-related potentials between medication responders and non-responders. International Journal of Psychophysiology 1997; 27: 9– 14.

http://dx.doi.org/10.5772/53782

[21] Biederman J, Mick E , Fried R, et al. Are stimulants effective in the treatment of executive function deficits? Results from a randomized double blind study of ROS-methylphenidate in adults with ADHD. European Neuropsychopharmacology 2011 (21): 508–515.

Chapter 10

The Impact of Attention Deficit/Hyperactivity Disorder in African-Americans; Current Challenges Associated with Diagnosis and Treatment

Rahn Kennedy Bailey and Ejike Kingsley Ofoemezie

Additional information is available at the end of the chapter

http://dx.doi.org/10.5772/54276

1. Introduction

ADHD constitutes a serious issue in the African-American community. The Center for Disease Control and Prevention lists the African American males as leading other racial groups and gender in the diagnosis of learning and behavioral disorders, incarceration rates, new HIV infections, homicide and poverty. Although the reason for these observations are quite complex and multidimensional, some of the comorbidities found in untreated African Americans patients with ADHD include conduct disorder, oppositional defiant disorder, depression, anxiety disorders, learning disabilities, and alcohol or drug addiction. In addition, even though African American males living in poverty are most likely to be referred to mental health agencies for mental health services, they are the least likely to receive mental health services. In 2006, the number of children in the United States aged between 5 and 7 who were diagnosed with ADHD was 4.5 million. In the last decades the number of children diagnosed with ADHD who are on psychotropic medication continues to rise steadily. However, the impact of this steady rise has been skewed and not evenly distributed by ethnicity, socioeconomic status and gender as minorities (African Americans and Hispanics) are most often diagnosed or misdiagnosed. The incidence of ADHD appears to be similar in African-Americans and White populations. ADHD is diagnosed in 4.1% of all children with the greatest prevalence among Caucasian children (5.1%). However, when the prevalence of ADHD among male children are considered by race, African American children and adolescents are disproportionately diagnosed with ADHD, with an estimated prevalence rate of 5.65%, 4.3% for Hispanics, 3% for Whites; and 1.77% for females of all races. The prevalence of ADHD in African-Americans is most likely similar to that in the general population (3-5%); nevertheless, minority children have lower likelihood of receiving a diagnosis of

ADHD and of receiving any treatment. Reasons for this disparity are multifaceted and diverse and have not been fully elucidated. Among some of the identifiable barriers that attempt to explain these disparities are family-driven (parent, patient, and family) and Policy-driven (healthcare system and physician bias) obstacles.

The primary goals of treatment of ADHD are to decrease disruptive behaviors, enhance academic performance, improve interpersonal relationships with peers, family and friends, improve self-esteem, and promote independence. There are difficulties inherent in the diagnosis of ADHD. These include absence of specific diagnostic tests, the lack of specificity of symptoms, inability to observe symptoms that may not be present in an office setting, low rate of concordance in symptom-reporting among various informants (i.e. parents, teachers and parents) and a lack of a standard evaluative process. Although medical professionals may use different diagnostic routes to diagnose ADHD, most agree that the Diagnostic and Statistical Manual of Mental Disorders (DSM-IV) is the basis for an appropriate diagnostic process. Others have suggested the use of multiple methods of assessment which are culturally-sensitive and, which involves several people with varying degrees of relationship to the child to be the most effective way to reduce the bias associated with diagnosis. Whaley & Geller observed that the use of informal interviews and methods of assessment seem to increase the bias towards more diagnosis of ADHD towards African Americans. In recent years, following extensive research in this subject by major medical organizations such as the American Academy of Pediatrics (AAP) and the American Academy of Child and Adolescent Psychiatry (AACAP), guidelines have been published to assist physicians in making the diagnosis of ADHD. Efforts must be made to identify these barriers of the diagnosis and treatment of ADHD, awareness among healthcare providers, and the African-American and other Minority communities. The objective of this chapter is to examine the disparities in the diagnosis and treatment of ADHD in the minority groups in America, especially the African-American community, the factors associated with disparities and the impacts of these disparities. The strategies and interventions to address the issue will also be outlined.

2. Challenges in diagnosis and treatment of ADHD in African-Americans

2.1. Parent-driven barriers to care

2.1.1. Lack of knowledge/awareness about ADHD

Perceptions of ADHD-related symptoms among parents of African American children appear to differ in important ways from those of parents of White children. African American families from low to middle class incomes, compared with Whites, tend to view behavioral and emotional difficulties as problems of and for families, institutions and communities rather than as constituting individual psychopathology. It is not uncommon for African-American parents to perceive many of the symptoms and behaviors associated with ADHD to be variants of normal behavior and not in need of professional intervention. When compared with parents from other ethnic backgrounds, many African-American parents are not well-informed about the symptoms and treatment of ADHD. Indeed, studies suggest that African-American parents may be even more uninformed about ADHD, its causes, diagnosis and treatment than are parents form other ethnic and racial backgrounds. Bussing and colleagues (1998) conducted a study that sought to identify the differences in ADHD knowledge between 224 African-American parents and 262 White parents. They reported that only 69% of African-American parents compared with 95% of White parents had ever heard about ADHD ($p<0.01$), and that 36% of African-Americans knew "a lot", "some" or "a little" about ADHD, compared with 70% of White parents ($p<0.01$). In addition, as reported by African-American parents, only 18% of them received information about ADHD from their physician, compared with 29% of White parents ($p<0.01$). Equally important, the study found the effects of ethnicity on ADHD familiarity were independent of other covariates, such as socioeconomic status. Furthermore, the lack of knowledge about ADHD among the African-American community has been described as a "vicious cycle" that may be caused when members of this community seek medical advice from other individuals within their own ethnic background who are equally uninformed about ADHD.

2.1.2. Fear of over-, under-, and misdiagnosis

ADHD in African-American children is associated with comorbid disruptive behavior; mood and anxiety disorders. However, African-American families may not attribute the symptoms of ADHD to the disorder itself and are less aware than White families about the etiology of ADHD. For example, sugar intake has been reported as a common explanation for the symptoms of ADHD among members of the African-America community. ADHD symptoms in African-Americans are frequently missed or incorrectly diagnosed and comorbid disorders go unattended. African-American parents feel more uneasy than White parents about treating their children with pharmacologic interventions. Dos and other investigators evaluated parental perceptions of stimulant medication for the treatment of ADHD; they demonstrated that significant numbers of non-whites parents (63%) than white parents (29%) thought that counseling was the best choice of treatment, whereas 59% of white parents of white parents preferred medication over counseling compared with 36% of non-white parents. In addition, 16% of non-whites compared with 5% of white parents believed that the use of stimulants would lead to drug abuse. School officials are more likely to assign African-American children to special education classes (which is the only educational resource employed to address many black children with ADHD), although many of the symptoms they display may be resolved with proper treatment that would allow them to remain in their regular classes. Between 1980 and 1990, black children were placed in special education at more than twice the rate of whites.

2.1.3. Fear of social stigma

African-American parents (57%) are more likely to believe that their children's race or ethnicity and fears of being "labeled" remain one of the important factors preventing acceptance of the diagnosis and treatment of children with ADHD. Many parents fear the perceived social stigma of ADHD diagnosis, and some fear overdiagnosis and misdiagnosis.

The stigma of ADHD and lack of information about ADHD were found to be significant barriers to treatment of ADHD among African Americans [Table 1]. In their survey study, Omolara and colleagues (2007) found evidence of racial concerns about the stigma of ADHD diagnosis among African American participants. While some believe that a diagnosis of ADHD "gives children a label for the rest of their lives', others viewed that medicalization as a form of social control with historical roots.

In addition, pressures from family and friends to refrain from seeking treatment, fear of jeopardizing future employment or ability to serve in the military, concerns that parental skills will be questioned, and fear of the unknown are other factors that have been described by patient and families and these are thought to impact the diagnosis and treatment of ADHD. The African-American population fear of the unknown may be related in part to the consequences of the Tuskegee Experiment, which caused many in the community to lose trust in the field of medical research. However, African American health professionals were even found to be less likely to diagnose ADHD or prescribe stimulant medication treatment due to their social and culturally constructed views of the disorder.

It has also been demonstrated from studies that a substantial proportion of children from all races who are at a high risk for ADHD drop out of care, and that adolescent perceived stigma about ADHD is influential, above and beyond the perspectives of parents.

	African-American	White
Familiarity with ADHD		
"Not at all familiar" with ADHD	10%	2%
ADHD is a "very serious" condition	36%	28%
Know someone diagnosed with ADHD	56%	78%
Have a child with ADHD who is receiving treatment	46%	60%
Cultural Perceptions and Beliefs		
African Americans are more likely than other ethnic groups to be diagnosed with ADHD	41%	13%
African-American children are told more often than children of other ethnic groups that they have ADHD	33%	8%
Teachers are more likely to suspect ADHD in African-American children with learning or behavioral problems than in other ethnic groups	45%	12%
Very concerned about what others may think	13%	5%
Concern about treatment based on race or ethnic background prevents parents from seeking proper treatment	36%	13%
Limited access to healthcare professionals knowledgeable about ADHD prevents children from receiving appropriate treatment	44%	39%
Aware of treatments that help to lessen the symptoms of ADHD	66%	84%
Have sought help from a medical professional for suspected ADHD	86%	94%
Would be very concerned if their child was diagnosed with ADHD	71%	53%
Know where to go for help if their child is diagnosed with ADHD	64%	79%

Table 1. Most prominent difference between African-American and white respondents in perceptions and attitudes about ADHD

http://dx.doi.org/10.5772/54276

2.2. Health system/clinician-driven barriers

A substantial number of obstacles to the successful diagnosis and successful treatment of ADHD overall are related to limitations in the diagnosis and treatment of ADHD in African-American patients. While some of these barriers are easier to remove, others may prove more difficult. Some of these barriers are race or ethnicity-related, while others may be attributable to limited access to healthcare or insurance coverage, low socioeconomic status of African-American patients and a dearth of culturally-competent mental healthcare providers. Bussing et al. (2003) found that African American children were less than half as likely to be assessed, diagnosed, and treated for ADHD as Caucasians. Their research survey among African American parents to determine common barriers to help seeking for their children with symptoms of ADHD found that across race, the most commonly cited barriers are system barriers, no perceived need and negative expectations of treatment outcomes.

2.2.1. Lack of culturally competent healthcare providers

It has been reported that during clinician-patient encounter, negative social stereotypes are known to shape behaviors and influence decisions made by healthcare providers. Race and ethnicity is known to adversely influence the medical care provided for other medical conditions. Minority patients with ADHD are likely to be affected by this practice as well. Historically, there has been a disproportionate pattern of diagnosis among minority populations in the category of disability. While some of this pattern of diagnosis may be related to minorities being disproportionately exposed to risk factors and psychosocial stressors and are more likely to be economically disadvantaged, the commonly used instruments of assessment which could provide misleading or invalid results when used alone to assess patients from various cultural backgrounds may explain the this phenomenon. Frequently, the quality of healthcare delivered is compromised when healthcare providers are culturally insensitive to patients. There are important cultural differences among individuals of diverse ethnic backgrounds pertaining to their attitudes and beliefs of illness, choice of care, access to care, and degree of trust toward authority figures or institutions and tolerances for certain behaviors. Investigators may have to use culturally sensitive diagnostic tools to assist them in uncovering important aspects about ADHD that may be unique to the African-American population.

2.2.2. Healthcare provider/teacher bias or prejudice

Humans have the inclination to perceive or label other people or things based on their initial impressions or due to harboring elements of discrimination and stigma. Healthcare workers and physicians who care for mental health patients are not exonerated from this attribute. Eack and colleagues (2008) reported that African-Americans were three times more likely as whites to receive a diagnosis of schizophrenia based on the physician perception of the truthfulness, suspicion of symptom denial, poor insight or "uncooperativeness" of their African-American patients. Without a good understanding of cultural nuances that may provide clues about other possible diagnoses and the stigma associated with a diagnosis of mental illness among the Black community, white physicians may view black patients with suspicion which may color or affect their clinical judgment. Interestingly, the same study reported that this disparity did not appear to affect other US minority groups, such as Hispanics.

Conscious (Explicit) or unconscious (Implicit) bias or prejudices held by healthcare providers and sometimes racially-motivated discrimination by mental healthcare personnel can cause the cross-cultural diagnosis of ADHD to be challenging. In addition, biases expressed by the evaluators, interviewers or the researcher may influence the outcomes of scoring the behavioral expressions of African-American children. Depending on this held biases or cultural expectations of what constitutes "normal behaviors", non-African American evaluators may rate American-American children with higher levels of hyperactive or disruptive behaviors even when the behavior is normal within the context of cultural expectations. It is not uncommon for parents and patients of ethnic minorities to report discrimination in receiving health care. Gingerich and colleagues (1998) reviewed several comparative studies in the 1970 which used teachers' ratings to compare the prevalence of hyperactivity, a component of ADHD among ethnic minorities and white children. They reported one large study conducted using 1700 elementary school children from rural and urban Texan locations in which African-American children were rated as more hyperactive than expected based on their representative population when compared with schools located in white, middle-class neighborhoods where they found that the frequency of hyperactivity was consistent across all ethnic groups. The biases held by health care workers or mental health service providers can result in either under or over-diagnosis of ADHD in African-American children.

2.2.3. Dearth of African-America healthcare providers

This factor may prevent the optimal care of Africa-American children with ADHD. More minority clinicians are needed to alleviate the intercultural issues of trust and communications that often arise. In 1985, out of the 30,000 Psychiatrists registered to practice in American, only about 600 were Black (Bell, Fayen & Mattox, 1998). In spite of the efforts and progress made in promoting diversity of healthcare professionals among the physician workforce, the concern about a lack of diversity continues to be an impediment to access and care, especially in the minority populations. Thus, despite some initial progress, African Americans, Latinos/Hispanics, and Native Americans continue to be underrepresented in the U.S. physician workforce. The American Medical Association Council on Medical Education Report 7 (2007) put the total number of US physicians involved in patient care in 2006 as 723,118. When categorized into Race/Ethnicity, 71.4% of these physicians were white, 15.8% were Asian, 6.4% were Hispanic, and 4.5% were Black/African-Americans. The American Medical Association report in 2012 puts the total number of Black physicians in the workforce at 3.5%, indicating a decline (Table 2). Complicating access to care, most of these physicians set up their practices in urban areas to the detriment of rural communities.

http://dx.doi.org/10.5772/54276

2.2.4. *Limited access to mental health care*

African-American families are less likely than their white counterparts to have access to the healthcare system. This may partly be due to the lower socioeconomic class and higher poverty levels among African-Americans. African-Americans tend to lack insurance coverage for psychiatric or psychological evaluations, behavior modification programs, school consultations, parent management training, and other specialized program. Substantial costs barriers exist resulting in out-of-pocket costs. Pastor and Reuben reported a significantly wide and long-standing gap in the rate of the diagnosis of ADHD based on the type of health insurance coverage. They reported that those with Medicaid insurance are most likely to be diagnosed with ADHD, followed by those with private insurance coverage, while those without insurance ended at a distant third. Even when they have insurance, the capitation imposed by the State Mental Health Services further makes access to care very difficult or inadequate, especially, for African Americans and other minority populations. Low income African American caregivers are often frustrated and feel helpless while trying to navigate the maze of the care system. There is no funded special education category specifically for ADHD. This limited access to healthcare system will contribute to less diagnosis of ADHD

Race/Ethnicity	Number	Percentage
White	519,840	54.5
Black	33,781	3.5
Hispanic	46,507	4.9
Asian	116,412	12.2
American Native/Alaska Native	1,594	.16
Other	13,019	1.3
Unknown	223,071	23.4
Total physicians by race/ethnicity – 2008		
(Total physicians = 954,224)		

Table 2. Source: Physician Characteristics and Distribution in the US, 2010 Edition. American Medical Association.

3. Impact of ADHD in African-Americans

Comorbidities associated with ADHD include Conduct Disorders, Opposition Defiant Disorders (ODD), Depressive Disorders, Anxiety disorders, Learning disabilities and Alcohol and Drug addiction. Samuel and colleagues (1999) stated that African-American children with ADHD have higher levels of comorbid psychopathology (Opposition Defiant Disorder, Severe Major Depression, Bipolar Depression, and Separation Anxiety) than in African-American controls. They also reported that when compared to their Caucasian counterparts,

African-American youths have a tendency to be more resistant or unable to seek treatment, only doing so when their symptoms are more severe. This may be responsible for a broader spectrum of the severity of ADHD symptoms in African-American youths. Epstein (2005) attributed the exhibition of more ADHD symptoms in African-American youths to fact that they are exposed to more ADHD-related risk factors. This concept was supported by Stein and colleagues (2002) who reported that African-American youth may be exposed to these risk factors at higher rates other than other youth, which may account for the higher prevalence of ADHD in African-Americans. In the general population, some of the risk factors associated with the development of ADHD and related pathology include low socioeconomic status (SES), juvenile detainee status, prenatal marijuana exposure and exposure to environmental toxins. Lead, one of the most thoroughly studied environmental toxins, is linked to impaired attention, hyperactivity, and aggression even at low levels of exposure. Bazargan and colleagues (2005) found that African-Americans living in Public Housing reportedly have higher incidence of ADHD than in the general population as a whole (19%) as compared to the pooled rate of 5%. The increased exposure resulted from paints used in housing before 1950s which contained a high percentage of lead. Other risk factors attributable to higher incidence of ADHD in African-Americans include low socioeconomic status, lack of access to healthcare (Kendall & Hatton, 2002) and high incidence of low birth weight (Breslau & Chilcoat, 2000). The higher incidence and symptomatology of ADHD in African-Americans has its consequences some of which will be further elucidated.

3.1. ADHD among African-American youth and the criminal justice system

There appears to be an epidemic of incarceration, especially of African-American males in the United States of America. Compared to the rest of the industrialized world, America has the highest rate of incarceration, currently at about 738 per 100,000. The Justice Department reports that there are about 2.3 million inmates incarcerated in America. In 2010, Dick and Sharon Kyle, a pair of citizen journalists and information activists reported (www.LAProgressive.com) in an article titled "More Black Men in Prison than Were Enslaved II" that by race, Black males continued to be incarcerated at an extraordinary rate. They pointed out that Black males make up 35.4 percent of the jail and prison population, even though they make up less than 10 percent of the overall U.S population. They also observed that four percent of U.S. black males were in jail or prison in 2009, compared to 1.7 percent of Hispanic males and 0.7 percent of white males. This translated to black males being locked up at almost six times the rate of their white counterparts.

Black and colleagues (2010) reported that although Attention Deficit/Hyperactivity Disorder (ADHD) is associated with comorbid psychiatric diagnoses and antisocial behavior that contribute to criminality, yet studies of ADHD in offenders are few. Out of the 319 offenders they evaluated using the Mini International Neuropsychiatric Interview and Medical Outcome Health Survey; ADHD was present in 68 (21.3%) subjects. Offenders with ADHD were more likely to report problems with emotional and social functioning and to have a higher suicide risk scores. Other psychopathologies identified in offenders with ADHD include higher rates of mood, anxiety, psychotic and somatoform disorders. They are also more likely to have antisocial and borderline personality disorders. To reduce the impact of ADHD on the rate of incarceration of African-American youth, they recommended that Prison Administrators be trained to recognize the symptoms of ADHD and recommend offenders for further intensive screening rather than commitment to prisons first.

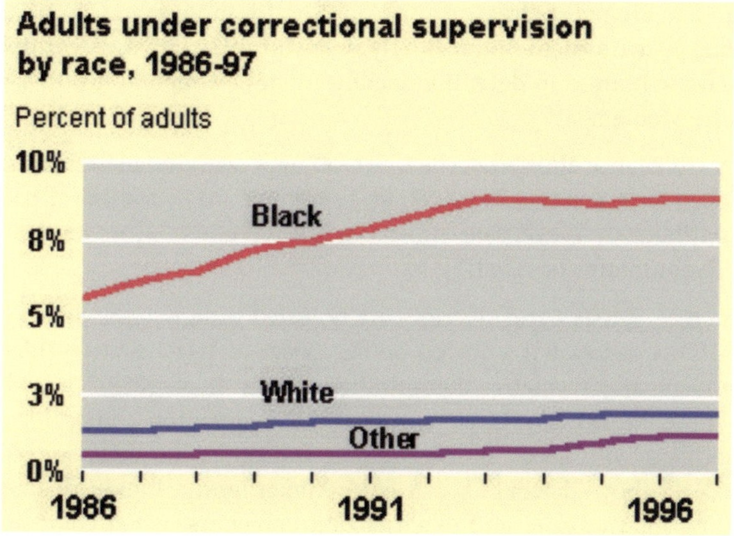

Figure 1. Source: www.prisonerhealth.org

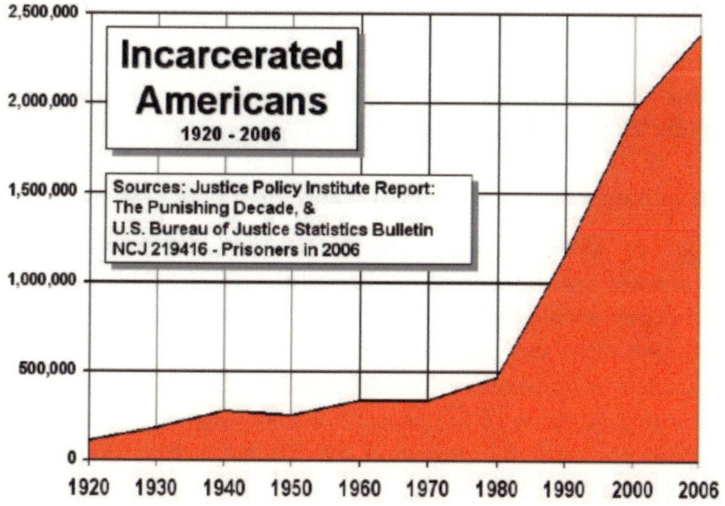

Figure 2. Source: Justice Policy Institute Report: The Punishing Decade, & U.S. bureau of Justice Statistics Bulletin. NCJ219416. Prisoners in 2006.

3.2. ADHD and substance abuse disorder in African-Americans

Records show that many American youth are caught up in our juvenile justice system. Significant proportions of the arrests are due to either possession of or use of substances, particularly marijuana and crack cocaine. The United States Department of Justice puts the estimate of yearly arrest of juveniles at 2.5 million with approximately over a 100,000 youth under the age of 18 years incarcerated daily. Minority youth in the African-America and Hispanic population are overrepresented, accounting for more than 60% of juvenile offenders in the juvenile justice system. Interestingly, many of these detained youth have psychiatric disorders and are housed in detention facilities that lack mental health services, thereby compounding the problem.

Individuals with substance abuse disorders exhibit hyperactivity, inattention and impulsivity which are core symptoms of ADHD. These symptoms may promote antisocial behaviors which may contribute or exacerbate substance use or abuse. Conversely, substance use could worsen the symptoms of ADHD.

Studies of substance abusers and delinquents revealed a higher prevalence of ADHD comorbidity. ADHD is associated with an earlier onset of psychoactive substance use disorders, independent of psychiatric comorbidities. Retz et al. (2007) stated that children with ADHD show higher levels of substance use disorder comorbidity, particularly when it is associated with social maladaptation and antisocial behavior. Addicted delinquents with ADHD showed worse social environment and a higher degree of psychopathology, including internalizing and externalizing behaviors, when compared to addicted delinquents without ADHD. Retz and coworkers (2007) systematically examined 129 young male prison inmates for ADHD and substance use disorder. They found that 64.3% showed harmful alcohol consumption and 67.4% fulfilled DSM-IV criteria for any drug abuse or dependence. Further analysis showed that 28.8% of the participants had a diagnosis of ADHD combined type and 52.1% showed ADHD residual type. The outcome of these results should suggest adequate therapeutic interventions for addicted young prison inmates, considering the ADHD comorbidity, which is associated with additional psychopathology and social problems.

3.3. ADHD, African-American children/youth, and the school system

The core symptoms of ADHD, hyperactivity, inattention and impulsivity, are associated with poor developments in several areas of normal functioning. This may be reflected in African-American children with ADHD as poor academic achievements and comportment at school. Biederman and other investigators found that while hyperactivity declines over the course of the disorder, inattention symptoms persist into adulthood. Currie and Stabile, (2006) stated that this persistence of the inattention component of ADHD may be associated with numerous functional deficits, including educational failure. ADHD symptoms affect social functioning, interactions with teachers, peers, siblings and overall quality of life. Non-African-American teachers are more likely to rate African-American children as more hyperactive and disruptive in class than children from other ethnic backgrounds. The Office of Special Education Report (2005) revealed that although African-American children represent

http://dx.doi.org/10.5772/54276

only 15% of the US population in 2001, they were overrepresented in specific learning disabilities (18%), mental retardation (34%) and are more likely to be emotionally disturbed (28%). The National Center for Education Statistics (2001) documented that African-American males make up the majority of students described as "emotionally disturbed" and are more likely to be suspended, expelled from school or subjected to corporal punishment than their white or female peers. In addition to living in extreme poverty and other social dysfunctions, it has been suggested that ADHD may be contributory to the high rates of school drop-out among African-American youth

3.4. The economic impacts of ADHD on African-American families

There is evidence that ADHD places a substantial economic burden on patients, their families and third-party payers. Pelham and his colleagues (2007) projected that the economic impact of education and medical services for children diagnosed with ADHD as at 2005 was conservatively estimated at $36-$52 billion per year, which makes ADHD an important economic and social issue. It is also true that most African-American families live in poverty and are less likely to be insured or have access to mental health services. ADHD leads to increased costs in healthcare and other domains, which is likely to have economic implications for African-American families, their children with ADHD diagnosis and the society in general. Das and colleagues documented a correlation between ADHD, employment status and financial stress in middle-age individuals with ADHD. They also reported significant impairment in health, personal and social domains in their study group.

The economic implications of ADHD on African-America families may include the costs related to common psychiatric and medical comorbidities of ADHD, the indirect costs associated with work loss among adults with ADHD, the costs of managing accidents among individuals with ADHD and the costs associated with the legal issues engendered by the criminality and deviant behaviors among individuals with ADHD. Chow and colleagues (2003) reported that the economic difficulties imposed on African-Americans due to poverty and lack of health insurance makes it more likely that African-Americans resort to the use of emergency services when they receive mental health care.

3.5. ADHD and the risk of sexually transmitted diseases among African-Americans

A comparative study on self-reported risky sexual behaviors was conducted by Flory and colleagues (2006) in young adults (ages 18 to 26) with and without childhood attention deficit/hyperactivity disorder diagnosis. Among the participants were 175 males with a Pittsburg Longitudinal Study (PALS) diagnosis of childhood ADHD. The controls were 111 demographically similar males without childhood ADHD diagnosis. The conclusion drawn from this study is that childhood ADHD predicted earlier initiation of sexual activity and intercourse, more sexual partners, more casual sex, and more partner pregnancies. Although they pointed out that childhood conduct problems did contribute significantly to risky sexual behaviors among participants with ADHD, they also observed an independent contribution of ADHD, which suggested that the characteristic deficits of the disorder or other associated features may be useful childhood markers of later vulnerability. White and colleagues (2012) reported that ADHD symptoms were associated with greater sexual victimization during adolescence and engagement in risky sexual behaviors. The same study also found a strong association between ADHD symptoms, sexual victimization as well as risky sexual behaviors which is stronger for black women than their white counterparts. Risky sexual behaviors result in increased incidence of Sexually Transmitted Diseases (STDs), HIV/AIDS and unplanned teen pregnancies among African-American youth. Currently, The Center for Disease Control and Prevention (CDC) ranks African-American males as leading other races and gender groups in incarceration rates, new HIV infections, homicide deaths, poverty rates, and diagnosed learning disorders. In addition, the 2011 CDC Report on "African Americans and sexually Transmitted Diseases" showed that STDs take an especially heavy toll on African Americans, particularly young African American women and men. Although African Americans represent just 14 percent of the U.S. population, yet they account for approximately half of all reported chlamydia and syphilis cases and almost three-quarters of all reported gonorrhea cases.

3.6. Impact of ADHD on family structure and cohesion among African-Americans

Das and colleagues reported that inattention symptoms associated with ADHD significantly affects multiple life domains in mid-life. Marriages, spousal relationships, social interactions and health-related quality of life are all negatively impacted by ADHD symptoms. The families of children with ADHD have to contend with a greater number of behavioral, developmental and educational disturbances which often requires that more time, commitment, logistics and energy be spent. ADHD can put a strain on family relationships, especially for partners that have different views on discipline and parenting styles. The stress may be elevated if either parent feels they are bearing the burden of dealing with the child with ADHD, like taking time off to deal with behavioral problems, school attendance, medical consultations or meeting as part of ADHD management. Parents can feel overwhelmed or find it challenging to cope with their child's disruptive behaviors. Parents may feel socially isolated if they start avoiding social events or family gatherings in hope of avoiding behavioral problems associated with their child's diagnosis. The child with ADHD may unintentionally hurt other kids or their siblings during plays or damage property, thereby causing strained relationships. Spousal relationships may be strained. There is the danger of both or either parents spending so much time on the child with ADHD that they do not spend enough time cementing their relationship as couples. This may lead to domestic conflicts, violence and sometimes divorce. The level of attention paid by parents to the child with ADHD may engender sibling jealousy and rival with the family

4. Conclusion

Strategies and interventions

A number of strategies and interventions have been suggested to improve outcomes and reduce the impact of ADHD in African-Americans. These should be targeted at early diagno-

http://dx.doi.org/10.5772/54276

sis and treatment of ADHD, increasing awareness about ADHD, removing the stigma of mental illness, elimination of healthcare disparities, enabling access to healthcare and teaching the benefits of ADHD treatment. The importance of early diagnosis and prompt treatment cannot be overemphasized. Instead of using one-size-fits-all or the traditional diagnostic parameters, clinicians should incorporate ethnically-sensitive structured parent questionnaires or rating scales to aid in the diagnosis of ADHD in African American children. It is also suggested that care be tailored to suit the needs of African-American children with ADHD and their care-givers. This may engender more corporation and acceptance of a diagnosis of ADHD in their children and compliance with treatment programs. It is important to have an integrated health care system where patients and their families can have greater access to culturally sensitive materials or programs that will educate them about the symptoms of ADHD and the benefits of proper treatment that will improve behaviors. Parents, caregivers and mental health counselors should be involved in all the stages of diagnosis and treatment planning of African-American children with ADHD. This strategy will enable them to become partners in their own care and secure their cooperation as much as possible. This will also decrease the rate of discontinuity of care since management of ADHD of ADHD requires adherence to treatment regimens and medical appointments.

Odom and colleagues evaluated and demonstrated the usefulness of increasing awareness of ADHD through educational intervention in mothers, predominantly African Americans and reported increase in parental confidence and satisfaction among those who were taught about ADHD; since these qualities are needed in coping with this chronic illness. Same education and training should be provided to teachers who serve the African American populations.

As earlier stated, clinicians may consider using ethnically sensitive, structured questionnaires or rating scales to aid in the diagnosis of ADHD in African Americans. Obtaining a thorough medical history, conducting a thorough physical examination and utilization of guidelines on the diagnosis and evaluation of ADHD is imperative rather than relying too heavily on questionnaires for the diagnosis of ADHD.

Substantial strides at improving outcomes can be made by clinicians and healthcare providers by initiating pilot programs that will track the efficacy of a longitudinal care model whereby primary care physicians will collaborate with mental healthcare professionals. Furthermore, schools, primary care providers and service agents should be incorporated into this collaborative effort to monitor symptoms of ADHD and the response to treatment since a successful management of ADHD is contingent on cooperation and open communication among these caretakers. It is very important that adequate numbers of minority healthcare providers be accessible in schools, clinics and hospitals to address the potential issues of cross-cultural bias and mistrust. Thus, healthcare organizations must recruit and retain a diverse staff whose demographic characteristics are representative of the service area

Healthcare institutions must consider ways of offering improved access to medical services and raising the level of awareness in the community. For example, community events, churches and day care centers could be used to disseminate information and teach about

ADHD in order to raise awareness regarding the importance of treatment and to lessen fears of stigmatization in the community.

It is important that care be tailored to suit the needs of various ethnic groups, such the African American community. Culturally competent medical care ensures that all patients will receive care that is compatible with their cultural beliefs and practices. The need to increase cultural competence in healthcare is described in detail in "Healthy People 2010", which is a statement of national health objectives that are designed to identify the most significant preventable threats to health and to establish national goals to reduce these threats. The criminal code of sentencing and guidelines for African-Americans with a diagnosis of ADHD needs to be reviewed with a view to the elimination of the zero tolerance policy. Instead of confining African American youths to the prison In conclusion, healthcare providers must be diligent in their commitment to reduce or remove barriers to the proper diagnosis and treatment of ADHD in African Americans. There is the need to increase awareness in the African American community regarding the symptoms of ADHD and its treatment, and to improve cultural awareness and sensitivity towards African-American patients among clinicians to reduce the challenges involved in the cross-cultural diagnosis.

Author details

Rahn Kennedy Bailey* and Ejike Kingsley Ofoemezie

*Address all correspondence to: rkbailey@mmc.edu; kofoemezie@mmc.edu; ofoemezie@msn.com

Department of Psychiatry & Behavioural Sciences, Meharry Medical College, Nashville, Tennessee, U.S.A.

References

[1] Abram KM, Teplin LA, McClelland GM, Dulcan MK.Comorbid psychiatric Disorders in Youth in Juvenile Detention. Arch Gen psychiatry. (2003)., 60, 1097-1108.

[2] American Academy of Pediatrics. Clinical practice guideline: diagnosis and evaluation of the child with attention-deficit/hyperactivity disorder.Pediatrics.(2000)., 105, 1-158.

[3] American Psychiatric Association.Diagnostic and Statistical Manual of Mental Disorders, 4th ed. Washington, DC: American Psychiatric Association; (1994).

[4] Anderson LA, Scrimshaw SC, Fullilove MT, et al.Culturally competent healthcare systems. Am J Prev Med. (2003)., 24, 68-79.

[5] Anonymous.National Institutes of Health Consensus Development Conference Statement: diagnosis and treatment of attention-deficit/hyperactivity disorder (ADHD). J Am Acad Child Adolesc Psychiatry. (2000).

[6] Ayalon, L., & Alvidrez, J. The experience of Black consumers in the mental health system: Identifying barriers to and facilators of mental health treatment using the consumer's perspective ((2007). Issues in Mental Health Nursing, , 28, 1323-1340.

[7] Bach PB, Cramer LD, Warren JL, et al.Racial differences in the treatment of early-stage lung cancer. N Engl J Med. (1999). , 341, 1198-1205.

[8] Black, DW et al.Int Journal of Offender Ther Comp Criminology June (2010). , 54(3)

[9] Burgess, D. L., Ding, Y., Hargreaves, M., van Ryn, M., & Phelan, S. The association between perceived discrimination and underutilization of needed medical and mental health care in a multi-ethnic community sample. J. Health Care Poor Underserved. (2008). , 19(3), 894-911.

[10] Bussing, R., Gary, F. A., Mills, T. L., et al. Parental explanatory models of ADHD: gender and cultural variations. Soc Psychiatr Epidemiol. (2003). , 38, 563-575.

[11] Bussing, R., Schoenberg, N. E., & Perwien, A. R. Knowledge and information about ADHD: Evidence of cultural differences among African-American and white parents. Soc Sci Med. (1998). , 46, 919-928.

[12] Bussing, R., Zima, B., Garry, E., & Garvan, C. (2003). Barriers to detection, help-seeking, and service use for children with Attention deficit Hyperactivity symptoms. Journal of Behavioral Health Services and Research, , 30, 176-189.

[13] Bussing, R., Zima, B. T., Mason, D. M., Porter, P. C., & Garvin, C. W. Receiving treatment for Attention Deficit Hyperactivity Disorder: Do the Perspectives of Adolescents Matter? Journal of Adolescent Health. (2012). , 49(2012), 7-14.

[14] Carpenter-Song, E. Caught in the Psychiatric Net: Meanings and experiences of ADHD, Pediatric Bipolar Disorder and Mental Health Treatment among a Diverse Group of families in the United States. Cult Med Psychiatry ((2009).

[15] Casangrande SS, Gary TL, LaVeist TA, Gaskin DJ, Cooper LA.Perceived discrimination and adherence to medical care I a racially integrated community. J. Gen Intern Med. (2007). , 222, 389-395.

[16] Center for Disease Control and Prevention(2006). Racial and Ethnic Disparities in the Diagnosis of HIV/AIDS...33 States, 2001-2004. Morbidity and Mortality Week Report, , 55, 121-125.

[17] Center for Disease Control and Prevention (CDC).African Americans and Sexually Transmitted Diseases. CDC Fact Sheets. April (2011). , 1-4.

[18] Center for Disease Control and Prevention (CDC).Racial and ethnic disparities in the diagnosis of HIV/AIDS, in 33 States, 2001-(2004). Morbidity and Mortality Weekly Report. , 2006(55), 121-125.

[19] Cuffe, S., Moore, C., & Mc Keown, R. Prevalence and correlates of ADHD symptoms in the National Health Interview Survey. Journal of Attention Disorders. (2005). , 2005(9), 392-401.

[20] Das, D., Cherbuin, N., Butterworth, P., Anstey, K. J., Easteal, S. A., Population-Based, Study., of, Attention., Deficit, Hyperactivity., Disorder, Symptoms., Associated, Impairment., in-Aged, Middle., Adults, P., & Lo, . PLoS ONE. www.plosone.orgFebruary (2012). e31500, 7(2)

[21] Davison JC, Ford DY,(2002). Perceptions of attention deficit hyperactivity disorder in one African American community. Journal of Negro education. 70(4); , 264-274.

[22] Dos, Reis. S., Zito, J. M., Safer, D. J., et al. Parental perceptions and satisfaction with stimulant medication for attention-deficit hyperactivity disorder. J Dev Behav Pediatr. (2003). , 24, 155-162.

[23] Eack, S. M., & Newhill, C. E. (2008). An investigation of the relations between student knowledge, personal contact, and attitudes toward individuals with schizophrenia. Journal of Social Work Education, 44(3), 77-95.

[24] Flory K, Molina BS, Pelham WE, Gnagy E, Smith B . Childhood ADHD Predicts Risky Sexual Behavior in Young Adulthood. Journal of Clinical Child & Adolescent Psychology. Volume 35, Issue 4, 2006. Pages 571-577. DOI:10.1207/s15374424jccp3504_8

[25] Foy, J., Earls, M. A., process, for., developing, community., consensus, regarding., the, diagnosis., management, of., attention, deficit., & hyperactivity, disorder. Pediatrics. (2005). , 115

[26] Geiger JH.Racial stereotyping and medicine: the need for cultural competence. Can Med Assoc J. (2001). , 164, 1699-1700.

[27] Giles WH, Anda RF, Casper ML, et al.Race and sex differences in rates of invasive cardiac procedures in US hospitals. Data from the National Hospital Discharge Survey. Arch Intem Med. 1 995; , 1, 55-318.

[28] Gingerich, K. J., Turnock, P., Litfin, J. K., et al. Diversity and attention deficit hyperactivity disorder. J Clin Psychol. (1998). , 54, 415-426.

[29] Greenhill LL.Diagnosing attention-deficit/hyperactivity disorder in children.Clin Psychiatry. (1998). , 59, 31-41.

[30] Harris Interactive Poll, Barriers to the Diagnosis and Treatment of ADHD among African American and Hispanic Children, 3(7):1-3, April 2003

http://dx.doi.org/10.5772/54276

[31] Hillemeier, Foster. E. M., Heinrichs, B., Heier, B., Conduct, Problems., Prevention, Research., & Group, . Racial differences in parental report of attention deficit/hyperactivity disorder behaviors. J. Dev Behav Pediatr. (2007). Oct; , 28(5), 404-5.

[32] Kellison, I., Bussing, R., Bell, L., & Garvan, C. Assessment of stigma associated with attention deficit hyperactivity disorder: Psychometric evaluation of the ADHD stigma questionnaire. Psychiatry Res. (2010). , 178, 363-9.

[33] Kendall, J., & Hatton, D. Racism as a source of health disparity in families with children with Attention-Deficit Hyperactivity disorder. Advances in Nursing Science: December (2002). , 25(2), 22-39.

[34] LeFever GB, Dawson KV, Morrow AL.The extent of drug therapy for attention deficit-hyperactivity disorder among children in public schools. Am J Public Health. (1999). , 89, 1359-1364.

[35] Lewitt, E. M., & Baker, L. S. Children in Special Education. The Future of Children: Special Education for Children with Disabilities. Spring (1996). , 6(1)

[36] Livingston, R. Cultural issues in diagnosis and treatment of ADHD. J Am Acad Child Adolesc Psychiatry. (1999). , 38, 1591-1594.

[37] Mattox, G. African American youngsters inadequately treated for ADHD.Psychiatric News. (2001).

[38] Miller, T., Nigg, J., & Miller, R. Attention deficit hyperactivity disorder in African American children: What can be concluded from the past ten years. Clinical Psychology Review. (2009). , 2009(29), 77-86.

[39] Monroe, C. R. Why Are "Bad Boys" always Black? Causes of Disproportionality in School Discipline and Recommendations for Change. The Clearing House. Classroom Management for Middle and Secondary Schools (Sep.- Oct., (2005). , 79(1), 45-50.

[40] Odom SE.Effects of an educational intervention on mothers of male children with attention deficit hyperactivity disorder. J Community Health Nurs. (1996). , 1, 3-207.

[41] Omolara, O., dos, Reis. S., Garriet, V., Mychailyszyn, M. P., Anixt, J., Rowe, P. C., & Cheng, T. L. Community Perspectives of Childhood Behavioral problems and ADHD among African American Parents. Ambulatory Pediatrics (2007). , 7, 226-231.

[42] Pastor PN, and Reuben CA.Diagnosed attention deficit hyperactivity disorder and learning disability: United States, (2008). National Center for Health Statistics. Vital Health Statistics, 10 (237), 2004-2006.

[43] Pastor PN, Reuben CA.Attention deficit disorder and learning disability: United States, National Center for Health Statistics. Vital Health Stat.(2002). , 1997-1998.

[44] Pelham, W. E., Foster, M., & Robb, J. A. The Economic Impact of Attention-Deficit/ Hyperactivity Disorder in Children and Adolescents. Journal of Pediatric Psychology 32(6) (2007). doi:10.1093/jpepsy/jsm022, 711-727.

[45] Reid, R., Du, Paul. G. J., Power, T. J., et al. Assessing culturally different students for attention deficit hyperactivity disorder using behavior rating scales. J Abnorm Child Psychol. (1998)., 26, 187-198.

[46] Rowland, Umbach. D. M., Stallone, L., et al. Prevalence of medication treatment for attention deficit-hyperactivity disorder among elementary schoolchildren in Johnston County, NC. Am J Public Health. (2002)., 92, 231-234.

[47] Sabin JA, Greenwald AG.The influence of implicit bias on treatment recommendations for 4 common Pediatric conditions: Pain, Urinary Tract Infection, Attention Deficit/hyperactivity Disorder, and Asthma. American Journal of Public Health. May (2012)., 102(5)

[48] Safer DJ, Zito JM.Psychotrophic medication for ADHD. Ment Retard Dev Disabil Res Rev. (1999)., 5, 237-242.

[49] Samuel, V. J., Biederman, J., Faraone, S. V., et al. Clinical Characteristics of Attention Deficit Hyperactivity Disorder in African American Children. Am J Psychiatry 155:5, May (1998).

[50] Shavers VL, Lynch CF, Burmeister LF.Knowledge of the Tuskegee study and its impact on the willingness to participate in medical research studies. J Natl Med Assoc. (2000)., 92, 563-572.

[51] Shiefer SE, Escarce JJ, Schulman KA.Race and sex differences in the management of coronary artery. Am Heart J. (2000)., 139, 848-857.

[52] Snowden, J., Wallace, N., Kang, S., Cheng, J., & Bloom, J. Capitation and Racial ethnic differences in use and cost of mental health services: Administration and Policy in Mental Health and Mental Health Research. (2007)., 456-464.

[53] Stevens, J., Harman, J. S., Kelleher, K. J., & Race, . Race/Ethnicity and insurance status as factors associated with ADHD treatment patterns. J. Child Adoles. Psychopharmacol. (2005).

[54] The National Health Survey: ADHD Prevalence and Service Use.Abstract A6. Presented in the 50th Anniversary Meeting of the Academy of Child and Adolescent Psychiatry. October 15, (2003). Miami Beach, Florida.

[55] Todd, N., Samaroo, N., & Hoffman, J. R. Ethnicity as a risk factor for inadequate emergency department analgesia. JAMA. (1993)., 269, 1537-1539.

[56] Tucker, C., & Dixon, A. L. Low-income African American male youth with ADHD symptoms in the United States: Recommendations for the Clinical Mental Health Counselors. Journal of Mental Health Counseling. (2009)., 1040-2861.

[57] Tucker, C. Low income African Americans caregivers' experiences of being referred to mental health services by school counselor. Professional School Counselor. (2009)., 2009(12), 240-252.

[58] U.S.Department of Health and Human Services. Healthy People (2010). nd ed. Washington, DC: U.S. Government Printing Office; 2000.

[59] United States Department of Health and Human Services (USDHHS)(2005). Minority Health and Health Disparities. Available at: http://www.hrsa.gov/OMH/.

[60] Whaley AL, Gellar PA.Ethnic/Racial differences in Psychiatric disorders: A test of four hypotheses. Ethnicity and Disease. (2003)., 2003(13), 499-512.

[61] White, J. W., Buchler, C., Adolescent, Sexual., Victimization, A. D. H. D., Symptoms, , Risky, Sexual., & behaviors, . JW, Buchler C. Adolescent Sexual Victimization, ADHD Symptoms and Risky Sexual behaviors. J Fam Viol ((2012)., 123-132.

[62] Young, Klap. R., Sherbourne, C. D., et al. The quality of care for depressive and anxiety disorders in the United States. Arch Gen Psychiatry. 200 1; , 58, 55-6.

[63] Zito, J. M., Safer, D. J., dos, Reis. S., et al. Racial disparity in psychotropic medications prescribed for youths with Medicaid insurance in Maryland. J Am Acad Child Adolesc Psychiatry. (1998)., 37, 179-184.

Section 5

Outcome

Chapter 11

Attention-Deficit/Hyperactivity Disorder (ADHD) as a Barrier to Learning and Development within the South African Context: The Perspective of Teachers

Zaytoon Amod, Adri Vorster and Kim Lazarus

Additional information is available at the end of the chapter

http://dx.doi.org/10.5772/53784

1. Introduction

Attention-Deficit/Hyperactivity Disorder (ADHD) is a universal condition transcending cultural, socio-economic and racial barriers. It is considered to be the most common psychiatric disorder amongst children in the United States and Europe, with an estimated 3-10% of children being affected [1]. The situation in Africa does not appear to be much different and although there is a lack of knowledge with regards to ADHD on the African continent, it is believed that the disorder is as prevalent as it is in Western countries [1]. In South Africa specifically it is considered to be the most prevalent psychiatric disorder amongst children with a prevalence rate of approximately 10% [2]. As this has not been confirmed officially, it raises issues relating to possible over-identification of the disorder in South Africa. However, it is feasible that children present with comorbid attention difficulties, when taking into consideration the huge backlog in the education system and the high incidence of learning disorders and language difficulties as additional barriers to learning.

The South African education system is still struggling with the aftermath of Apartheid, which promoted exclusion in schools, not only based on race, gender, class, and ethnic background, but also on disability. This lead to the creation of a dual education system and learners, who did not meet the requirements of mainstream education, were placed in special education when educationalists considered it to be in the best interest of the learner [3]. With the abolition of Apartheid and the advent of the Constitution of the Republic of South Africa, Act No. 108 of 1996 [4], respect for the rights of all children regardless of variables such as race, gender, ethniticity, religion and ability was emphasised. This lead to the adaption of a new South African Education Policy, embedded in the philosophy of inclusive education and with its primary focus on "meeting the needs of all learners and actualising the full potential of all learners" [5, p.344].

Inclusive education is not uniquely South African and emerged as a key international policy when UNESCO's Salamanca Statement was adopted in 1994, at the World Conference on Special Needs Education in Salamanca, Spain [6]. The emphasis at the Salamanca Conference was on the development of an inclusive education system that would

> ...accommodate all children, regardless of their physical, intellectual, social, emotional, linguistic or other conditions. This should include disabled and gifted children, street and working children, children from remote or nomadic populations, children from linguistic, ethnic, or cultural minorities and children from other disadvantaged or marginalised areas or groups. [7]

It was further noted that inclusive education systems, must not only recognise and respond to the diverse needs of learners, but also make room for different learning styles and rates. In addition, it is important that education systems ensure the quality of education through the design of appropriate curricula and teaching strategies, whilst also using and involving appropriate community and other resources. [7]

Although inclusive education therefore has a universal philosophy and universal practices, in the South African context it needed to be indigenised to meet the needs of the South African education system. This was done partially through the adoption of an eco-systemic framework in viewing barriers to learning and development.

2. Eco-systemic framework

> Seen in different contexts, human nature, which I had previously thought of as a singular noun, became plural and pluralistic; for the different environments were producing discernible differences, not only across, but also within societies, in talent, temperament, human relations, and particularly in the ways in which the culture, or subculture, brought up its next generation. (Bronfenbrenner, 1979:p.xiii as cited in [8])

Urie Bronfenbrenner is widely known for his development of the eco-systemic theory which looks at the manner in which different environments and social contexts, including political, socio-economical, and cultural patterns, produce distinct differences in the way in which children develop. He argues that to truly understand a child, as well as his/her developmental difficulties, one must view the child holistically within his/her context [9]. The eco-systemic theory, which forms part of the broader social ecological model to understanding learning barriers and more recently titled the bio-ecological perspective [10], amalgamates ecological and systems theories to exemplify how a person's physical environment and the different levels of the person's social context are linked in dynamic, interacting, and interdependent relationships.

Therefore, on the one hand the eco-systemic perspective emphasises the importance of the impact that a person's physical environment can have on the development of the person. On the other hand, systems theory examines the multiple levels and groupings of a person's social context that function interdependently so that the whole is reliant upon the interaction of the parts and can only be understood if the different parts are examined. Furthermore, as the different levels of a person's social context is linked in every-changing, interacting and interdependent relationships; a shift in one system will impact the whole in a cyclical fashion.

Applied to ADHD within the South African context, the eco-systemic theory assists us in understanding how environmental factors such as lead poisoning [11], which are prevalent in the South African context [12-13], can have on the development of the disorder. Other environmental factors that are of particular importance in the development of ADHD [11] and prevalent in the South African context [14], include poverty and insufficient living conditions. In addition, the eco-systemic theory also assists us in understanding how the child's micro-, meso-, exo-, macro-, and chronosystems [10] can have on the developmental course of ADHD. Here factors such as family discord, a maternal history of psychiatric disorders and a particular parenting style, are of importance [11]. Therefore, applied to ADHD, the eco-systemic perspective helps us to understand that children cannot be viewed in isolation, but as part of the bigger whole and in a reciprocal relationship with it. Taking this into consideration, one of the major challenges in effectively addressing ADHD within the South African context is to understand the complexity of the disorder as seen in a particular context and environment [9].

3. Barriers to learning and development

Although the predominant paradigm in understanding learning barriers such as ADHD, used to be the medical-deficit model, a more social-ecological approach is applicable when introducing inclusive education into an education system as it shifts attention from viewing psychiatric disorders as caused by or located within the individual, to viewing the child as being part of a broader system that contains many risk and protective factors that either contribute to the development and maintenance of a particular difficulty, or the prevention thereof. The World Health Organisation [15] defines environmental factors such as poor socio-economic status and high crime rates that can increase the risk of the developmental of externalising difficulties such as ADHD, as risk factors. In contrast, factors such as supportive parenting styles and educational support that moderate the effects of ADHD and assist in the appropriate adaptation of children with this to the school environment, are seen as protective factors.

In adopting a more socio-ecological paradigm, there will therefore be a shift from using labels such as special needs to applying terminology such as risk and protective factors, or as it is noted in the South African policy documentation; barriers to learning and development [16]. Barriers to learning and development are defined as all factors that can impact upon learning

[17]. These barriers can occur within all levels of the eco-system and can be placed on a continuum; from intrinsic barriers that can be found within the individual, to extrinsic barriers which refer to factors outside the individual [17]. Some of the most prominent extrinsic barriers within the South African context include socio-economic barriers, negative attitudes towards difference and psychiatric disorders, inflexible curricula, inaccessible and unsafe building environments and schools, inappropriate and inadequate provision of support services, lack of enabling and protective legislation and policy, lack of parental recognition and involvement, and lack of human resource development strategies [16]. Some of the most prominent intrinsic barriers include language and communication difficulties, health difficulties such as HIV and tuberculosis, sensory impairments, intellectual and learning difficulties, and pervasive developmental disorders [17].

ADHD would be considered an intrinsic barrier as research has shown that genetic and biological factors such as an imbalance in the neurotransmitters noradrenalin and dopamine play an important role in the development of the disorder. It is however important to also take cognisance of the role that extrinsic barriers such as those noted above, as well as poor socio-economic circumstances, high crime rates, repeated trauma, parenting styles and parent-child interactions play in the maintenance and further developmental course of the disorder [15].

4. Teachers: A pivotal part of the eco-system

From an eco-systemic perspective, teachers can act as extrinsic barriers to learning and development when they act as risk factors in the developmental course of ADHD in particular learners in their classrooms. Likewise, teachers can also act as protective factors when their understanding of ADHD and support offered to the learners in their classrooms, positively impact on the developmental course of the disorder.

Teachers are often the primary source of identification and play a pivotal role in the diagnosis, management and intervention of ADHD. They have firsthand experience of the learner in the classroom situation; a setting which requires the learner to sit still, pay attention, adhere to instructions and interact with peers and adults in an appropriate manner. Teachers' knowledge and understanding will determine how they engage with and manage learners experiencing ADHD. Furthermore, their attitudes towards different forms of ADHD intervention would affect their support of these treatment methods and the learners in their classrooms. Early identification and intervention by teachers is vital, especially as a large percentage of individuals continue to have symptoms in adolescence and adulthood [18], which can impede their future wellbeing. It is important to take cognisance of the manner in which teachers' perceptions, knowledge and attitudes are influenced by contextual and socio-cultural factors, as shown in previous studies [1, 19-20].

It has however been found that teachers' understanding of ADHD is often based on myths and false beliefs. It has been reported that some teachers believe that ADHD is a direct cause of the intake of certain food additives and eating too many sweets [21]. Others are of the idea that ADHD is mainly as a result of biological abnormalities [11], or as a direct result of bad parenting and a lack of parental supervision [22]. It is essential to understand that if teachers have an incorrect understanding of ADHD and its causes and symptoms, it may lead them to actually support the presence of behaviours associated with ADHD, which can lead to inaccurate diagnosis [23].

Over the past decade, many research studies have been done on teachers' perceptions and knowledge of ADHD. In the United States, a sample of primary school teachers watched a video of a student displaying ADHD-like behaviours as well as those behaviours that are characteristic and unique to Oppositional Defiant Disorder (ODD). When examined, teachers were accurate in their evaluations of ADHD-like symptoms such as inattention and hyperactivity. However, when students displayed behaviours that belong solely to the domain of ODD, such as opposition and non-compliance, teachers automatically assumed that these behaviours were indicative of ADHD. Thus, teachers mistakenly assumed that children who displayed only ODD-like behaviours also exhibited ADHD-like behaviours [23]. A study conducted in Australia likewise revealed that teachers often provide parents and professionals with incorrect and inappropriate advice and information regarding the child who is displaying ADHD-like symptoms [21]. A study conducted in South Africa by [24] revealed that teachers are actually over identifying children with ADHD, as in the study 11.9% of the learners actually had ADHD, whilst teachers identified 15.4% of the learners to have ADHD. Thus, misunderstandings and misperceptions held by teachers may lead to inaccurate information being passed onto professionals, who carry out the task of making an actual ADHD diagnosis.

In support of these findings, further evidence reveals that teacher knowledge of ADHD tends to be very narrow and limited and even incorrect [21]. Three studies, as discussed in [21] were conducted in Australia over the last decade, which explored this area. One of the studies revealed that the teachers in the selected sample group were able to answer 60.7% of items in a questionnaire on ADHD. In a different study, the researchers administered the Knowledge of Attention Deficit Disorders Scale (KADDS) to a group of teachers. The findings of this study reflected that teachers knew more about the causes of ADHD, but possessed less information regarding treatment interventions for ADHD [21].

In South Africa, a study conducted in the peripheral areas of the Cape Town Metropole in the Western Cape, also employed the KADDS to assess 552 teachers' knowledge of ADHD [2]. Their study revealed that the participants did not have an adequate understanding of ADHD. An overall score of correct responses of 42,6% was obtained. An overall percentage of 35.4% was gathered for "don't know" responses, and 22% for incorrect responses [2].

These above results are consistent with a study conducted by [25]. In this South African study teachers' perceptions of their ability to identify and manage learners diagnosed with ADHD were investigated. Four out of five teachers did not consider themselves able to adequately manage ADHD symptoms, and some of the teachers misidentified and misunderstood certain symptoms of this condition. In a further study, [26] revealed that teachers do not have a sound understanding of the symptoms of ADHD, and the majority of teachers in the sample were unable to distinguish between inattention and ADHD. According to Venter (2011, as cited in [27]), teachers from poor black communities that teach at rural South African schools are the ones who possess the most limited knowledge on the condition. Consequently, these children are physically and verbally punished as a result of their ADHD behaviour.

Conversely, a South African study conducted by [28], which included five schools situated in economically deprived areas and three school situated in economically affluent areas, showed different results to those yielded by [2]. It was revealed that the majority of teachers in this sample group in fact had in-depth knowledge and understanding of ADHD, and were acutely aware of the symptoms of ADHD. The teachers believed that their role in the classroom was crucial to the management of the condition. Furthermore, teachers in this study were very eager to learn and gain more information on the condition. However, this study consisted of a very small sample group and the results garnered appear to be more of an exception and stronger evidence exists for the fact that teachers generally have a poor understanding and lack of knowledge on the condition [2].

Research in the past decade, has explored if older teachers and those teachers who have had more years of teaching experience have better knowledge and understanding of ADHD. An Australian study conducted by [29], where 120 teachers completed a survey on what they thought and knew about ADHD, showed that teachers with more years of teaching experience perceived themselves to have greater knowledge on the condition than the less experienced teachers. However, the number of years of teaching experience of these teachers was not related to their actual levels of knowledge. The age of the teachers was also not linked to the teachers' level of knowledge and understandings of the condition. These results are confirmed by the findings by [2].

However, other research [30] reported that in fact younger teachers know more about ADHD than older ones, a finding which is confirmed by [31]. One explanation for this may be the fact that younger teachers notice the condition more in their classrooms compared to their older counterparts who have developed effective classroom behaviour management strategies. One researcher [32] believes that older teachers are much more rigid and set in their ways as compared to younger teachers, who are willing to be open, honest and adaptable to the needs of ADHD learners.

The question arises as to whether a teacher, who has obtained a more advanced level of education, consequently knows more about ADHD. A study [33] conducted in the United States, which aimed to investigate preschool teachers' past educational practices and their knowledge and understanding of ADHD, revealed that those teachers that obtained higher levels of academic training, such as a university education, performed on a superior level and obtained higher scores on the administered questionnaire than those teachers that only obtained a high school level of education.

The study by [29] also indicated that having taught a student with ADHD is related to that teacher's actual knowledge of the condition. Then the question arises as to whether training and exposure in the area, such as the reading of articles on the topic and the attendance of workshops, contributes to a teacher's level of understanding and knowledge on ADHD. A study by [34], answers this question in the affirmative, and revealed that the attendance of workshops on ADHD has a positive relationship with teacher knowledge and understanding of ADHD. In the study by [2], teachers' exposure to ADHD, which includes the number of workshops attended as well as the number of articles read was positively correlated to their overall knowledge and understanding of the condition.

In the study by [29] older teachers were more likely to attend workshops and engage in ADHD training than the younger teachers. Teaching experience and exposure to ADHD also increased the likelihood of teachers attending workshops. The more workshops the teachers attended, the more knowledge they had on the disorder, compared to the teachers who did not attend workshops. This was confirmed by the South African study conducted by [2]. Teachers' confidence levels in their ability to teach and deal with a child with ADHD was positively related to their overall knowledge of this condition. As every teacher will experience at least one learner with ADHD per year, it may become essential for teachers to receive pre-service training in the area of ADHD [35].

5. Knowledge and perceptions of ADHD held by a sample of South African foundation phase township teachers

Whilst understanding the pivotal role that teachers' knowledge and perceptions play in the identification and treatment of ADHD, this chapter aims to integrate the information from the studies above, with one particular South African study [36] that focussed on the knowledge and perceptions held by a sample of South African Foundation Phase township teachers.

A range of mainstream and special education schools exist in South Africa, which include private and government funded schools. Of the government funded schools, formally white schools were better funded and resourced in comparison to the black township, rural and informal settlement schools. There is no previous documented research on township teachers' perceptions of ADHD in South Africa, which prompted the current study. The study was conducted in Alexandra Township in Gauteng, which is one of the oldest townships in South Africa. It was proclaimed as a township for black persons in 1912, by the Apartheid regime which classified South Africans into four racial groups. Alexandra Township, with a population of about 350 000 people, covers an area of over 800 hectares of land. It consists of persons of different cultures and varying degrees of income and education and has a history of poverty, overcrowding as well as high levels of unemployment and crime.

5.1. Aim of the study

The overall aim of this study was to explore and assess the knowledge and perceptions of ADHD held by a sample of Foundation Phase (Reception year to Grade 3) teachers within a township setting. More specifically, the research aimed at exploring the teachers' general knowledge as well as their inadequate knowledge and misconceptions regarding ADHD, with emphasis paid to its' associated features, symptoms/diagnosis and treatment. Teachers' knowledge of ADHD was also investigated in relation to their demographic group.

In fulfilling the aim of the study, the following research questions were posed:

- What is the teachers' general knowledge of the content areas of ADHD in terms of:
  - Associated Features
  - Symptoms/Diagnosis
  - Treatment
- What are teachers' specific areas of inadequate knowledge and misconceptions in the content areas of:
  - Associated Features
  - Symptoms/Diagnosis
  - Treatment
- Is teachers' knowledge of the ADHD content areas different by demographic group in terms of:
  - Associated Features
  - Symptoms/Diagnosis
  - Treatment

5.2. Research design and methodology

This research was exploratory in nature as there is very limited documented research on ADHD in South Africa. The study garnered both qualitative and quantitative material which was analysed using numerical and descriptive statistics. For logistical and practical reasons, nine primary schools situated within the Alexandra Township were selected. Non probability, convenience sampling was employed as participation by the teachers depended on their availability and willingness to respond. As a result, the final sample of 100 female teachers who consented to participate in the study was not random in nature [37-38]. Foundation Phase teachers were chosen as the sample for this study due to the fact that they play an integral and primary role when it comes to the identification and recognition of ADHD-like symptoms [39]. Permission to undertake the investigation was sought from the Gauteng Department of Education and the ethics committee at the University of the Witwatersrand. A detailed information sheet detailing issues of anonymity and confidentiality regarding the particulars of the study was distributed to the principals of the schools and their teachers.

Clear instructions were given to the respondents during administration of the instrument and assistance was provided if they did not understand what was required. A questionnaire was chosen as the preferred instrument as it allowed for administration to a large group of subjects [38]. The questionnaire which was administered to the 100 participants was threefold in nature. It included; demographic/biographical questions, the Knowledge of Attention Deficit Disorders Scale (KADDS), as well as open-ended questions. Permission to use the KADDS measure was obtained from Professor Mark Sciutto.

In the first section of the questionnaire teachers were asked demographic questions such as their gender, age, educational level and number of years of teaching experience. Teachers were also asked to provide the number of hours of ADHD training that they had received (if any), as well as the number of evaluations and assessments that they had requested for children in their classes that they thought may have ADHD. Teachers were required to indicate the number of children that they had taught with a medical diagnosis of ADHD, how many workshops that they had attended on the topic as well as the number of articles that they had read on the condition. The teachers were also asked to rate their confidence levels to teach a child with ADHD. Lastly, teachers were required to indicate whether they had been asked for feedback by a professional, such as a doctor or psychologist, regarding a child in their class with ADHD in order to assess the child's medication. These questions were based on a questionnaire that was administered in the previously reported South African study conducted by [2].

The second section of the questionnaire consisted of the Knowledge of Attention Deficit Disorder Scale (KADDS). This scale was developed by [31] and was previously used in similar studies in South Africa, see [2] and Australia, see [40]. It was designed and consequently published to assess teachers' knowledge, of the symptoms, associated features and treatment of ADHD. The KADDS is a 39 item rating scale which elicits true and correct answers (T), false, incorrect and misperceived answers (F) and don't know answers (DK). Previous research conducted on the internal consistency of the KADDS total score, based on the original 36 items that constituted this scale, revealed high internal consistency ranging from.81 to.86 [31,41-42]. A similarly high internal consistency for the KADDS was found in the present study, with the Cronbach's alpha for the total score being.88. In terms of validity, KADDS scores are sensitive to teacher characteristics such as exposure to and interaction with a child with ADHD and prior training on this condition [31].

The last section of the questionnaire contained open- ended questions, where participants were given the opportunity to provide any additional comments or ideas that they had regarding ADHD. This information served to substantiate and support the quantitative results garnered by the research. In research terms, this method of using multiple sources of data to strengthen the trustworthiness of the data, is referred to as the triangulation of data [43].

5.3. Data analysis

Descriptive and inferential statistics and graphs were used to describe the sample respondents and the measurement scales, and to address the aims of the research study. In order to investigate the areas of inadequate knowledge and misconceptions held by teachers, summary statistics for the central tendency, variability and shape were computed at the item level of the KADDS subscales. These results were tabulated using a robot- type colour coding scheme whereby higher mean scores were shaded in deep green and shades of yellow through to red were used for relatively lower and low means respectively. Furthermore, the responses to each item were categorised as "don't know", incorrect responses or misconceptions, and correct responses, thereby enabling the examination of the extent of teachers' misconceptions versus poor knowledge at the item level of each of the subscales. This analysis was depicted graphically in the form of a stacked bar graph for the items of each subscale of the KADDS. In order to address the teachers' general knowledge of ADHD content areas in terms of their demographic group, a 1-way Analysis of Variance (ANOVA) was used. This was used to compare the mean responses of the respondents across the levels within each demographic variable on the three KADDS subscales. Line graphs were used to portray the differences between means in the case of significant ANOVA comparisons. Furthermore, the post hoc Scheffe test was used to indicate pairwise significances for significant analyses of demographic variables with more than two levels. In view of the non-normality of the score distributions, the parametric ANOVA tests were validated using the non-parametric equivalent Kruskal-Wallis test. Finally, the Chi squared test was used to compare the demographic characteristics of the respondents who opted versus those who did not opt for a future workshop on ADHD and profile line graphs were plotted to describe the two groups of these demographic variables. In addition, the t-test was used to compare the mean knowledge scores on the three KADDS subscales of these two groups. These analyses were complemented by the researcher's thematic analysis of the qualitative responses.

5.4. Findings

All of the 100 respondents, who agreed to participate in this study, were female. The average learner to teacher ratio in the schools include in the schools, were 50:1. Almost two-thirds of the teachers in the sample were older than 40years, with a negligible number of them in the 20-25 year category. Consistent with the age distribution of the teacher respondents, the majority (60%) had more than 11 years of teaching experience, 20% had 6-10 years teaching experience and 20% had 5 years or less. Almost a quarter of the sample had a university level of education, while the remaining individuals had college level training. Over half of the respondents expressed no confidence in their ability to teach children with ADHD. Regarding their knowledge of ADHD, two thirds of the teachers had received no ADHD training. Over half of the respondents (52%) claimed that they had taught children diagnosed with ADHD and had assisted with ADHD evaluations (59%). Almost 40% claimed that they had been asked for feedback by a doctor regarding a child with ADHD in their classroom.

The overall results of the KADDS questionnaire revealed that there is a substantial lack of knowledge about ADHD amongst the participants. Based on the results of Table 1 the overall percentage of correct responses to the 39 KADDS items was 34.9%. Nine of the 100 educator respondents scored zero on all 39 items of the scale.

	Mean	95% Confidence Interval for mean		Median	Standard deviation	Skew Ness
Associated features	30.4%	27.0%	33.8%	31.3%	17.2%	-0.21
Symptoms/ Diagnosis	47.9%	43.3%	52.5%	50.0%	23.3%	-0.51
Treatment	30.6%	26.5%	34.8%	30.8%	20.9%	0.10
Overall	34.9%	31.3%	38.6%	37.2%	18.2%	-0.33

Table 1. Summary descriptive statistics of the three content areas of ADHD

Regarding the teachers' knowledge in terms of the Associated Features subscale, a mean score of 30.4% was garnered which was lower than the overall scale score of 34.9%, and based on the median score reflected in Table 1, half of the respondents answered fewer than 31.3% of these items correctly. The minimum scores of zero on the Associated Features subscale show 10 teachers who either did not know and/or who answered all the items of the subscale incorrectly. Of the three subscales, the highest mean (percentage correctly answered items) is for Symptoms/Diagnosis (47.9%). Even on this subscale, the average respondent answered approximately half of the items incorrectly. Nine of the 100 teachers scored zero on this Symptoms/Diagnosis subscale. The mean score of 30.6% on the Treatment subscale is comparably low in relation to the mean score on the Associated Features subscale which was lower than the overall KADDS score of 34.9%. The minimum scores of zero on this subscale show 15 teachers who either did not know and/or who answered all the items of the subscale incorrectly.

In order to determine the specific areas of poor knowledge and misconceptions of the content areas of ADHD, the scores of the educator respondents were examined at the item level for the three KADDS subscales. The low internal consistency reliability and low average inter-item correlation for the Associated Features subscale (Table 2) imply that some items of the subscale were answered correctly by teachers who answered other items incorrectly, and thus some items would be expected to have vastly different means from others. To reflect the items on which low and poor correct responses were obtained, a robot-type colour coding system was used whereby lower means were shaded red and highest means were shaded dark green with shades of orange for items in between. Item 1, which suggests that ADHD occurs in approximately 15% of school age children, item 27, which states that children with ADHD generally experience more problems in novel situations rather than familiar ones, item 30, which states that the problem behaviours in children with ADHD are distinctly different from the behaviours of non-ADHD children and item 39, which states that children with ADHD display an inflexible adherence to routine, all have very low percentage correct responses with means between 4% and 12%. These percentages are particularly low compared to items 13, which states that it is possible for an adult to have ADHD, item 31, which refers to the idea that children with ADHD are more distinguishable from normal children in a classroom setting as opposed to a free play situation and item 32, which states that the majority of children with ADHD evidence some degree of poor school performance during their early school years, which all have relatively high percentage correct responses with means between 60% and 62%. Apart from these three items, the mean score on the rest of the items of this subscale were all below 42%, and thus the standard deviations were low on these items and as a result on the whole subscale. This low response variability would have impacted negatively on the internal consistency reliability as Cronbach's alpha was dependent on the variability in the responses.

In order to investigate the low item scores, a distinction was made between misconceptions, i.e., incorrect responses, versus "don't know" responses. This distinction is displayed graphically for the Associated Features items in Figure 1 where bars shaded in blue indicate the percentage of misconceptions and bars shaded in red indicate incorrect responses for each item. Figure 1 shows that teachers have the greatest extent of misconception of ADHD on items 27, 1, 39 and 24, which states that a diagnosis of ADHD by itself makes a child eligible for placement in special education. These items arranged in decreasing order of incorrect responses from 53% to 40% and the least extent on items 31, 13 and 32 (these items similarly arranged in decreasing order of incorrect responses from 14% to 11%).

Items	Mean	Median	Std.Dev	95% Confidence Interval for mean		Skewness
1: Most estimates suggest that ADHD occurs in approximately 15% of school age children.	4%	0%	20%	17%	23%	4.77
4: ADHD children are typically more compliant with their fathers than with their mothers.	22%	0%	42%	37%	48%	1.37
6: ADHD is more common in the 1st degree biological relatives (i.e. mother, father) of children with ADHD than in the general population.	34%	0%	48%	42%	55%	0.69
13: It is possible for an adult to be diagnosed with ADHD.	62%	100%	49%	43%	57%	-0.50
17: Symptoms of depression are found more frequently in ADHD children than in non- ADHD children.	41%	0%	49%	43%	57%	0.37
19: Most ADHD children "outgrow" their symptoms by the onset of puberty and subsequently function normally in adulthood.	25%	0%	44%	38%	51%	1.17
22: If an ADHD child is able to demonstrate sustained attention to video games or TV for over an hour, that child is also able to sustain attention for at least an hour of class or homework.	32%	0%	47%	41%	54%	0.78
24: A diagnosis of ADHD by itself makes a child eligible for placement in special education.	32%	0%	47%	41%	54%	0.78
27: ADHD children generally experience more problems in novel situations than in familiar situations.	5%	0%	22%	19%	25%	4.19
28: There are specific physical features which can be identified by medical doctors (e.g. paediatrician) in making a definitive diagnosis of ADHD.	20%	0%	40%	35%	47%	1.52
29: In school age children, the prevalence of ADHD in males and females is equivalent.	33%	0%	47%	41%	55%	0.73
30: In very young children (less than 4 years old), the problem behaviours of ADHD children are distinctly different from age-appropriate behaviours of non-ADHD children.	10%	0%	30%	26%	35%	2.71
31: Children with ADHD are more distinguishable from normal children in a classroom setting than in a free play situation.	60%	100%	49%	43%	57%	-0.41

Items	Mean	Median	Std.Dev	95% Confidence Interval for mean		Skewness
32: The majority of ADHD children evidence some degree of poor school performance in the elementary school years.	66%	100%	48%	42%	55%	-0.69
33: Symptoms of ADHD are often seen in non-ADHD children who come from inadequate and chaotic home environments.	28%	0%	45%	40%	52%	0.99
39: Children with ADHD generally display an inflexible adherence to specific routines or rituals.	12%	0%	33%	29%	38%	2.37

Table 2. Associated Features item statistics

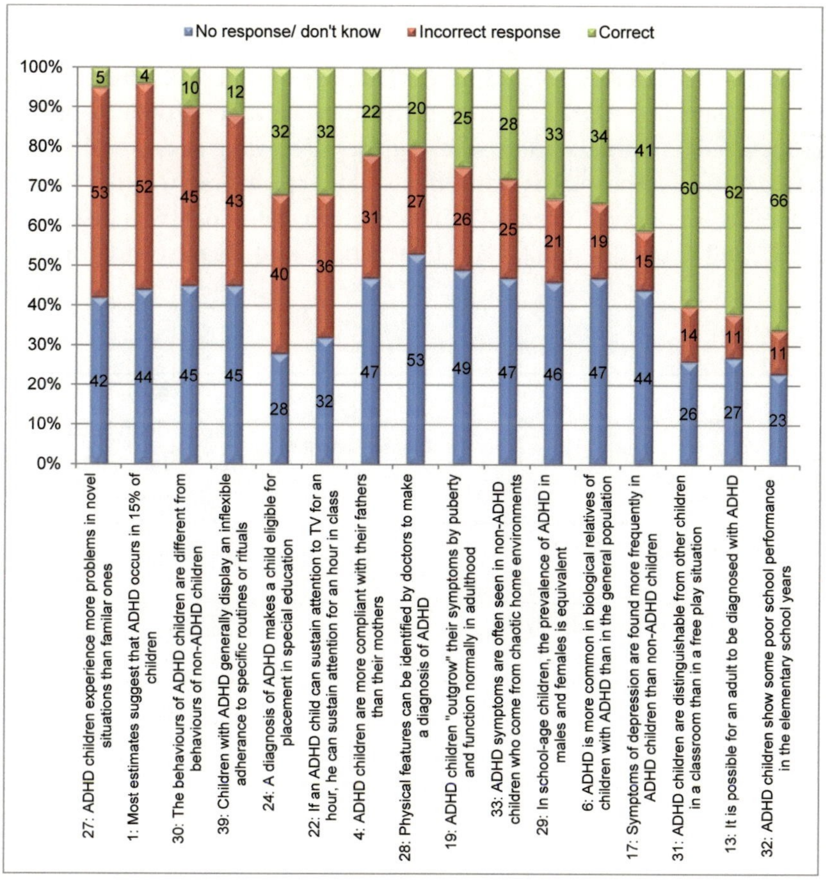

Figure 1. Categorised responses to Associated Features items

In line with the relatively higher mean score of the Symptoms/Diagnosis subscale compared to the other subscales (Table 1), the item means presented in Table 3 for this subscale are generally higher than those of the Associated Features subscale. The items that the teachers found most difficult were 11, which state that it is common for ADHD children to have an inflated sense of self-esteem or grandiosity and 38, which states that if a child responds to stimulant medications then they probably have ADHD, as the mean correct responses obtained were 18% and 23%, respectively. More than two-thirds of the teachers scored the following items correctly: item 3, which states that ADHD children are frequently distracted by extraneous stimuli; item 9, which states that ADHD children often fidget or squirm in their seats; item 21, which states that a child must present with symptoms in two or more settings to obtain an ADHD diagnosis and item 26 which states that ADHD children often have difficulties organising tasks and activities.

Once again, in order to investigate the low item scores for Symptoms/Diagnosis, a distinction was made between misconceptions, that is, incorrect responses, versus "don't know" responses. This distinction is displayed graphically for the Symptoms/Diagnosis items in Figure 2 where bars shaded in blue indicate the percentage of misconceptions and bars shaded in red indicate incorrect responses for each item. The figure shows that teachers have the greatest extent of misconceptions of ADHD Symptoms/ Diagnosis on item 7, which states that one of the symptoms displayed by ADHD children is that they are cruel to other people and item 14, which states that ADHD children often have a history of stealing or destroying other peoples' things (48% and 47% misconceptions respectively). Figure 2 also shows that teachers have the least extent of misconceptions on items 21 and 16; which states that two clusters of symptoms exist for ADHD, and items 3, 9 and 26 have between 9% and 5% misconceptions.

Items	Mean	Median	Std. Dev.	95% Confidence Interval for mean		Skewness
3: ADHD children are frequently distracted by extraneous stimuli.	70%	100%	46%	40%	54%	-0.89
5: In order to be diagnosed with ADHD, the child's symptoms must have been present before age 7.	36%	0%	48%	42%	56%	0.59
7: One symptom of ADHD children is that they have been physically cruel to other people.	31%	0%	46%	41%	54%	0.83
9: ADHD children often fidget or squirm in their seats.	78%	100%	42%	37%	48%	-1.37
11: It is common for ADHD children to have an inflated sense of self-esteem or grandiosity.	18%	0%	39%	34%	45%	1.69
14: ADHD children often have a history of stealing or destroying other people's things	21%	0%	41%	36%	48%	1.45

http://dx.doi.org/10.5772/53784

Items	Mean	Median	Std. Dev.	95% Confidence Interval for mean		Skewness
16: Current wisdom about ADHD suggests two clusters of symptoms: One of inattention and another consisting of hyperactivity/impulsivity.	57%	100%	50%	44%	58%	-0.29
21: In order to be diagnosed as ADHD, a child must exhibit relevant symptoms in two or more settings (e.g., home, school).	68%	100%	47%	41%	54%	-0.78
26: ADHD children often have difficulties organizing tasks and activities.	77%	100%	42%	37%	49%	-1.30
38: If a child responds to stimulant medications (e.g., Ritalin), then they probably have ADHD.	23%	0%	42%	37%	49%	1.30

Table 3. Symptoms/Diagnosis item statistics

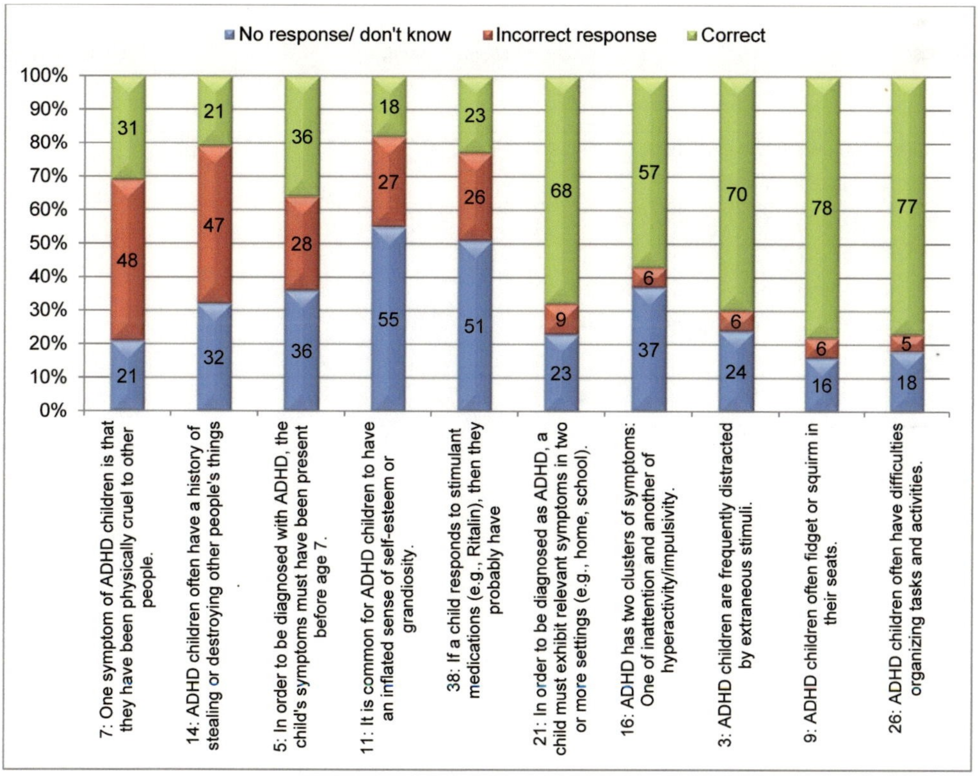

Figure 2. Categorised responses to Symptoms/ Diagnosis items

As for the Associated Features subscale, the knowledge level on the treatment subscale was poor (Table 4), with 14% or fewer of the teachers responding correctly to item 23, which states that the reduction of sugar intake leads to the reduction of ADHD symptoms; item 34, which states that behavioural interventions for children with ADHD focus primarily on the child's problems with inattention; item 35, which states that Electroconvulsive Therapy has been found to be an effective treatment for severe cases of ADHD and item 37, which states that research has shown that the prolonged use of medications leads to increased addiction in adulthood. Only on item 10, which states that parent and teacher training in managing an ADHD child are generally effective when combined with medication, did the majority of the teachers answer correctly.

Once again, the categorised responses of "don't know" versus misconceptions and correct responses are displayed in Figure 3 for Treatment items. This figure shows greatest misconceptions for items 23 and 34, which relate to dietary intake and ADHD and behavioural/psychological interventions for children with ADHD (53% and 47% incorrect responses respectively), and fewest misconceptions on item 35; which relates to electroconvulsive therapy as a treatment approach for ADHD and item 20, which states that medication is often used before other behaviour modification techniques are attempted.

Items	Mean	Median	Std. Dev.	95% Confidence Interval for mean		Skewness
2: Current research suggests that ADHD is largely the result of ineffective parenting skills.	37%	0%	49%	43%	56%	0.55
8: Antidepressant drugs have been effective in reducing symptoms for many ADHD	46%	0%	50%	44%	58%	0.16
10: Parent and teacher training in managing an ADHD child are generally effective when combined with medication treatment.	65%	100%	48%	42%	56%	-0.64
12: When treatment of an ADHD child is terminated, it is rare for the child's symptoms to return.	26%	0%	44%	39%	51%	1.11
15: Side effects of stimulant drugs used for treatment of ADHD may include mild insomnia and appetite reduction.	43%	0%	50%	44%	58%	0.29
18: Individual psychotherapy is usually sufficient for the treatment of most ADHD children.	19%	0%	39%	35%	46%	1.60
20: In severe cases of ADHD, medication is often used before other behavior modification techniques are attempted.	36%	0%	48%	42%	56%	0.59
23: Reducing dietary intake of sugar or food additives is generally effective in reducing the symptoms of ADHD.	7%	0%	26%	23%	30%	3.42
25: Stimulant drugs are the most common type of drug used to treat children with ADHD	34%	0%	48%	42%	55%	0.69

Items	Mean	Median	Std. Dev.	95% Confidence Interval for mean		Skewness
34: Behavioral/Psychological interventions for children with ADHD focus primarily on the child's problems with inattention.	12%	0%	33%	29%	38%	2.37
35: Electroconvulsive Therapy (i.e. shock treatment) has been found to be an effective treatment for severe cases of ADHD.	14%	0%	35%	31%	41%	2.11
36: Treatments for ADHD which focus primarily on punishment have been found to be the most effective in reducing the symptoms of ADHD.	47%	0%	50%	44%	58%	0.12
37: Research has shown that prolonged use of stimulant medications leads to increased addiction (i.e., drug, alcohol) in adulthood.	12%	0%	33%	29%	38%	2.37

Table 4. Treatment item statistics

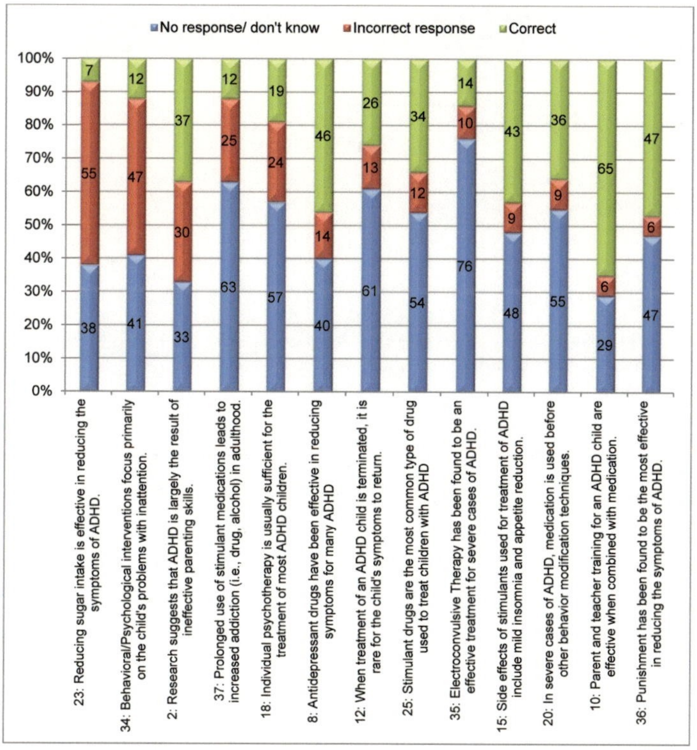

Figure 3. Categorised responses to Treatment items

In order to investigate whether the teachers' general knowledge of the content areas of ADHD differed in terms of their demographic group,their scores on the three ADHD content areas were compared across the levels of each of the demographic variables (Table 5) using 1- way Analysis of Variance (ANOVA).

	df	Associated Features – F	Associated Features - p	Symptoms/ Diagnosis - F	Symptoms/ Diagnosis – p	Treatment - F	Treatment – p
2. Age group	2	2.114		2.126		2.674	
3. Education level	1	15.780	***	13.919	***	6.409	*
4. Number of years of teaching experience	2	1.485		1.174		0.092	
5. Hours of ADHD training received	2	9.035	***	8.521	***	15.924	***
6. Evaluations/ assessments of children you thought may be ADHD	1	0.071		0.432		0.059	
7. Number of children taught with a medical diagnosis of ADHD	1	0.347		0.919		1.431	
8. Number of workshops attended on ADHD	1	11.508	**	13.928	***	20.087	***
9. Number of articles read on ADHD	2	6.538	**	18.290	***	20.170	***
10. Confidence to teach a child with ADHD	3	3.275	*	8.298	***	5.629	**
11. Teachers asked by a DR to assess the medication of a child with ADHD	1	12.506	***	21.961	***	16.809	***

Table 5. ADHD content areas compared across levels of demographic variables

Education and training is the common theme underlying these items reflecting significant differences on knowledge levels of the three ADHD content areas. Based on the direction of the means and the Scheffe post hoc tests for the significant ANOVA comparisons, the general trend of the means is that the more educated and trained teachers are more knowledgeable in each of the three ADHD content areas than are the less educated and trained teachers. Specifically, teachers with a university education score significantly higher than those with a college education [$F(1;93) = 15.780$, $p < 0.001$; $F(1;93) = 13.919$, $p < 0.001$; and $F(1;93) = 6.409$, $p < 0.05$], teachers with more than ten hours of ADHD training score higher than teachers with none or few hours, [(F (1; 93) = 9. 035, $p < 0.001$; F (1; 93) = 8.521, $p< 0.001$; and F (1; 93) = 15. 924, $p <0.05$]. Those teachers that have attended ADHD workshops score higher than those who have not [(F (2; 93) = 11. 508, $p < 0.001$; F (2; 93) = 13. 928, $p< 0.001$; and F (1; 93) = 20. 087, $p <0.05$]. Those teachers who have read more than five ADHD articles score higher than those who have not read any ADHD articles [(F (2; 93) = 6. 538, $p < 0.001$; F (2; 93) = 18. 290, $p< 0.001$; and F (2; 93) = 20. 170, $p <0.05$]. In addition, those teachers who have been asked by a doctor to assess medication of a child with ADHD, and those who feel more confident to teach children with ADHD have significantly higher scores on the three ADHD content areas than other teachers (F (3; 93)= 3.275, $p < 0.001$; F (3; 93) = 8.298, $p < 0.001$ and F(3; 93) = 5.629, $p< 0.05$) and (F (1; 93)= 12. 506, $p < 0.001$; F (1; 93) = 21. 961, $p < 0.001$ and F(1; 93) = 16. 809, $p< 0.05$). Finally, it should be noted for all the significant comparisons of the demographic variables, knowledge levels on the Symptoms/ Diagnosis content area were significantly higher than on the Associated Features and Treatment content areas. The qualitative results from the questionnaire revealed that teachers are willing and eager to participate in workshops on ADHD, substantiated by 73% of the sample group indicating that they were in favour of this. Interestingly, the 27% of teachers who did not opt to attend the workshop tended to be older, less confident (Pearson Chi-square(3) = 6.41, $p<0.10$), tended to have attended fewer ADHD workshops, read fewer ADHD articles and had been less often asked by a doctor to assess the medication of a child with ADHD (Pearson Chi-square(1) = 5.00, $p<0.05$). However, although the mean scores on the three content areas of ADHD of the respondents who opted for the workshops were marginally higher than those who did not opt to attend, these differences were not significant.

Teachers were given the opportunity to provide additional comments at the end of the questionnaire. Four teachers commented that there exists a lack of resources at the disposal of teachers and that schools should have special classes for children with ADHD, and that schools have a dire need for psychologists to help identify the children who are displaying ADHD - like symptoms as soon and early on as possible. Some of the teachers explained that there is often a misdiagnosis of ADHD; and often an over diagnosis made by teachers of this condition. Teachers expressed that they would like to learn more about the identification, treatment and possible classroom interventions for learners with ADHD children.

5.5. Discussion

This study sought to investigate the knowledge and perceptions of ADHD held by Foundation Phase teachers within a township setting in South Africa. The results of the study suggested that there exists a substantial lack of knowledge about ADHD among this sample group. These findings are consistent with the body of literature which states that teachers generally lack knowledge and hold certain misconceptions in the area of ADHD [21]. Teachers in the present study were the most knowledgeable about the symptoms of ADHD, less knowledgeable about the associated features and the least knowledgeable about treatment for this condition; which supported the results reported in an Australian study [21].

Teachers' generally good understanding of the symptoms of ADHD which was shown in this research study, is supported by several other South African studies which were conducted using a range of different teacher and school samples [2, 26, 28, 44]. Even though teachers in this study obtained the highest percentage of correct responses for the symptoms/diagnosis subscale of the KADDS, there were two specific items which resulted in the greatest extent of teacher misperception. Physical cruelty to other people and a history of stealing and destroying other people's things were perceived by the teachers as features of ADHD. The behaviours included in these two items are those that are characteristic of a Conduct Disorder and suggestive of an Oppositional Defiant Disorder [45], which the teachers in the present study may not have been aware of. These findings are consistent with the results of a study that was conducted in America [23].

In the present study, teachers were less knowledgeable about the associated features of ADHD, than they were about the symptoms, as half of the respondents answered less than 31% of the items on this subscale correctly. However, teachers obtained the lowest scores on the treatment subscale. Teachers in the present study possessed very poor and even incorrect knowledge regarding the treatment of ADHD. This finding has an important implication for teacher pre-service and in-service training, as teachers play an important role in the identification, management and treatment of ADHD [21]. Teachers in this study seemed to possess limited and even incorrect knowledge on the after effects of medication, and many of them believed that stimulant medications lead to drug and alcohol addictions in adulthood. Nevertheless, the majority of the teachers in the current study were aware that parent and teacher training in managing a child diagnosed with ADHD combined with medical treatment, was generally an effective and preferable method of treatment for this condition.

In line with the results of a number of other studies [2, 46], a large number of teachers in the present study incorrectly believed that the alteration of diet and the reduction of sugars and food additives would lead to the alleviation of ADHD symptoms. Few studies have supported the idea that the alteration of one's diet alleviates symptoms of ADHD, and in fact labels this belief as a common myth [15].

Among the sample group in this study, there existed a clear lack of knowledge on the epidemiology of ADHD, as a very low percentage of correct responses was obtained for the item which stated that most estimates suggest that ADHD occurs in approximately 15% of school age children. As pointed out by the study conducted by [23], if teachers are unaware of how many students in their classrooms have ADHD, it may lead to the condition being overlooked and unidentified, or conversely, it may lead to the teacher attributing many of a child's unruly and uncharacteristic behaviours to ADHD resulting in incorrect referrals [2].

Poor academic performance is often considered as one of the most prominent factors associated with ADHD, and students with ADHD are at an increased risk for grade retention and school failure [15]. Teachers in the present study seemed to be aware of this, and results revealed a large number of correct responses for the questionnaire item which looked at the idea that the majority of ADHD children evidence some degree of poor school performance in the elementary school years.

In this study, while the age of the teachers was unrelated to their overall level of ADHD knowledge, their educational level was positively related to this variable. The higher their level

http://dx.doi.org/10.5772/53784

of education, the more knowledge they possessed on ADHD, possibly as a result greater exposure to this condition. Unlike the findings of [31], teachers' knowledge of ADHD was unrelated to their number of years of teaching experience in this study. An important finding for school administrators is the result that teachers who previously attended training programmes and workshops and those that were exposed to ADHD by means of written articles, all knew more about the condition than those teachers with less training and exposure in the area. Furthermore, teachers who felt more confident to teach a child with ADHD obtained higher scores on the KADDS, and thus knew more about the condition. This finding supports the results of studies conducted by [2, 31], where the more confident teachers had more knowledge on ADHD.

It was noted in this study, that it was the younger, more confident, more experienced teachers who wanted to participate in workshops on ADHD. The teachers also suggested that the workshops include a section on treatment, which is an area where knowledge is seemingly lacking. The older, more inexperienced teachers were those who were reluctant and disinterested to partake in workshops. One reason for this may be because the older teachers are more set in their ways, and are thus more reluctant to engage in and learn new material.

The finding may be related to what Martin Seligman calls learned helplessness. This is once an "individual learns that he or she is not in control, the motivation to seek control may be shut down, even when control later becomes possible [47, p.252]. Due to the lack of resources within the townships in South Africa and the possible lack of options that some of these teachers are faced with, they may have come to learn that they are not in control of the situation, and often what they do is to no avail. Thus, when a workshop is offered to them, they may have learned that they are not in control, and consequently they do not believe that the workshop will be of assistance and benefit to them.

5.6. Implications of the research

Results of the study imply that South African Foundation Phase teachers do not have adequate knowledge or sufficient understanding of ADHD. Teachers seem to have some information on the symptoms of ADHD, and less on the associated features and treatment for the condition. It is therefore important that training programmes or workshops address these gaps in the teachers' knowledge regarding the condition. Overall, the majority of teachers in this study expressed willingness to participate in workshops and training programmes on ADHD. Teachers also indicated that there is a lack of resources at the township schools to aid in the recognition and management of the condition. It is essential that the South African Department of Education becomes aware of these issues and provides teachers with the necessary training and ongoing support to facilitate the learning and schooling experience and holistic development of children with ADHD. This is of particular importance if inclusive education is to be implemented successfully.

5.7. Limitations of the study

The following were some of the limitations of the present research study:

- The sample for the study was obtained on a strict voluntary basis; using a purposive, non probability sampling method. The current sample is not representative of the entire population of Foundation Phase township teachers. Responses to the questionnaire were very much dependent on the teachers' availability and willingness to participate in the study. A sample of 100 teachers from a specific geographic location was obtained, and there were no male participants. Thus, the sample used in the study was small and narrow. For these reasons, issues with generalisability arose and therefore widespread conclusions from the results cannot be drawn.
- English is not a first language for many of the teachers that participated in the research study. It is unknown to what extent the teachers' responses to the questionnaire were hampered by language related issues, which similar research studies conducted in the future would have to consider. The construct validity of the measuring instrument used was therefore a possible limitation of the study.
- There is limited local literature and research on ADHD. Further work is necessary to develop and contextualize international developments in relation to the unique South African context.

5.8. Suggestions for future research

The following suggestions are made for future research:

- The majority of teachers in this study were willing to participate in workshops related to ADHD training. Future researchers could focus on creating and providing training programmes that would bridge the gaps in knowledge about ADHD and its causes, symptoms and treatment.
- After the implementation of teacher training and workshops, follow up programme evaluation studies and longitudinal research would be beneficial. This research could serve as a springboard for future workshops and educational programs to be implemented at schools at a national level.
- Broader teacher samples from public, private, rural and township schools need to be considered in future ADHD studies.
- Future research could focus on creating awareness and gathering resources to aid in the recognition and management of the condition at schools. It is essential that teachers receive the necessary training and ongoing support to facilitate the learning and schooling experience of children with ADHD.

6. Conclusion

This chapter primarily focused on one particular South African study [36] that sought to investigate the knowledge and perceptions of ADHD held by Foundation Phase teachers in a township in Gauteng. The results of the study were compared to local and international

http://dx.doi.org/10.5772/53784

research conducted in the last decade. After an in depth analysis of the results of the study and other research conducted, the chapter highlighted that the lack of knowledge that teachers has, as well as the misperceptions they hold regarding ADHD, need to be addressed as teachers play a vital role in the identification, diagnosis, referral and treatment process of ADHD. Inaccurate information about ADHD can lead to inaccurate referrals, resulting in the incorrect information being relayed to parents and doctors, which in itself has negative effects and consequences for individuals' diagnosed with the condition. In addition the chapter also noted the need for more workshops and programmes to become available to teachers to aid them in the recognition and management of ADHD in their classrooms. Overall, the chapter highlighted the need for more research to be conducted in the area of ADHD in South Africa, in order for every learner to maximise his or her potential and to succeed within the South African inclusive education classroom environment.

Author details

Zaytoon Amod[1], Adri Vorster[1] and Kim Lazarus[2]

*Address all correspondence to: adri.vorster@wits.ac.za

1 Department of Psychology, University of the Witwatersrand, Johannesburg, South Africa

2 Epworth Children's Village, Johannesburg, South Africa

References

[1] Meyer A. Cross-cultural issues in ADHD research. Journal of Psychology in Africa 2005;10 101-106.

[2] Perold M., Louw C., Kleynhans S. Primary school teachers' knowledge and misperceptions of attention deficit hyperactivity disorder (ADHD). South African Journal of Education 2010;30 457-473.

[3] Naicker SM. From Apartheid education to inclusive education. International Education Summit for a Democratic Society, 26-28 June 2000, Detroit, Michigan.

[4] South African Government. Constitution of the Republic of South Africa, Act No. 108 of 1996. Pretoria: South African Government; 1996.

[5] Prinsloo E. Working towards inclusive education in South African classrooms. South African Journal of Education 2001;21(4) 344-348.

[6] Engelbrecht P., Green, L. Responding to the challenges of inclusive education in southern-Africa. Pretoria: Van Schaik Publishers; 2011.

[7] UNESCO. The Salamanca statement and framework for action on special needs education. World Conference on Special Needs Education: Access and Quality, 7-10 June 1994, Salamanca, Spain.

[8] Donald D., Lazarus S., Lolwana P. Educational psychology in social context: Challenges of development, social issues and special need in southern Africa. Cape Town: Oxford University Press; 1997.

[9] Vorster A. Developmental Psychopathology. In: Burke A. (ed.) Abnormal psychology: A South African perspective. Cape Town: Oxford University Press; 2009. p420-463.

[10] Swart E., Pettipher R. Perspectives on inclusive education. In: Landsberg E., Krüger D., Swart E. (eds.) Addressing barriers to learning: A South African perspective. Van Schaik Publishers; 2011. p3-26.

[11] Havey J.M., Olson J.M., McCormick C., Cates G.L. Teachers' perceptions of the incidence and management of Attention-Deficit Hyperactivity Disorder. Applied Neuropsychology 2005;12(2) 120-127.

[12] South African Medical Research Council & Department: Minerals and Energy Republic of South Africa. Blood lead levels in South African children at the end of the leaded petrol era. http://www.mrc.ac.za/healthdevelop/BloodLevels.pdf (accessed 21 September 2012).

[13] Mathee A., Von Schirnding Y., Montgomery M., Röllin H. Lead poisoning in South African children: The hazard is at home. Reviews on Environmental Health 2004;19(3-4) 347-361.

[14] South African Human Rights Commission and UNICEF. South Africa's children: A review of equity and child rights. http://www.sahrc.org.za/home/21/files/SA%20CHILDREN%2024%20MARCH%202011%20SAHRC%20_%20UNICEF%20REPORT.pdf (accessed 16 July 2012).

[15] Vorster A. Developmental Psychopathology. In: Burke A. (ed.) Abnormal psychology: A South African perspective. Cape Town: Oxford University Press; 2012. p512-557.

[16] National Commission on Special Needs in Education and Training (NCSNET) & National Committee on Education Support Services (NCESS). Quality education for all: Overcoming barriers to learning and development. Pretoria: Department of Education. http://www.education.gov.za/LinkClick.aspx?fileticket=BNWeQZpNO14=&tabid=97&mid=400 (accessed 16 July 2012).

[17] Nel N., Nel M., Hugo A. Learner support in a diverse classroom: A guide for foundation, intermediate and senior phase teachers of language and mathematics. Pretoria: Van Schaik Publishers; 2012.

[18] Kerig P.K., Ludlow A., Wenar C. Developmental Psychopathology (6th ed.). McGraw-Hill; 2012.

[19] Meyer A., Eilertsen D.E., Sundet J.M., Tshifularo J., Sagvolden T. Cross-cultural similarities in ADHD-like behavior amongst South African primary school children. South African Journal of Psychology 2004; 34(1) 122-138.

[20] Nonvilitis J.M., Fang P. Perceptions of ADHD in China and the United States: A preliminary study. Journal of Attention Disorders 2005; 9(2) 413-424.

[21] Efron D., Sciberras E., Hassell P. Are Schools Meeting the Needs of Children with ADHD? Australasian Journal of Special Education 2008; 32 187-198.

[22] Peacock J. ADD and ADHD: Making sense of confusion. USA: Capstone Press; 2002.

[23] Reid R., Johnson J. Teacher's guide to ADHD. USA: The Guilford Press; 2011.

[24] Kern A., Seabi J. Educators' perceptions of attention deficit hyperactivity disorder: An exploratory study. The Journal of Psychology in Africa 2008; 18641-644.

[25] Strous L. Teachers' perceptions of the role they play in the identification and management of children with Attention Deficit Disorder with and without hyperactivity. Honours dissertation. University of the Witwatersrand Johannesburg; 2000.

[26] Kern A. Foundation phase educators' perceptions of attention deficit hyperactivity disorder (ADHD) at private and public schools. Masters research report. University of the Witwatersrand Johannesburg; 2008.

[27] Graham W. Is your ADHD child being picked on? IOL Lifestyle 2011. http://www.iol.co.za/lifestyle/family/parenting/is-your-adhd-child-being-picked-on-1.1053935 (accessed 21 September 2011).

[28] Durbach C. Dealing with scattered minds: Teachers' perspectives on attention deficit hyperactivity disorder in the classroom. Masters research report. University of the Witwatersrand Johannesburg; 2001.

[29] Kos J. What Do Primary School Teachers Know, Think And Do About ADHD? 2008. http://research.acer.edu.au/tll_misc/8 (accessed 03 August 2012).

[30] Schultz B.K. Teacher behavior ratings of adolescents with Attention Deficit Hyperactivity Disorder (ADHD): Inter-tater reliability and sources of rater bias. PhD thesis. University of Pennsylvania Philadelphia; 2008.

[31] Scuitto M.J., Terejesen M.D., Bender-Frank A.S. Teachers' knowledge and misperceptions of attention deficit/hyperactivity disorder. Psychology in the Schools 2000; 37 115-122.

[32] Jensen P.S. Making the system work for your child with ADHD: How to cut through red tape and get what you need from doctors, teachers, schools and healthcare plans. USA: The Guilford Press; 2004.

[33] Stormont M., Stebbins M.S. Preschool teachers' knowledge, opinions and educational experiences with Attention Deficit Hyperactivity Disorder. The Journal of Teacher Education Division of the Council for Exceptional Children 2005; 28 52-61.

[34] Vereb R.C., Diperma J.C. Teacher's knowledge of ADHD, treatment of ADHD and treatment acceptability: An initial investigation. School Psychology Review 2004; 33 421-428.

[35] Du Paul G.J., Stoner G.D. ADHD in the schools: Assessment and intervention strategies. USA: The Guilford Press; 2003.

[36] Lazarus K.J. The knowledge and perceptions of Attention Deficit Hyperactivity Disorder: An exploratory study. Masters research report. University of the Witwatersrand Johannesburg; 2011.

[37] [37]Cottrell RR., McKenzie J.F. Health promotion and education research methods: Using the five-chapter thesis/dissertation model. USA: Jones and Bartlett Publishers Inc; 2005.

[38] Gravetter F.J., Forzano L.B. Research methods for the behavioral sciences (3rded.). USA: Wadsworth Cengage Learning; 2006.

[39] Goldstein S., Goldstein M. Managing ADHD: A guide for practitioners. USA: John Wiley & Sons Inc; 1998.

[40] Kos J.M., Richdale A.L., Jackson M.S. Knowledge about attention deficit hyperactivity disorder: A comparison of in-service and pre-service teachers. Psychology in the Schools 2004; 41 517-526.

[41] Bender A.S. Effects of active learning on student teachers' identification and referrals of Attention Deficit Hyperactivity Disorder. PhD thesis. Hofstra University Hempstead; 1996.

[42] Sciutto M.J., Nolfi C.J., Bluhm C. Effects of child gender and symptom type on referrals for ADHD by elementary school teachers. Journal of Emotional and Behavioural Disorders 2004; 12(4) 247-253.

[43] Mills G. E. Action Research: A guide for the teacher researcher (2nd ed.). NJ: Merrill/ Prentice-Hall; 2003.

[44] Economou N. Facilitating a distracted mind: Teachers' experience of attention deficit hyperactivity disorder. Masters research report. University of the Witwatersrand Johannesburg; 2002.

[45] Mash E.J., Wolfe R.A. Abnormal child psychology (4th ed.). California: Wadsworth; 2009.

[46] Dennis T., Davis M., Johnson U., Brooks H., Humbi A. Attention deficit hyperactivity disorder: Parents' and professionals perceptions. Community Practitioner 2008; 81(3) 24-28.

http://dx.doi.org/10.5772/53784

[47] Friedman H.S., Schustack M W. Personality: Classic theories and modern research (3rd ed.). USA: Person//Allyn and Bacon; 1999.

Chapter 12

ADHD Children's Emotion Regulation in FACE© – Perspective (Facilitating Adjustment of Cognition and Emotion): Theory, Research and Practice

Smadar Celestin-Westreich and
Leon-Patrice Celestin

Additional information is available at the end of the chapter

http://dx.doi.org/10.5772/54422

1. Introduction

Children with ADHD are known to display primary features of impulsivity, inattention and/or hyperactivity [1]. They also constitute a diverse group, encompassing predominantly inattentive (ADHD-I), hyperactive/impulsive (ADHD-HI) and combined (ADHD-C) subtypes with multiple comorbidities and developmental paths [2]. ADHD children's cognitive functioning and outcomes have been investigated extensively. Remarkably, much less research and prevention efforts have been devoted to their emotional processes and outcomes [2-4]. Consistent with a surge in research placing emotions at the centre of various psychopathologies over the past decade, a start has been made toward gaining a more balanced view of ADHD children's functioning.

This chapter discusses why emotion research is important for ADHD children (§2), presents the FACE©-model (Facilitating the Adjustment of Cognition and Emotion, [5, 6]) (§3) as a comprehensive framework through which to identify the major components and levels of emotional and associated cognitive functioning covered by the broad concept of emotion regulation (ER) (§4) and critically reviews which of these issues have been investigated in the context of ADHD (§5). The chapter pursues with identifying cautions and conditions for translating research into practice and reformulating these into a resiliency perspective on ADHD children's emotional functioning, after which implications are drawn from the evidence-base to inform intervention and prevention efforts with ADHD youth and their families (§6). The chapter briefly rounds out by outlining a strengths-based perspective on further emotion-oriented research and practice with ADHD youth (§7).

2. Why emotional functioning matters in children with ADHD

ADHD children's frequent learning and academic difficulties have received ample attention [1,2]. Programs destined at helping children with ADHD typically focus on alleviating the behavioural components that contribute to such difficulties in order to facilitate their school and subsequent professional curriculum. Less extensively investigated yet widely documented is ADHD children's often complicated social, relational and family functioning [7-9]. Children with ADHD are known, for example, to have more negative peer relationships [10], be subject to bullying [11], engage in risk-taking and antisocial behaviour [12], and experience family difficulties [4, 13, 14]. While these risk factors have led to underscoring the importance of social skills training for children with ADHD, relatively few studies to date have investigated these issues from an emotion perspective that may shed light on their underlying mechanisms.

Children with ADHD are also diagnosed more often than not with comorbid disorders [1], such as conduct disorder (CD) and oppositional defiant disorder (ODD) in 40 to 60% of cases [15-17], as well as anxiety and depression (including suicide risks) [17-20]. Attachment problems [21, 22] and posttraumatic stress symptoms/disorder are also frequently associated with ADHD [12, 23]. Furthermore, Bipolar Disorder (BD) constitutes a major possible comorbidity with emotional implications for ADHD children [5, 24-26]. Pointing to yet another line of potential deficits in emotion processing, it is also increasingly acknowledged that children may concurrently present with ADHD and autism spectrum symptoms or disorder (ASS/D) [27-29].

When evaluating the impact of ADHD on children's developmental course, research therefore typically grapples with the issue of disentangling to what extent their relational and social problems are a mere consequence of their core behaviour regulation difficulties, or whether and when these problems reflect more fundamental facets of their emotional functioning. In addition, the pervasiveness of emotion-related difficulties throughout the spectrum of ADHD subtypes and comorbidities questions the extent to which such difficulties are ADHD (subtype) specific or represent overarching mechanisms of emotional dysregulation that broadly put children at risk for experiencing clinical problem behaviour.

3. ADHD children's behaviour in FACE©-perspective: Cognitive and emotional adjustments within a risk-resiliency context

While diverse areas of research address the above-cited issues separately, there is a need to move toward a comprehensive, integrated view of ADHD children's cognitive and emotional functioning, so as to inform research as well as prevention and intervention efforts in this context. Stated in a nutshell and schematized in Figure 1, the FACE©-model aims to respond to this need by focusing on ADHD children's reciprocal adjustments of cognitive control and emotion regulation on a micro-level, while accounting for biopsychosocial risk and resiliency dynamics on a macro-level [4-6].

http://dx.doi.org/10.5772/54422

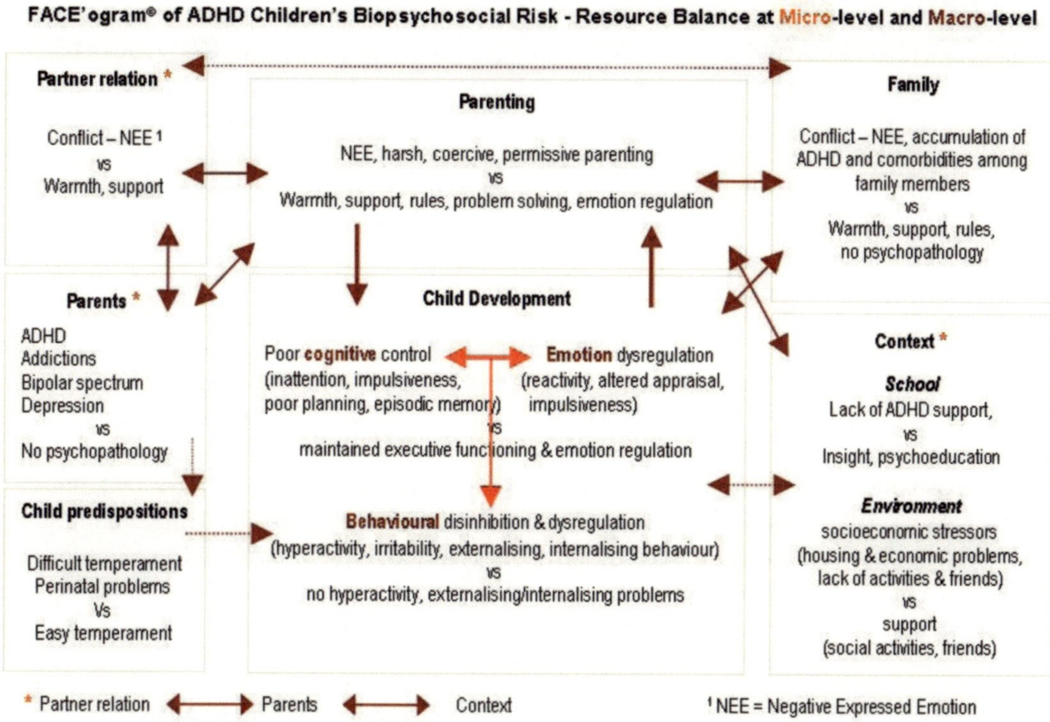

Figure 1. ADHD Children's Functioning in FACE©-perspective, at Cognitive-Emotional Micro-level and at Biopsychosocial Macro-level

The FACE©-model thus posits that in order to constructively apprehend and act upon ADHD children's behavioural and relational challenges, it is necessary to gain insight into their cognitive-emotional adjustment processes within the ecological context of their experienced allostatic load [30]. Importantly, systematically accounting for the risk and resiliency balance operating in the ADHD child's life should also contribute to a strengths-based approach that fosters the 'positive faces' of ADHD and thereby pave the way for effective prevention and intervention programs [4, 31, 32]. Figure 1 illustrates this model at micro-level [6, 25, 33-35] and at macro-level [4, 6, 30], as discussed hereafter.

3.1. The role of reciprocal cognitive and emotional adjustments on a micro-level

The notion that successful coordination of cognitive control and emotion regulation is pivotal to adaptive behaviour has been increasingly recognised over the past decade.

From a predominantly *cognitive* perspective, ADHD's cardinal characteristics of impaired sustained attention and impulsiveness provide grounds per se for expecting so-called top-down disturbances of emotional functioning. Attentional fluctuations for example may interfere with how and when the child notices emotional cues, both internal and interpersonal [36-39]. Similarly, poor behavioural control and planning typical of ADHD are likely to hamper, amongst others, the child's ability to postpone emotional responses or to adequately modulate their form and intensity [40-43]. High-order cognitive processes such as behavioural inhibition, sustained attention, attention allocation and cognitive switching indeed are critical to flexibly responding to emotional interactions in everyday life. Neuroscience studies have allowed to quite consistently link ADHD children's problems with these processes to distinct underactivation of inferior frontal cortex (IFC) and dorsolateral prefrontal cortex (DLPFC) circuitries. In comparison, evidence suggests that conduct disordered children display underactivation of paralimbic system areas and bipolar children of ventral frontostriatal circuitry [44, 45].

Even within this top-down perspective, the reciprocal directions of cognitive and emotional effects in behavioural (dis)adjustments need to be underscored. For example, in a five-year follow-up of preadolescent girls with ADHD, the association between childhood executive functioning skills such as planning and adolescent internalising and externalising comorbidity was partially mediated by social functioning in adolescence, and vice versa [46]. Studies in this vein yet still focus on behavioural manifestations of interpersonal functioning rather than on underlying emotional processes. Moreover, although the above predominant 'cognitive-toward-emotional' pathways have been only partially investigated to date, it has become apparent that they do not suffice to fully explain the range of emotional dysfunction and comorbidity in children with ADHD [47, 48].

More recently, ADHD theories have therefore turned to including an *emotion-centred* perspective. This perspective is supported by brain functioning studies on how underlying emotional mechanisms may be disrupted in their own right in the context of ADHD [47, 49]. Neuroimaging studies indeed demonstrate the complexity of the neurobiological circuitry of emotion regulation, which requires continuous adjustments and integration of limbic and prefrontal brain systems [19, 45, 50, 51]. The dorsolateral, orbitofrontal and anterior cingulate cortex in fact are part of complex interrelated networks that mediate emotional and cognitive information processing in relation with striatal, cerebellar, and parietal regions along with the amygdala and hippocampus [44, 45, 48, 51, 52]. More specifically, ADHD disruptions in IFC and DLPFC regions are found to be associated with prominent structural deficits in basal ganglia, deficient connectivity with reduced amygdala along with (possibly compensatory) enlarged hippocampus, all of which mediate emotion processing [44, 49]. Expectations of central emotional disruptions in ADHD children's functioning hereby are further supported by the convergence of certain early-onset ADHD manifestations and the developmental precedence of the emotional brain systems compared to a comparatively late maturing cognitive circuitry [37, 44].

In short, from a micro-level perspective, children with ADHD may be vulnerable to emotion dysregulation through predominant 'cognitive-toward-emotional' pathways as well as through primary disturbances in an intrinsically integrated 'emotional-with-cognitive components' circuitry. This intricacy of reciprocal emotion and cognitive processing provides a basis for neural understanding of the different emotion regulation levels detailed further on.

3.2. The role of the biopsychosocial risk and resiliency balance on a macro-level

Several fields of study, such as developmental psychopathology, trauma and stress-related as well as neurobiological investigations, converge to demonstrate that children's dysfunctional behaviour, cognition and emotion do not occur in isolation but relative to an immediate and larger environment [7, 31, 53]. Children's direct and long-term outcomes are determined by a dynamic balance of risks versus resources across several domains throughout their development, as illustrated in Figure 1 [6].

Children with ADHD are known to be at increased risk of confronting additional stressors that even further diminish their perceived resources, notably as regards their parents' (e.g. ADHD, substance abuse, stress, anxiety) and siblings' functioning (e.g. ADHD or behavioural problems) [13, 54, 55], along with the quality of their parenting (e.g. harsh or inconsistent) [56, 57] and family environments (e.g. high levels of negative expressed emotions) [14, 58, 59] as well as school or leisure context (e.g. peer rejection) [10, 11, 60]. In other words, assessing ADHD children's emotional functioning without considering the scope of stressors versus resources operating in their immediate and larger environment will generate only a limited understanding of the processes at hand.

Investigating this risk-resiliency load furthermore may be particularly pertinent to understanding ADHD children's emotional functioning given their peculiar arousal balance. Children with ADHD are indeed documented to struggle simultaneously with being overburdened and under-challenged when processing information [2]. While these features have been demonstrated in predominantly cognitive situations, and while clinical accounts do tend to reflect issues with emotional overburdening in ADHD children's day-to-day interpersonal functioning [4, 61, 62], there is a need for empirical evidence to this regard.

In short, ADHD children's emotion regulation skills may be extra challenged given the potential level of additional stressors that they tend to face. Their emotional functioning therefore deserves to be examined against the broader backdrop of cumulative *risks* operating in their lives. Inversely, assessing the impact of contextual *resources* on ADHD children's emotion regulation skills is likely to provide precious leads for enhancing intervention and prevention efforts.

Taking into account these conceptual foundations, the FACE©-model hereafter first more specifically guides our focus on the emotional and associated cognitive components implied in the emotion regulation process (§4). The evidence-base with regard to how these components present in children with ADHD is then primarily discussed on a micro-level (§5, 5.1-5.3). Macro-level parenting and family influences on ADHD children's emotional functioning are briefly reviewed in relation to their cognitive-emotional adjustments (§5.4).

4. Which aspects of emotion regulation merit investigation in ADHD children and why?

The field of emotion regulation research is unwieldy and potentially confusing as illustrated hereafter (§4.1). To clarify the evidence-base regarding ADHD children's emotion regulation, the next paragraphs first disentangle its major operational components (§4.2) and then integrate these in the micro-level of the model introduced with Figure 1 (§4.3).

4.1. Investigating ADHD children's emotion regulation: A complex issue

The adequate recognition and expression of emotions is fundamental to a child's development, and emotion regulation is instrumental to the personal and relational as well as the cognitive fulfilment of the child [42, 63]. Despite this knowledge, few empirical studies among children with ADHD (or adults for that matter) are specifically dedicated to their emotion regulation skills. It has not helped that emotion regulation tends to be approached in a broad variety of ways, regardless of the investigated population. The focus of ER research with ADHD children notably ranges from physiological mechanisms and neurobiological circuits to questionnaire-based and observational behavioural measures; and from laboratory to ecologically pertinent studies. Furthermore, emotional functioning consists of autonomic, automated and implicit responses [16, 48, 50] as well as deliberate, effortful regulation [20, 37], which adds to the investigation range [42]. In fact, the transient, elusive and subjective nature of emotions has complicated the process of generating an encompassing and yet precise definition of emotion since centuries, and has probably contributed to empirical research shying away from the subject [51, 64]. The conceptualisation history of ADHD thus has moved away during the second half of the 20th century from emotional features that were previously included in its core descriptions, only to return to addressing their pervasiveness in the contemporary literature [47]. In recent years, a more pragmatic approach involves focussing on the typical or core features of ER that allow setting a framework with working definitions to guide emotion research [63].

4.2. Major operational components and levels of emotion regulation

Three operational specifications of emotion regulation appear particularly pertinent to the present purpose of clarifying the investigation of emotional processes in children with ADHD.

First, *emotions* are bio-psycho-social phenomena that consist of (unconscious, autonomic) physiological reactions, which are accompanied by subjective experiences and behavioural expressions within a given context [48, 63, 65]. Emotion research with ADHD children therefore deserves to include at least three levels of interest, namely a biological, an (introspective) experiential and a behavioural-interpersonal level.

Second, competent *emotional functioning*, which appears to be challenged in children with ADHD, consequently comprises at least three core, interconnected components that merit examination, namely the adequate appraisal, modulation and expression of emotions [42,

http://dx.doi.org/10.5772/54422

50, 63, 64, 66]. Cognitive and emotional processes are intricately interwoven in these components. This is the case, for instance, as thoughts and feelings jointly constitute the subjective experience accompanying a child's initial physiological reactions (appraisal); or as memory intervenes along with emotional reactivity in how the child regulates emotional intensity (modulation); or as attention allocation, planning and attributed feeling reciprocally determine the behaviour through which the child exhibits an emotion (expression).

Third and in line with the above, a more detailed working definition of the *process of emotion regulation* has been proposed by Eisenberg and Spinrad (2004) as consisting of "initiating, avoiding, inhibiting, maintaining, or modulating the occurrence, form, intensity, or duration of internal feeling states, emotion-related physiological, attentional processes, motivational states, and/or the behavioural concomitants of emotion in the service of accomplishing affect-related biological or social adaptation or achieving individual goals" [67, p.338]. This definition further highlights the important range of processes at work in emotion regulation. Taking into account this working definition, ADHD children's important levels of externalising (CD, ODD, BD) as well as internalising comorbidity (anxiety, depression, BD) imply that their emotional arousal, appraisal and expression might carry both 'hot' and 'cold', as well as 'approach' and 'avoidance' features as detailed further on [60].

4.3. ADHD children's emotion regulation conceptually revisited

Closing in on the micro-level of the FACE©-model allows summarising the aforementioned multiple facets and levels of emotional, and associated cognitive, functioning covered by the concept of emotion regulation, as visualised in figure 2.

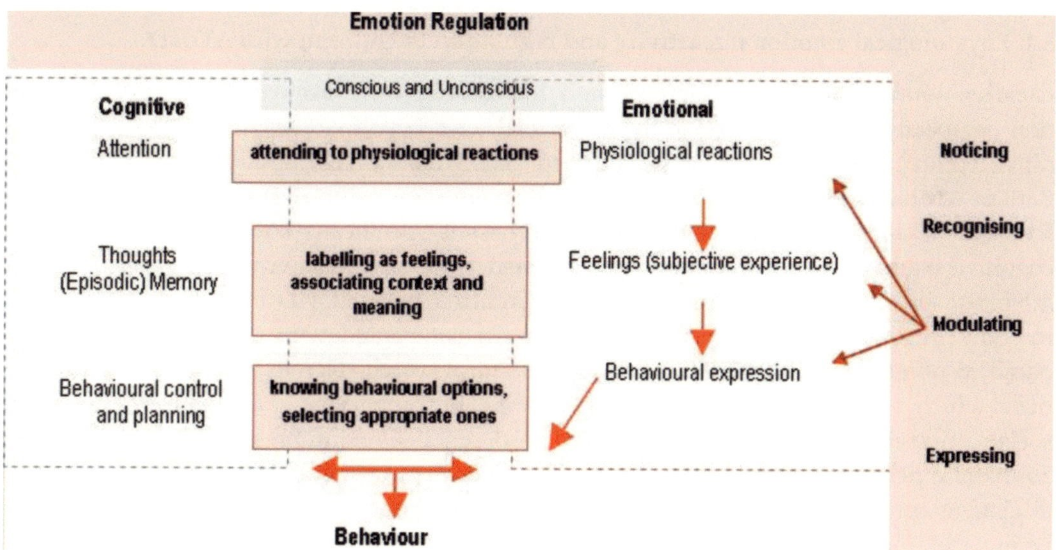

Figure 2. ADHD children's cognitive, emotional and behavioural ER components

Given this broadness of the emotion regulation concept, it could be argued that much research has in fact touched upon ADHD children's emotional functioning in one way or another. Diverse perspectives, such as parent- and self-reported accounts of affective lability and comorbidities, social information processing or temperament can be conceived as questioning the role of emotions in ADHD children's outcomes [3, 11, 68]. However, only a limited number of studies to date have effectively investigated the emotion-centred theory in children with ADHD as a means of understanding underlying mechanisms of their behavioural expressions [69, 70].

In what follows, our focus consequently will be on studies that have explicitly undertaken to test hypotheses about ADHD children's functioning through the lens of emotion regulation. Given our focus, the discussion will more specifically highlight the fields of ADHD children's emotional functioning that have remained relatively neglected to date, namely their physiological reactivity, basic and contextual emotional appraisal skills, along with, to a lesser extent, deliberate emotion regulation efforts.

5. Emotion regulation in ADHD children according to the evidence-base

Consistent with the aforementioned facets of emotion regulation (see figure 2), the review of the evidence-base hereafter is organised into arousal, basic appraisal and expression research. Thus, we focus primarily and successively on studies examining how children with ADHD physiologically regulate emotions (§5.1), how they process basic or contextualised emotional cues, mainly in facial expressions (§5.2), and how they deliberately modulate emotional experience and expression (§5.3); this with a priority on recent findings.

5.1. Physiological emotional reactivity and regulation in children with ADHD

Children with ADHD's hyperactivity and impulsivity have been posited from an emotion perspective to reflect a basic hyper-arousal tendency, apart from later maturing cognitive control [47]. This tendency has been called emotional impulsiveness, notably by Barkley (2010), and considered to constitute in its own right a core feature of children with ADHD [42, 47, 48]. Emotional impulsiveness is specifically conceived, relative to its cognitive equivalent, as consisting of heightened emotional reactivity along with lessened inhibition of emotional expression [47, 61]. Children with ADHD thus may be expected to show increased physiological reactivity when confronted with affective stimuli compared to non-clinical children. On the other hand, research relative to externalizing disorders, which are often concomitant with ADHD, has suggested that children with antisocial, oppositional-defiant and conduct disordered behaviour present an underaroused autonomic nervous system in general baseline [65, 71] as well as in physical or emotional change conditions [16, 48]. ADHD children's emotional reactivity may therefore also be expected to vary according to the nature of their comorbidities.

On a physiological level, *emotional arousal* reflects in sympathetic nervous system mobilisation, for example through increased heart rate, sweating, muscular tightening and so forth, which puts the body in basic 'approach/fight' versus 'avoidance/flight' readiness. The *regulation* of emotional arousal additionally involves activation of the parasympathetic nervous system, either unconsciously or through deliberate efforts. Emotional reactivity therefore is often operationalised by confronting children with emotionally evocative material, such as pictures, stories or movies and measuring their changes from baseline in heart rate (HR), blood pressure (BP) or skin conductance (SC) levels [48, 65, 71, 72]. Blood pressure and skin conductance levels hereby provide information about sympathetic activity, whereas heart rate is linked to both sympathetic arousal and parasympathetic physiological inhibition [65, 71, 72]. Furthermore, to obtain a dynamic assessment of effortful emotion regulation, research may present children with emotional challenging tasks while measuring their reciprocal adjustments of sympathetic and parasympathetic responses (see below).

Only a handful of studies to date have directly examined the first component of emotional impulsiveness, namely ADHD children's autonomic nervous system reactivity [48, 65, 71, 73-76]. Most of these studies, moreover, were not emotion-driven, but pertained to physical positional changes [76], cognitively challenging tasks [71, 72] or daily routine conditions [74, 75]. Only one published study appears to have addressed the issue in an explicit emotion regulation context as detailed further on [48].

The findings regarding ADHD children's autonomic reactivity have remained inconclusive so far, depending on comorbidity, selected physiological measures and laboratory paradigms [74-76]. For instance, a naturalistic study of circadian arousal variations revealed heightened diurnal and nocturnal heart rate levels in primary school age children with ADHD compared to non-clinical controls [75]. In contrast, a laboratory study examined whether school-aged children with ADHD had lower autonomic functioning and reactivity relative to those with an anxiety disorder. This was tested during and after a cognitively challenging task requiring mental arithmetic, as indexed by alteration of SC and HR levels [71]. ADHD children's skin conductance did not differ from anxious ones in baseline, stress or recovery conditions. Their heart rate yet showed a decreased response when recovering after the cognitively challenging task. These findings suggest a relative parasympathetic dominance in children with ADHD that was even more pronounced in those without comorbid CD or ODD [71].

Moreover, one early study by Beauchaine et al (2001) used a two-phase paradigm with (indirect) emotional elements, namely a reward and extinction based repetitive response task, that was followed by the viewing of a two minute video portraying escalating conflict between peers [73]. Skin conductance, cardiac pre-ejection periods (PEP) and respiratory sinus arrhythmia (RSA) were investigated as respective indices of sympathetic and parasympathetic responses in adolescents aged 12 to 17 with ADHD (n=17) and ADHD with CD (n=20) compared to non-clinical controls (n=20). Although both ADHD groups displayed lower SC than controls during baseline, no differences emerged during the reward/extinction condition. However, the comorbid ADHD children exhibited more sympathetic reactivity (PEP) compared to the ADHD and control groups at baseline, and relative to the controls only during the reward/extinction phase. They also showed lower baseline parasympathetic activity (RSA) relative to the ADHD-only and control children, but the groups did not differ in

RSA during the video condition. The SC and PEP findings of this study were essentially replicated in a more recent investigation with four to six year old preschoolers at risk for having ADHD and ODD (n=18) [77]. Changes in at-risk preschoolers' heart rate in this study further pointed to a predominance of parasympathetic mediation of their autonomic responses in behavioural reward/extinction conditions.

In all, one published study could be identified that explicitly investigated whether children with ADHD display a particular sympathetic and/or parasympathetic reactivity in manifest emotional conditions and whether this differs according to emotions. In a rare laboratory paradigm using active emotion induction and suppression conditions, Musser et al. (2011) indeed examined 66, seven to nine-year old, ADHD and non-clinical control children's autonomic responses [48]. Children were first instructed to facially mimic emotions of a main character viewed in a developmentally appropriate film clip (active emotion induction), and subsequently to imagine the main characters' feelings yet while not expressing any facial emotion (active emotion suppression). The children's sympathetic cardiac PEP and parasympathetic RSA were recorded throughout positive and negative emotion induction and suppression conditions. ADHD and control children's autonomic responses did not differ in baseline or neutral conditions. No significant group differences emerged either in children's sympathetic (PEP) responses. However, ADHD children exhibited a slight yet significant parasympathetic augmentation (RSA), and this inflexibly across all emotional conditions (positive and negative, induction and suppression). Moreover, when expressing deliberate positive facial emotion, the ADHD group responded with a more pronounced ineffective parasympathetic increase in contrast to control children's RSA decrease, suggesting an inadaptive emotional approach response.

ADHD children's physiological reactivity has furthermore been investigated along an additional line of questioning concerning alterations in their hypothalamic-pituitary-adrenocortical (HPA) axis. Consistent with the initially outlined expectations, ADHD children have been expected to show blunted cortisol responses to stress [78-80]. Again, studies in this respect have as yet seldom focused specifically on emotional contexts and have yielded mixed results across ADHD heterogeneity. In essence, predicted blunted cortisol responses are evidenced in children with ADHD and comorbid disruptive behaviour disorders. However, children with ADHD and comorbid anxiety disorders tend to show increased cortisol reactivity [78, 79]. Furthermore, one study compared cortisol responses during a public speaking situation among children with ADHD-C (n=52), ADHD-I (n=23) and non-clinical controls (n=25) [80]. In this more manifest psychosocial stress condition, ADHD children's HPA functioning showed subtype distinctions along similar externalising versus internalising lines as above, with ADHD-C children displaying blunted and ADHD-I increased cortisol responses. Finally, one study explicitly examined whether ADHD children's oppositional behaviour would be mediated by their cortisol reactivity to expressed emotions during a family emotion provocation task [58]. High levels of parental negative expressed emotion were indeed associated with both oppositional behaviour and increased cortisol responses in children with ADHD. Cortisol reactivity hereby mediated the emotion-to-behaviour pathway in all children.

Taken together, findings remain mixed as regards several aspects of ADHD children's autonomic reactivity. The earlier indications of a heightened sympathetic responsiveness in comorbid ADHD and CD children in a reward-based condition contrast with both underarousal expectations and with ADHD-only children's similar-to-control sympathetic reactivity in an active emotion induction/suppression context. A convergent tendency yet appears to come forward regarding ADHD children's inadaptive parasympathetic responses across different investigation contexts (deliberate emotion induction/suppression versus spontaneous responses to cognitively challenging tasks). This tendency would lend support to behavioural observations that children with ADHD especially have difficulty adequately adjusting their emotional responses [42, 61]. Moreover, ADHD children tend to show altered HPA-functioning, as evidenced in blunted versus intensified cortisol reactivity in respectively externalising (ADHD-C and conduct disorder comorbidity) and internalising (ADHD-I and anxious comorbidity) children. Thus, ADHD children's cortisol reactivity might mediate their emotional responses in emotionally challenging situations. Evidently, however, given the scant number of available studies, further specific examination is required of ADHD children's physiological arousal in emotional conditions. Variations herein according to ADHD comorbidities and subtypes merit further clarification, with the latter remaining largely unaddressed as regards sympathetic and parasympathetic physiological regulation.

5.2. ADHD children's processing of basic (facial) emotional cues

Emotion research in children with ADHD has emerged in part through a select number of 'early' studies examining their facial emotion recognition (FER) skills. Research on FER questions the ability of the child to adequately process or appraise basic emotional cues, a skill that is instrumental to its survival and interactions with others [40, 41, 81]. Although such cues can be verbal as well as non-verbal, especially the latter are recognised to be forceful communication elements and this early-on in development [82]. FER research paradigms thus generally consist of recording children's proficiency in labelling facial emotions, which are either viewed in isolation or within a broader visual or verbal context.

Given the discussion so far, at least four basic questions apply to ADHD children's FER, namely 1) are ADHD children's FER skills compromised compared to those without ADHD?, 2) if so, for which emotions is this the case?, 3) are ADHD children's FER skills linked to their (interpersonal) behavioural functioning?, and 4) which underlying mechanisms may explain ADHD children's FER difficulties?

Altogether, fourteen published studies were identified from 1998 on in Pubmed and through further reviewing of references that have directly addressed (facial) emotion recognition and understanding in children diagnosed with ADHD, besides one study on 'at-risk' children [83] and an ongoing study by our FACE©-ADHD program [30, 84]. As summarised in Table 1 and discussed in paragraph 5.2.1, two-third of these studies [28, 36, 39, 40, 85-89] have focused on simple FER and mostly pointed toward ADHD children experiencing significantly more FER difficulties compared to non-clinical controls. The investigated samples however remain relatively small and diverse in terms of context and comorbidity. Furthermore, precise indications regarding which facial emotions are more challenging for ADHD children to process remain inconsistent. As reviewed in Table 2 and discussed in paragraph 5.2.2, six studies also focused on emotion understanding in context and/or simultaneously compared ADHD children's simple versus contextualised emotion recognition [39, 41, 81, 90-92].

Authors[1,2] Year Country	**ADHD Comparison Age Sex**	**Type Comorbidity Medication Setting**	**Measures (primary)**	**Findings**
Ahmadi 2011 Iran	35 A / 31 NC 6-11 Boys	? ? no school	(initial) visual orientation to negative-neutral face pairs	no group differences in initial attention allocation expected orientation tendency to negative emotions in controls
Brotman 2010 USA	18 A / 37 NC 43 BD / 29 SMD 8-17 Boys	? ?(SA,SP) no clinical	fear, hostility, & nose-width ratings in happy, angry, fearful, & neutral faces; RT amygdala fMRI	Fear: BD & SMD more fear ratings neutral faces:ADHD no difference Hostility, nose-width: no differences ADHD left amygdala hyperactivation vs SMD hypoactivation for fear – nose-width contrasts
Cadesky 2000 USA	68 A / 27 NC 63 ADHD+CP 24 CP 7-13 Boys / Girls	? (ODD) no clinical	DANVA facial & oral happy, angry, sad, fear	Controls; ADHD+CP least errors Fear errors: ADHD+CP 23% vs NC 27% Sadness errors: ADHD+CP 33% vs NC 29% ADHD mostly random errors ADHD; CP more errors, sig for sad, marginal for happy & fear; not for anger ADHD vs CP similar (CP more sad errors)
Guyer 2007 USA	35 A [3] / 92 NC 42 BD / 39 SMD 44 Anx-Dep 7-18 Boys / Girls	? CD yes clinical	DANVA n° errors labelling happy, angry, sad, fear	Most errors by BD and SMD patients All: errors angry > fear > sad > happy Happy: ADHD+CD more errors than controls, less than BD and SMD Angry, sad, fear: ADHD+CD least errors compared to clinical groups and NC
Krauel 2009 Germany	30 A / 25 NC 12-15 Boys	? 16 ODD/CD 40% ?	IAPS, 50% neutral, 25% neg, 25% pos immediate recognition & memory (new / old picture)	All: faster response to positive pictures All: memory negative > positive > neutral ADHD neutral pictures memory < controls (unengaged when no salience) ADHD+CD+ODD memory positive pics lower than controls & ADHDonly

Authors[1,2] Year Country	ADHD Comparison Age Sex	Type Comorbidity Medication Setting	Measures (primary)	Findings
Pelc 2006 Belgium	30 ? 30 NC 7-12 Boys / Girls	HI no no	Ekman, morphed intensities happy, angry, sad, disgust 7-point rating difficulty (7point)	ADHD general deficit & specific difficulties for anger (high intensity) & sadness (all intensities), not for happiness & disgust poor awareness errors for anger and disgust ADHD FER errors inversely linked to interpersonal problems
Shin 2009 Korea	42[a] / 95[b] A 6-10[a] / 6-15[b] 27 NC Boys	? no no clinical	[a] ERT: pos / neg; context matching; [b] attention	[a] sample 1, [b] sample 2 No difference in pooled positive (happy, surprise) or negative (angry, sad, fear, disgust) FER between ADHD and controls See table 2
Sinzig 2008 Germany	21 auti+ADHD 19 autism 30 A / 29 NC 6-18 Boys / Girls	I / C CDD/ODD no clinical	FEFA: FER, eye pairs Happy, angry, sad, fear, disgust, surprise, neutral Sustained attention, Inhibition, Set shifting	Autism+ADHD and ADHD poorer facial & eye pair recognition than autism and controls Joy, surprise: ADHD < Autism+ADHD < controls and autism FER linked with sustained attention and inhibition deficits in ADHD children
Williams 2008 Australia	51 A / 51 NC 8-17 Boys	I / C Opp/Anx/Dep no(T1) / yes(T2) clinical	FER Happy, angry, sad, fear, disgust, neutral ERP during 2nd FER naturalistic open design, pre-/post MPH	ADHD(anx/dep) poorer FER anger & fear than controls; no ADHD subtype effects reduced initial occipital activity, followed by exaggeration, & reduced temporal activity during contextual processing After MPH normalized brain activity but no mood changes

[1] First author, see references for full author list | [2] Legend: ? = unspecified, A = ADHD, NC = Non-clinical controls, BD = Bipolar Disorder, SMD = Severe Mood Dysregulation, CP = Conduct problems, CD = Conduct Disorder, ODD = Oppositional Defiant Disorder, Anx = anxiety, Dep = deptression, SA = separation anxiety, SP = social phobia, opp = oppositional; I = ADHD Inattentive subtype, C = ADHD Combined subtype, HI = ADHD Hyperactive-Impulsive subtype; MPH = Methylphenidate; RT = reaction times; DANVA = Diagnostic Analysis of Nonverbal Accuracy; ERT = Emotion Recognition Test; ;JACFEE = Japanese & Caucasian Facial Expressions of Emotion | [3] Sample comprising 18 ADHD, 7 CD, 10 ADHD+CD children

Table 1. Published studies on basic FER skills in children with DSM-IV diagnosed ADHD

Authors[1,2] Year Country	Groups Comparison Age Gender	Type Comorbidity Medication Setting	Measures (primary)	Findings
Corbett 2000 USA	37 A / 37 NC 6-12 Boys / Girls	C no no clinical	JACFEE: happy, angry, sad, fear, disgust, surprise, neutral Prosody Test (identify happy, angry, sad, neutral from speech intonation) Inhibition: Go No-Go Task (verbal); Matching Familiar Figures Test (nonverbal) Attention: Memory for Sentences (verbal); Knox Cube Test (nonverbal)	ADHD children significantly less proficient than controls on all measures (visual and verbal emotion recognition, verbal & non-verbal attention, and impulse control with non-verbal stimuli), except for the Go No-Go task where they scored better. FER skills explain 85% of variance in discriminating ADHD from control children.
Braaten 2000 USA	24 A/ 19 NC 6-12 Boys	HI C ? no community	Empathy to fictitious story with positive vs negative and simple vs complex feelings (match between labelling characters' emotion and labelling own emotion; explaining characters' emotion) Parent-reported emotional behaviour Self-reported emotional intensity and reactivity to reward / punishment situations	ADHD children less match between characters' and own emotion than controls ADHD less character-centred explanations of characters' emotions than controls More parent-reported emotional behaviour in ADHD children than controls No sign. differences in child-reported emotional intensity and contingency reactivity
Da Fonseca 2008 France	27 A / 27 NC 5-15 Boys / Girls	C 6ODD 1CD no clinical	(1) Magazine pictures (face / body) (2) Similar pictures, masked face (emotional) or object (non-emotional) Happy, angry, sad, fear Non-verbal labelling (Smiley)	ADHD children less efficient in recognising simple and contextualised emotions than controls, no emotion specificity ADHD no significant difficulties in recognising objects in context All: FER happy, angry > fear, sad
Singh 1998 USA	50 - 34 boys 16 girls	? ? no SP[3]	JACFEE: happy, angry, sad, fear, disgust, surprise;	74% mean correct identification for ADHD Errors: Fear>Anger/ Surprise>Disgust>Sad>Happy

http://dx.doi.org/10.5772/54422

Authors[1,2] Year Country	Groups Comparison Age Gender	Type Comorbidity Medication Setting	Measures (primary)	Findings
			to be linked with emotion stories comprising target emotion word	Confusions: fear-surprise, anger-disgust
Shin 2009 Korea	42[a] / 95[b] 27 NC 6-10[a] / 6-15[b] Boys	? no no clinical	[a] Study 1, ERT: see table 1; Match situational cartoon to facial picture [b] Study 2, Attention: ADS continuous performance target / non-target (omission, commission errors, RT, RT variability)	FER: See table 1 (no differences) ADHD lower contextual understanding (face to situation match) than controls Only omission attentional errors account significantly for ADHD children's contextual understanding (not verified in controls)
Yuill 2007 England	19[a] / 17[b] 5-11[a] / 5-6[b] Boys	? ?ODD no clinical	[a] Study 1, Match facial expression to emotional situation sentence; match object picture to non-emotional situation sentence [b] Study 2, Same task, with inhibitory scaffolding (impulsive inhibition)	All: non-emotion task easier than emotion task ADHD overall poorer performances; Emotional: 30-40% correct (21% for suprise) vs 79-95% in controls; Non-emotional: mostly 40-50% correct vs 94-100% in controls No age effects; no ODD effects

[1] First author, see references for full author list. | [2] Legend: ? = unspecified, A = ADHD, NC = Non-clinical controls, CD = Conduct Disorder, ODD = Oppositional Defiant Disorder, C = ADHD Combined subtype, HI = ADHD Hyperactive-Impulsive subtype; RT = reaction times; JACFEE = Japanese & Caucasian Facial Expressions of Emotion | [3] Summer program

Table 2. Published studies on contextual emotion understanding by DSM-IV ADHD-children

5.2.1. ADHD children's simple facial emotion recognition skills

Children generally are able to identify basic facial emotions (happiness, anger, sadness and fear) by early childhood and gain in accuracy to accomplish fuller emotion classification by middle childhood [86]. In children with ADHD, brain imaging studies have documented (posterior) right hemispheric specificities, such as an enlarged right hemisphere structure and hypofused functioning, along with possibly reduced amygdala and compensatory enlarged hippocampus [44, 49]. Since such deficits are profoundly linked to impairments in evaluating emotional stimuli, children with ADHD may be expected to have difficulties in adequately perceiving or processing emotions at an appraisal level [41]. Additionally, ADHD children's fluctuating attentional deployment raises questions as to whether impaired sustained attention also contributes to difficulties in processing affective cues [83].

More precise expectations about differential emotion recognition difficulties have been difficult to formulate. For instance, joy and surprise tend to be more easily recognised by children overall compared to fear, sadness and disgust [86]. Yet, negative facial expressions compared to neutral ones are also documented to mobilise typically developing children's attention; a tendency that is understood as an adaptive response toward potential danger [36, 15]. Children with CD/ODD, which are frequent ADHD comorbidities, for their part seem to display a marked increased bias toward processing negative emotional information in social situations. At the same time, CD/ODD children also appear less aroused by negative emotional stimuli [15, 85]. Thus, detailed expectations about ADHD children's FER skills may depend on their clinical constellation including their comorbidities.

Overall, the reviewed studies point to statistically significant *differences* in basic FER skills between children with ADHD and non-clinical controls or other clinical groups, as illustrated in Table 1 *(question 1)*. However, depending on comorbidity and comparison groups, differences are not necessarily to the disadvantage of the ADHD population and/or tend to vary widely as regards which emotions elicit more recognition difficulties *(question 2)*. Moreover, whenever performance percentages are specified, a majority of ADHD children (60% and up) still appear to exhibit accurate FER.

Thus, the right hemisphere hypothesis has been supported at least partially as several studies document children with ADHD to be less efficient at identifying *negative facial cues* compared to non-clinical controls [36, 40, 83, 84, 88, 89]. Specific negative FER difficulties, however, vary across studies and children's clinical status, with no clear pattern coming forward. For example, an expected dampened detection of anger and fear was found compared to non-clinical controls in a sample of 51 adolescent boys with ADHD and associated oppositional behaviour along with depressed and anxious mood [89]. This was also the case for anger and sadness, but not for fear, in a sample of hyperactive/impulsive ADHD children without comorbidities [88].

These findings partially converge with pilot results from an ongoing multi-method, multi-informant research that operationalises the above FACE©-model. In this research, a naturalistic group of medicated ADHD children in a special school setting is compared with gender- and age-matched non-referred children (ages 7-12, mean age 10, 80% boys) on correlates of emotion regulation [30, 84]. On a micro-level, children are examined on emotional components of ER (basic FER, emotion recognition in context, and self-reported experience) along with cognitive (Theory-Of-Mind), attentional (simple and modified emotional Simon tasks), and behavioural ones (multi-informant reports of problem behaviour including aggression and anxiety). Children's developmental risk-resiliency load is furthermore registered on a macro-level. Compared to controls (n=13), a preliminary sample of ADHD children (n=15) with comorbid learning problems and autism spectrum symptoms (ASS) (respectively 66% and 33%) made significantly more FER errors than controls (t (26) = -2,578, p = 0,016) and doubted more their choices (t (26) = -2,147, p = 0,041). These comorbid ADHD children were in particular marginally less efficient at identifying happiness and anger. A second subsample of ADHD children (n=20), also with mainly learning problems but no ASS, did not differ in basic FER compared to controls (n=20) but was less efficient in contextualising emotions, especially anxiety, during a verbal recognition task, as well as in Theory of Mind (also see §5.2.2). For all children, happiness was best recognised facially, followed by anger, and fear (sample 1) or sadness (sample 2) [4, 5, 30, 84].

The aforementioned less expected difficulties with the recognition of the *positive emotion* happiness were also found in children with ADHD and comorbid CD [86], as well as in a comparison among children (ages 6-18) with autism, autism and ADHD, and ADHD-only [28] (see Table 1). In the latter study, both groups with ADHD, namely ADHD-only and comorbid autism and ADHD, were less proficient in recognising happiness as well as surprise on faces and on eye pairs, relative to autism-only and non-clinical children [28].

In contrast, ADHD appears to be associated with *more* successful FER in some instances, as comes forward from a detailed analysis of studies examining whether FER patterns are distinct or cut across clinical conditions. This was the case, for example, in a rare study comparing FER among children and adolescents with BD, severe mood dysregulation (SMD), ADHD and/or CD, anxiety and/or depression and controls [86]. Markedly, the ADHD with CD group appeared to make least errors in angry, sad and fearful FER compared to all other groups, including non-clinical controls. Similarly, another study compared FER among children with ADHD, ADHD with conduct problems (CP) or CP (all with comorbid ODD), and controls. Along with controls, the comorbid ADHD with CP children also exhibited least errors except for sadness, while ADHD-only children mostly displayed random errors.

Findings tend to be clearer regarding the *behavioural and relational impact* of children's FER skills *(question 3)*. When this is examined, studies indeed report significant associations between ADHD children's FER skills and daily-life outcomes. For instance, in the pilot study of the FACE©-research, ADHD children's FER skills were inversely proportional to parent and teacher rated ADHD-specific (hyperactivity, inattention, impulsivity) and non-specific (oppositional and aggressive) problem behaviour [30, 84]. Similarly, the above-cited hyperactive/impulsive ADHD children without comorbidities investigated by Pelc et al. (2006) who made more FER errors also exhibited higher interpersonal problems [88].

Finally, some studies attempted to shed light on the neural basis of ADHD children's FER skills *(question 4)* (see table 2). One study examined contrasted amygdala responses when rating emotional cues (fear and hostility) versus non-emotional ones (nose-width) in happy, angry, fearful or neutral faces, and this among youth with BD, SMD, ADHD and non-clinical controls [85]. Interestingly, although ADHD youth did not differ from the other groups in fear, hostility or nose-width ratings, they manifested left-amygdala hyperactivation in fear – nose-width contrasts compared to healthy controls, bipolar and SMD children. Another study, by Williams et al. (2008), recorded ADHD youth's event-related potentials during a second presentation of facial emotion labelling, before and after methylphenidate (MPH) treatment in an open label trial spanning four weeks [89]. ADHD boys showed a pattern of reduced occipital activity during initial perceptual analysis that was associated with their disrupted FER and mood. This was followed by flow-on difficulties in emotion processing, such as an exaggerated structural encoding activity and finally reduced temporal contextual activity. In short, these findings lend further support to possible (compensatory) amygdala responses and specific temporal-occipital pathways in mood processing linked to ADHD.

5.2.2. Understanding of emotions in context by children with ADHD

While identifying simple facial emotions represents the most basic form of emotion recognition, real-life communication seldom consists of isolated facial expressions. Facial expressions are mostly if not always situationally embedded. From their earliest interactions, children learn to modulate their appraisal of facial emotions according to the context [66]. As experience develops, this skill increasingly involves (episodic) memory and associated hippocampal functions through which emotional stimuli are linked to (the remembrance of) contextual cues. Specifically, given disruptions in right hemispheric functioning and in the IFC/DLPFC to amygdala circuitry reported for children with ADHD, they may be expected to display difficulties in contextualising emotions over and above their simple FER difficulties [44, 49]. A next level in emotional assessment therefore consists of examining the child's ability to appropriately link facial expressions and (social) situations or to understand emotional cues in their context (e.g. in stories) [42, 64].

All six reviewed published studies (see Table 2) provide evidence that children with ADHD are less successful in reciprocally matching (facial) emotions and interpersonal situations than non-clinical controls *(question 1)* [39, 41, 81, 90-92]. Furthermore, as mentioned above (§5.2.1), the subsample of ADHD children with learning problems of the ongoing FACE©-ADHD research was significantly less efficient than non-clinical controls in identifying emotions in verbally presented stories [84]. Along the same line of thought, an early study by Braaten et al. (2000) stands somewhat apart by addressing a more sophisticated level of emotional understanding. Here, children's ER was further probed by assessing their ability to recognise characters' emotions in a story and to relate these to their own feelings [90]. Children with ADHD were less likely than controls to match their own feelings with those of the child in the story and to interpret the latter according to the characters' context.

Again, however, no clear pattern emerges as to whether ADHD children have more difficulty contextualising specific emotions *(question 2)*. For example, an early study with five to 13-year old ADHD boys and girls enrolled in a summer camp, using Ekman's facial affect pictures, suggested a mixed pattern of negative emotions as well as surprise to elicit more contextualisation errors than happiness [81]. Another mixed pattern of better contextualising of happy and angry, than fearful and sad feelings occurred for both ADHD-combined subtype and control children when asked to link symbolic facial expressions (Smiley's) to masked faces of people in popular magazine pictures [91].

Apparently, few of these studies furthermore examined the link between ADHD children's contextualised emotion recognition and their behavioural outcomes *(question 3)*. In our ongoing research, children's emotion recognition (and Theory-of-Mind) were found to be inversely related to reports of their externalizing and internalizing problem behaviour in both subsamples regardless of type of ADHD comorbidity [30, 84].

Some studies finally addressed possible underlying mechanisms of ADHD children's difficulties in contextualising emotions *(question 4)*. For instance, Da Fonseca et al's (2008) study also included the matching of objects to situational magazine pictures. In contrast to the emotional matching, ADHD children displayed no significant difficulties in replacing ob-

http://dx.doi.org/10.5772/54422

jects in their context, confirming an emotional rather than solely perceptual nature of their matching errors [91]. A study addressing the link between ADHD boys' continuous attentional performance furthermore found only omission errors to account significantly for ADHD children's matching of facial emotional expressions to situational cartoons [39]. Also, in an early yet thorough study involving FER, along with prosody, verbal and nonverbal impulse inhibition and attention tasks, ADHD children's significantly poorer performances on all tasks relative to controls where explained for 85% by their FER skills [41].

Still, findings on ADHD children's contextual emotion recognition seem to remain quite task and/or stimulus dependent. For instance, one study involved the matching of facial expressions to specifically designed emotion-situation sentences, and object pictures to non-emotional sentences [92]. In this case, ADHD boys exhibited exceptionally poor performances with only 20 to 40% of correct emotional and 40 to 50% non-emotional matchings. Control children, in turn, achieved 79 to 100% correct matchings across conditions. These findings contrast with a sensibly higher overall mean of 74% of correct contextual emotion identification by ADHD children documented in Singh's early study [81]. In the same line of stimulus-dependent ER variations, a condition of contextualised emotion recognition in verbal material yielded anger to be least well identified by both control and ADHD children, as opposed to being second-best recognised in a condition of FER [84].

Of note, studies comparing contextual emotion recognition among children with ADHD and *other clinical conditions* or different *subtypes* are still lacking. Simple or contextualised processing of *prosody* also has hardly been investigated in children with ADHD [15, 93]. In adults, emotional semantic processing has been found to be enhanced compared to controls, possibly through compensatory mobilisation of cognitive resources [94]. Similar investigations are needed in children with ADHD.

5.2.3. Summary

Overall, ADHD children as a group do appear to display specificities in FER skills that tend to set them apart from non-referred controls and children with other clinical conditions. In addition, the ADHD child and adolescent population also does seem to exhibit more difficulties in matching facial emotions to contextual clues, or recognising emotions in verbal context, compared to non-clinical controls.

The pattern of these basic and contextualised (facial) emotion recognition specificities yet remains unclear to date. ADHD children with or without comorbidities are diversely found to be less efficient in recognising simple negative as well as positive facial emotions compared to non-clinical controls and possibly also to children with different clinical conditions. However, the opposite occurs in some instances, with some large comparison studies documenting better FER skills in (comorbid) ADHD children relative to other clinical and non-clinical groups. Comorbidity or medication statuses do not appear to provide sufficient leads for explaining these contrasting outcomes. Potential influences of maturation (age) and ADHD heterogeneity (subtypes) still require further clarification given that half of the studies span child through adolescent populations, and that the majority leaves ADHD subtypes unspecified. Also needed are studies that address potential gender effects on simple or contextualised emotion recognition with sufficient participation of girls with ADHD. The effects of verbal versus non-verbal stimulus modes as yet remain underexplored too.

Furthermore, when FER difficulties are documented in ADHD children, these appear to be linked to adverse behavioural and interpersonal outcomes. Similar links remain to be further established for ADHD children's contextual emotion recognition.

Finally, there are some indications that ADHD children's basic and contextual emotion recognition skills are related to specificities in right hemispheric emotion-processing and (left) amygdala hyperactivity, while attentional impacts remain less well established. The intricacy of cognitive and emotional systems hereby points to the need of considering multiple pathways of underlying mechanisms instead of mutually exclusive ones, whereby probable compensatory functioning may contribute to explaining the absence of observed emotion processing deficits in some instances.

In sum, the heterogeneity of the population of youth with ADHD, the relative scarcity of current studies directly addressing their emotion recognition skills, and the contrasting outcomes so far all call for a research agenda that would more systematically examine the extent to which gender, age, ADHD subtypes, comorbidities and stimulus type account for variability in ADHD children's basic and contextualised emotion recognition skills.

5.3. How do children with ADHD (deliberately) modulate subjective experiences and behavioural expressions of emotional reactivity?

As defined previously, emotional impulsiveness consists of diminished inhibition of emotional expression besides heightened emotional reactivity (cf.§5.1) [47, 61]. ADHD children's difficulties with modulating their emotional expressions have been mostly documented indirectly through a vast literature attesting to their externalising problem behaviour. Specific examination of the behavioural component of ADHD children's emotional impulsiveness to date has mainly concerned their management of frustration, and this principally in cognitive task-interference contexts [61, 83].

On a behavioural level, children with ADHD are inclined to favour situations that provide immediate reward. They also tend to have difficulty persisting when gratification is delayed. This tendency has been described under the delay-aversion hypothesis [66]. Still, the question arises what makes it more difficult for children with ADHD than for their peers to delay reward and persist when positive reinforcement remains uncertain? From an emotion-centred perspective, ADHD children's difficulties with persisting under delayed reward conditions are thought to be mediated by the challenge of regulating negative emotions, and especially frustration.

Several studies have therefore explicitly investigated how children with ADHD modulate their emotional experience and expression in constrained task conditions that elicit frustration. Frustration is defined here as the emotion resulting from an absence of reward when such reward is expected [82]. Persistence can thus be conceived as the ability to adjust or modulate frustration perception so as to maintain task-oriented behavioural continuity.

http://dx.doi.org/10.5772/54422

Study paradigms consequently generally consist of manipulating children's reward expectancy and registering their self-reported and/or behaviourally observed emotional responses.

Most studies have confirmed children with ADHD to experience heightened frustration levels in association with persistence and behavioural control problems, this both in cognitive task conditions [66, 95, 82] and in less investigated emotional contexts [9]. Detailed accounts of their task-related emotional experiences however provide important nuance regarding ADHD children's emotional understanding and process insight [66, 82].

For instance, an early study compared how seven to nine year old, clinically-referred ADHD children (n=22) and non-referred controls (n=20) compared on performance, study-time, self-rated persistence (namely how much did the child feel like continuing), and facially recorded frustration levels during a nonsense word learning task [82]. Children were assigned to either a predetermined continuous reinforcement (CRF) or partial reinforcement (PRF) condition. The CRF and PRF conditions both consist of an acquisition phase followed by a non-reward extinction phase, yet PRF involves random instead of continuous reward during acquisition. Importantly, reinforcement pertained to persistence rather than task correctness in this study. As expected, learning occurred in both phases for both groups. Children with ADHD yet made more errors, expressed more frustration and felt less like persisting overall. Interestingly, especially the random reward (PRF) condition yielded three-fold frustration levels in ADHD children during the acquisition phase along with a persistence deficit. In turn, only children with ADHD (and not controls) in the CRF condition spent more study-time over the acquisition course [82]. Thus, children with ADHD displayed a marked difficulty habituating to initial frustration, while investing considerable effort in a consistent reward condition.

In the same vein, self-reported frustration was studied in medicated children with ADHD (n=21; mostly combined subtype) compared to non-clinical controls (n=43) using a blindfolded puzzle task [66]. This study moreover recorded detailed accounts of children's emotions, such as their self-reported mood after the task, general persistence and frustration tendency (likeliness of quitting and getting frustrated compared to peers), insight in the accompanying physical, emotional, or cognitive sensations of their frustration and how they dealt with it. Children additionally completed a structured emotional competence self-report measure, along with a mathematics task. Consistent with the previous findings, the present ADHD children were less persistent overall but invested as much time as control children in the tasks. This yielded them mixed results: they were more likely to quit the puzzle task and completed less mathematic problems than their peers, but the ones they completed were accurate. Of special interest for the present focus, the children with ADHD were likelier to report suffering frustration and give up compared to other children, were able to identify signs of their frustration and knew about ways of dealing with it. However, they were significantly less effective at acting upon this emotional understanding than controls.

Children with ADHD have also been demonstrated to have difficulty deliberately masking their emotions in an elicited frustration situation [95]. One study for instance examined ADHD boys' (n=26, ages 6 to 11) observed emotion regulation compared to that of controls (n=23), by explicitly asking them to hide their feelings even if they became upset during a competitive Stop Signal Task with peers. The boys with ADHD not only had more difficulty with regulating their emotions compared to their non-clinical peers, they were also less successful at hiding their emotions despite knowing that they were expected to do so [95].

Of note, the previous studies examined ADHD children's emotional expression in cognitively challenging contexts. Two other studies did so too in more explicitly emotion-related interpersonal contexts. One study used a prize paradigm with 8 to 11-year-old medicated children with ADHD-combined (ADHD-C, n=16) and inattentive (ADHD-I, n=14) subtypes (12 boys, 9 girls) compared to controls (n=17) [9]. Children's emotional responses were recorded in disappointing versus non-disappointing conditions, namely receiving an unwanted versus a desired prize, after they had been asked to rank prizes in order of desirability and told they would receive prizes for helping another examiner. Emotion-focused measures included children's facial and non-verbal reactions (classified as positive, negative, social monitoring or tension behaviour), along with self-rated affect (how they felt about the prize, how frustrated they felt and how they liked the prize). As expected, all children generally displayed condition-congruent behaviour, along with more intense self-reported affect following disappointment and more interest and effective ER in the non-disappointing condition. Children with ADHD-C additionally showed a trend toward more negatively behaving after disappointment, experiencing more prize interest and affect intensity as well as poorer ER than inattentive and control peers. Remarkably, children with ADHD-C also showed significantly more positive behaviour overall (regardless of condition) than their inattentive and control peers [9]. These findings concord with evidence stemming from physiological reactivity research (cf. §5.1), suggesting that children with ADHD, and among them mainly those with the combined subtype, experience difficulties in adjusting their emotions and related behaviours across shifting situational demands.

A study by Melnick & Hinshaw (2000) employed a more ecologically valid approach by using a videotaped frustrating family task to examine emotional reactivity and regulation among six to twelve year old, low aggressive (n=23) and high aggressive (n=25) ADHD boys compared to non-clinical controls and their parents (see §5.4 for the latter) [60]. Frustration, or negative emotion, was elicited by asking the child to complete a construction model with parental help while two building pieces were lacking. Children's behaviour was coded as regards the intensity of their emotional ventilation (or reactivity) and the appropriateness of their emotion modulation strategies (such as problem solving, seeking help, accommodating, negative focussing or shutting down). Interestingly, no generalised ER difficulty could be demonstrated for these ADHD children. Observer-rated aggression was also not related to children's emotion regulation strategies overall, nor was emotional reactivity a significant predictor of their behavioural and social (peer) outcomes in this study. However, within-population distinctions emerged whereby high-aggressive ADHD boys exhibited expected overreactive emotions and impaired problem solving, whereas low-aggressive ADHD boys showed either normal range or underresponsive emotional reactions [60].

It should be noted that, similar to (facial) emotion recognition evidence, findings on ADHD children's emotional intensity and behaviour may present measure-dependent variations. For instance, the early empathy study by Braaten et al. (2000) cited in paragraph 5.2.2 addi-

http://dx.doi.org/10.5772/54422

tionally assessed children's emotional behaviours, intensity and reactions to contingencies using reported responses to hypothetical reward and punishment situations instead of live laboratory paradigms [90]. The use of these formats yielded parent-reports of more manifest signs of sadness, anger and guilt in ADHD boys but no self-reported differences in emotional intensity or reactivity compared to controls.

Finally, the chronic and pervasive impact of emotional impulsiveness is documented in a rare longitudinal study that followed up on hyperactive (n=158) and community control (n=81) children, currently 27 years of age [47]. Participants reported on emotional impulsiveness (such as impatient, irascible, easily excited, frustrated, annoyed and emotionally overreactive behaviour) and were interviewed on multiple domains of functioning (e.g., home life and responsibilities, marital life, social interactions and leisure activities, occupation, and so forth). Emotional impulsiveness was highly correlated with the interrelated dimensions of inattention and hyperactivity-impulsivity in participants with persistent ADHD. The severity of emotional impulsiveness furthermore contributed uniquely to participants' overall impairment and multiple domain-specific adverse outcomes.

Taken together, these studies' findings lend credence to the emotion-centred expectations that ADHD children's (cognitive) abilities may become masked, not only by task modalities, but significantly so too by difficulties in modulating their emotional responses across tasks and situational demands. They also indicate that children with ADHD may especially benefit from support in translating mood- and mood-repair-knowledge into action. Still, there is ample room for further investigation of ADHD children's deliberate modulation of emotional responses in emotional contexts. The small number of studies and limited investigation scope leave more open questions than answers for the time being, notably regarding whether and to what extent children with ADHD experience differential emotion regulation difficulties depending on the type of emotions, their intensity, the interaction styles and the involved relational contexts, to name but a few. The longitudinal findings on the unique lifelong impact of emotional impulsiveness underline the importance of uncovering early intervention leads for supporting youth with ADHD to behaviourally modulate their emotions.

5.4. ADHD children's emotion regulation in the context of parenting and family risks and resources

The reviewed evidence-base suggests that children with ADHD differ from other children in their processing of facial affective clues, are less effective at matching (facial) affect and context, experience higher frustration levels in (cognitively) challenging situations and experience more difficulty habituating to negative feelings and/or modulating these by acting upon mood-repair techniques, despite some degree of insight into internal emotion-related signals. Importantly, these difficulties occur even though children with ADHD appear to invest considerable effort into 'doing well' and complying with external instructions.

From a theoretical viewpoint (see paragraph 3.2), these observations raise questions about contextual effects, and especially parenting and family ones, on ADHD children's emotion regulation skills. Several macro-level pathways may indeed influence the development of ER skills in children with ADHD, both directly and indirectly, as illustrated by the arrows in

Figure 1. Exploring these contextual pathways seems all the more pertinent given the observed discrepancies of ER findings within the ADHD youth population and apparently insufficient explanatory value of subtype, comorbidity or medication-statuses.

The most *direct* contextual effects on ADHD children's ER skills concern the way in which parents raise their children and run the family as regards these skills. Mediating and moderating effects of, for instance, parental depression, marital conflict, and critical and harsh parenting indeed already have been documented in general developmental studies and in research regarding predictors of early-onset conduct problems [53, 96, 97]. With the increased recognition of adult persistence of ADHD, many children with ADHD are acknowledged to grow up in families with at least one parent with ADHD [8, 43] and possibly siblings too [55, 96]. Emotional impairments in children with ADHD therefore are expected to be reciprocally shaped by their personal neurobiological predispositions and parenting- and family-related disruptions in emotion regulation [8, 14, 43, 57, 97, 98]. ER disruptions also involve *less direct* effects, such as ADHD children's observational, modelled learning of emotion expression through their parents and possibly siblings. Moreover, structural and functional contextual risks and resources are known to operate through *cumulative and relative principles*, also described as psychological allostatic load [7, 13, 30, 35, 53]. For example, an accumulation of family members with ADHD, internalising or externalising comorbidity, family conflict and an adverse school climate would expectedly culminate in mutually undermining effects on the ADHD child's ER skills. Conversely, the presence, for example, of family members with strong emotion regulation skills and a supportive school climate would constitute cumulative resources that stimulate the ADHD child's emotion regulation skills, or at least counterbalance its personal liabilities to this regard.

Unfortunately, to what extent parental, parenting and family ER difficulties affect specific ER components in ADHD offspring has hardly been empirically examined. A Pubmed search with the key-words 'ADHD', 'emotion regulation' and 'parenting' yields a mere five published articles, among which only the above-cited study of Melnick et al. (2000) directly tackled the subject (see §5.3) [60]. In this previously described videotaped frustrating family task, asides from child ER, parental behaviour was also observed as regards positive versus negative parenting (e.g. situational advice, warmth, structuring and empathy versus negativity, intrusiveness, withdrawal), along with personal (global) emotion regulation (e.g. anxiety, maintenance of focus on and interaction with the child). Mean levels of parenting behaviour did not differ significantly among the ADHD (sub)groups and control children. However, parental anxiety/nervousness and mother's negativity were significantly associated with child global emotion regulation difficulties overall; whereas father's global ER and advice-giving were marginally linked with child positive coping behaviour.

These findings are consonant with several other research reports linking parental negativity, sometimes in association with parental ADHD, to (self-reported) adverse outcomes on emotion regulation in ADHD offspring and this throughout the life span [21, 47, 99].

For instance, in the broader literature children with ADHD have been described to resort to overestimation of their social, behavioural or family-related self-perceptions, probably as a compensation mechanism for excessive emotionally negative interactions [98, 99]. This phenomenon, described as the positive illusory bias, was investigated in one study as regards its link with parental emotional expression among families with seven to ten year old children with ADHD compared to controls (N=56) [99]. Parental criticism was indeed associated with greater positive illusory bias, and parental warmth with lower bias regarding social functioning in children with ADHD. Such findings call for the investigation of comparable parenting effects on ER aspects such as ADHD children's physiological reactivity, basic or contextualised emotion appraisal and behavioural modulation.

Regarding behavioural modulation, a retrospective study for instance examined whether recalled parental ADHD and parenting behaviour related to current emotion regulation among adults with persistent ADHD (n=73, mean age 40, half combined/half inattentive subtypes) [21]. The ADHD adults whose mother possibly had ADHD recalled more maternal rejection and punishment, less paternal rejection and punishment, along with more emotional warmth. These retrospectively identified maternal parenting characteristics, as well as recalled maternal ADHD symptoms, were linked to current insecure emotional functioning and interpersonal relationships. ADHD adults' current attachment and emotion processing patterns were not similarly linked to recalled paternal ADHD and fathering characteristics.

To conclude on potential contextual influences on ADHD children's emotion regulation, it is noteworthy that the cultural component hereof has drawn little attention so far. While basic FER is considered to be relatively universal, this assumption is far less evident for the contextual embedment of emotions and for their behavioural correlates. One study for instance found parenting strategies among children with ADHD to differ by ethnicity, although this did not moderate treatment outcomes [100]. Potential effects of ethnicity and culture on ADHD children's appraisal and expression of emotions thus deserve examination.

In sum, the frequent cumulative presence of ADHD among family members by itself forms a considerable risk burden that may increase emotion dysregulation in children with ADHD or constitute critical obstacles toward their learning of effective emotion regulation. While these risks of parental ADHD, negative parenting and family interactions are easily conceived, there is a lack of empirical research that investigates when and how such cumulative risks versus resources specifically operate in the ADHD child's acquisition of emotion regulation skills.

5.5. Summary

Behavioural observations, neurobiological and brain imaging data have led to postulate that children with ADHD may experience disrupted emotion regulation. More specifically, ADHD children are expected to exhibit right hemispheric- and attention-related emotion recognition difficulties along with emotional impulsiveness, including heightened physiological reactivity and lessened control of behavioural emotional expression, as synthesised at micro-level of the FACE-model. ADHD children's emotion regulation consequently merits investigation as regards their physiological arousal levels, basic and contextualised appraisal of (facial) emotional cues and modulation of emotional behaviour.

Our review of the current evidence-base concerning ADHD children's emotion regulation reveals a still emerging field that involves a wide scope of ER components and operationalisations, which have only been investigated to a limited extent to date. This state-of-the-art prohibits drawing definite conclusions on the extent to which the ADHD youth population exhibits the expected ER difficulties, and the degree to which these apply to its heterogeneous subgroups as regards subtypes and comorbidities. Further empirical evidence is required too regarding how, precisely, parental, parenting and family dynamics hamper versus foster specific aspects of ADHD children's emotion regulation.

Taken together, the available studies nevertheless suggest that children with ADHD tend to differ from other children in their processing of facial affective clues and are at-risk for being less effective at adequately adapting their physiological arousal to situational demands, and at matching (facial) affect and context. Children with ADHD also appear vulnerable to experiencing higher frustration levels in (cognitively) challenging situations, and having more difficulties with behaviourally habituating to negative feelings and modulating these by acting upon mood-repair techniques. This happens despite indications that children with ADHD do demonstrate some degree of insight into internal emotion-related signals. Perhaps even more importantly, it appears that children with ADHD invest considerable effort into 'doing well' and attempting to control their negative emotions when requested to do so, yet these efforts are seldom acknowledged and/or accompanied by the expected results. The prevention and intervention implications hereof are discussed hereafter.

6. From studying to facilitating ADHD children's emotion regulation

Translating research into practice remains an important challenge for designing, implementing and evaluating ADHD prevention and intervention programs [6, 18, 57, 101]. Several characteristics of the extant ER research yet call for caution when attempting to move from the evidence-base toward one-on-one practice with ADHD children. We therefore first analyse conditions for a cautious interpretation of the evidence-base that also foster a strengths-based approach, this along three related lines pertaining to the individual, the proportional and the clinical relevance of the empirical findings (§6.1). Several potential implications of the ER evidence-base for emotion-oriented intervention with ADHD children and their families are considered subsequently (§6.2).

6.1. Cautions and conditions for an evidence-based, resiliency-oriented practice

A *first* and fundamental challenge when relying on the evidence-base for practice consists of deciphering its potential relevance for the individual child with ADHD and its family. Empirical research indeed mostly reports on statistically significant differences between groups of children with and without ADHD; or on *group-level* correlations between the ADHD status and several emotion regulation aspects. Such mean differences or group-wise correlations evidently do not concern all investigated ADHD children. Most of the current research data thus critically leave open questions as to which children within the investigated ADHD

http://dx.doi.org/10.5772/54422

groups are more particularly concerned by specific ER difficulties [19, 28, 37, 46]. Moreover, cross-sectional research, which is currently dominant, informs little to none about children's personal trajectories, while understanding these trajectories is crucial to guiding prevention and intervention efforts with individual ADHD children and their families.

A *second*, related challenge consists of clarifying the proportions of children with ADHD who are vulnerable to exhibiting ER difficulties. Percentages of ADHD versus control children concerned by the observed ER differences indeed are not systematically provided in many studies. A clear view of the proportion of the investigated ADHD children facing emotion regulation challenges consequently does not automatically emerge from the evidence-base. Closer analysis nevertheless reveals that oftentimes only a minority or a subgroup among the children with ADHD presents deficits in the investigated emotion regulation components, while a majority successfully accomplishes the tasks at hand. Practice relevance would consequently be enhanced if empirical research were oriented to a larger extent on identifying the subsets of ADHD children who account for the differences in emotion regulation observed between investigated groups.

A *third* challenge concerns the clinical relevance of statistical findings. Group-level *statistically* significant differences or correlations do not naturally equal *clinically* significant levels of emotion dysregulation in (all) children with ADHD [6]. When studies report statistical ER differences between groups of controls and children with ADHD, it therefore still remains to be specified to what extent these *differences* correspond to clinically relevant functional *impairments* in the latter. This challenge is compounded by the inherent chiasm between, on the one hand, striving toward as 'pure' as possible research conditions, and on the other hand, obtaining ecologically valid insights of how ADHD children's emotion regulation efforts unfold when cognitive, emotional and behavioural stimulus input and output occur simultaneously in a continuous loop of adjustment processes.

Additionally, and contrasting with a voluminous parenting literature and demand, very little empirical research has been devoted to the potential emotional strengths that may come with ADHD [13]. A growing resiliency-oriented literature yet suggests that the aim of helping ADHD children better deal with their personal and interpersonal challenges may be more difficult to attain when weighing in on 'what goes wrong' without simultaneously trying to understand 'what goes right' [102]. The macro-level of the FACE-model indeed reminds that solely assessing ADHD children's emotion-related problems does not provide a valid view of day-to-day dynamics. Importantly, it creates the risk of overlooking child- and family strengths that contribute to compensating, alleviating or avoiding negative emotional outcomes in the ADHD child's development [31]. This omission of strengths, or of at least a balanced risk-resiliency assessment, may contribute to accounting, for instance, for the proportions of children with diagnosed ADHD in which no significant emotion regulation deficits are found in the discussed studies.

Altogether these factors add to necessary caution when linking empirical data to real-life implications for ADHD children and their families. Given a generalised tendency to overgeneralisation, evidence-based practice would benefit from studies adding more ecologically valid indices in their conclusions regarding the profiles of ADHD children to which observed emotion processing and regulation characteristics apply, and to which degree these correspond to clinically relevant impairments [6, 19]. Even when considering that emotion regulation training probably constitutes a valuable asset to any prevention and intervention effort, the main preoccupation for children with ADHD still consists of tailoring such efforts as closely as possible to their particular ER challenges. The current knowledgebase hereby points to potentially relevant prevention/intervention avenues that merit individual tailoring when addressing ADHD children's emotional functioning in practice.

6.2. How to face emotion regulation in children with ADHD and their families: Prevention and intervention keys

Bearing the discussed cautions in mind, an integrated theory-grounded, evidence-based and strengths-oriented approach offers several instrumental leads for accompanying children and their parents towards facing emotionally disruptive facets of ADHD and equipping them with emotion regulation strengths.

On a *micro-level*, it appears key to help at-risk ADHD children with adjusting their emotional reactivity, with appraising how emotions relate to particular contexts, with recognising negative emotions, and with acquiring problem solving, mood-adjustment knowledge and techniques to act upon this knowledge.

On a *macro-level*, parents with ADHD are likely to find solace in the same focuses, while parents of ADHD children in general may benefit from psychoeducation about the aforementioned ER specificities in their children (and partners) and from tailoring emotion regulation and problem solving techniques to these specificities.

Given the most directly influential impact of parenting on the child's life, it appears particularly important for practice to identify parental ADHD as well as parental emotional resources. Indeed, adults who suffer emotional disruptions themselves confront a significant parenting burden when rearing one or more children with ADHD. Parents with ADHD, but also with other affective issues such as depression, may be particularly vulnerable toward disrupted emotion regulation [43]. Conversely, since not all parents of ADHD children present with ADHD and not all ADHD parents suffer (the same extent of) emotional impairments, recognising ER resources in parents represents a valuable asset for building resiliency in their children. Identifying the ER strategies acquired by parents with ADHD hereby especially offers added value because this simultaneously allows drawing on experience-tested insights, promoting empathy with the ADHD child and engaging in uncovering existing strengths in the family.

An illustration of these principles can be found and is currently evaluated in the ongoing FACE©-ADHD program, which consists of thirteen weekly, 2-hour sessions combining child and parent intervention [4, 5, 30]. Sessions evolve from psychoeducation through problem-solving activities and cognitive-oriented parenting support, toward more specific targeting of (negative) emotions, building emotional skills and training in emotion regulation so as to reduce negative and increase positive experiences and interactions by and among ADHD children and their parents. In a preliminary evaluation, this approach yielded significant pre- versus posttest improvements in child- and parent-reported experiential and behavioural outcomes after program completion [4, 5, 30]. The FACE©-program hereby also involves stimulating the transfer of clinic-based activities through home activities during which parents and children use self-report versions of the FACE'ogram© illustrated in Figure 1 to map perceived stressors and resources. Micro-challenges in daily adjustments are also monitored through the use of a cognitive-emotional diary (FACE©-CEM) [6]. Similar diary methods have been found useful for identifying ADHD families' daily challenges [103].

Despite a growing range of evidence-based interventions for ADHD children and their families, emotion-centred insights yet still remain sparsely applied in this context [104]. To date, many of these interventions also have more broadly concerned children with oppositional behaviour and conduct problems, whereby ADHD symptoms may be involved but not necessarily amount to formal ADHD diagnoses. Most interventions thus still tend to focus primarily on behavioural and/or cognitive modification techniques, even if emotion-related management is more or less implicitly involved in parent-training intervention components [56, 104-106]. A recent meta-analysis of 40 ADHD-oriented parent-intervention studies hereby showed parenting competence to be the only parent-intervention outcome with a large-to-moderate effect from immediate assessment to follow-up, among otherwise generally moderate-to-small outcome effects [104]. Training outcomes seem to follow comparable trajectories for mothers and fathers, consisting of immediate efficacy followed by limited generalisation and waning longer term effects, although it should be noted that fathers typically have been less implicated and thus less investigated [106].

Interestingly, two interventions that do include a more explicit emotion-centred focus, one of which was aimed at ADHD children, are reported to yield firmer long-term outcomes. Thus, one study assessed whether limiting negative emotional control through the training of parental positive behaviour in a family-centred intervention would amend the growth of children's early behaviour problems [107]. An effortful increase in proactive parenting was indeed significantly associated with lower levels of toddlers' general behavioural problems through age two to four. Another study more specifically evaluated the efficacy of the Incredible Years (IY) interventions for children with a primary ADHD diagnosis [108]. The IY interventions involve emotion-focused techniques, besides more traditional child and parent behaviour modification and parenting support, and have been found effective in reducing negative parenting and externalising behaviour among children with ODD and CD in a series of randomized control group studies [96, 108]. An updated program version was used to more precisely examine IY efficacy with four to six-year-old ADHD children (n=49) and their parents who participated in six intervention months. Emotion-focused targets included emotional coaching and teaching of ER strategies, reducing parental depression and anger and increasing family support. Statistically and clinically significant post-treatment effects were found for most outcome variables; including parent-reported and observed parenting, child social, externalising and ADHD-specific behaviours. Significantly, ADHD children's treatment progress was maintained after one year [108].

Finally and for the sake of exhaustiveness, it deserves to be noted that, given space-constraints, the present discussion did not extensively review medication effects on ADHD children's emotion regulation. Briefly considered, the additive value of combining medication and psychosocial treatments has been demonstrated especially for children with intense ADHD symptomatology [2, 105, 108]. It is therefore likely that medication may benefit the efficacy of emotion-focused interventions with these children too, albeit because a normalisation of behavioural activity levels is expected to improve learning conditions and family communication [38]. For instance, a study on 43 elementary-school-age children with ADHD documents the positive impact of amphetamine medication on child and family dynamics [59]. Furthermore, Williams' et al.'s study (2008) on youth's event-related potentials before and after MPH treatment [89], evoked in paragraph 5.2.1, specifically showed that improved brain activity after MPH treatment predicted diminution of emotional lability although not of negative mood. Medication has however also been reported to result in blunted, flattened, restricted and dysphoric emotional expression along with passive and even submissive behaviour among children with ADHD [109]. Optimising medication doses may therefore be crucial, as evidenced by one study reporting curvilinear MPH dose effects on ADHD children's visual focusing and variability of facially expressed emotions [38]. Suboptimal medication protocols might in turn interfere with the process of training ADHD children's emotion regulation skills. Investigating the impact of ADHD medication on emotion-centred intervention outcomes and its differential effects according to symptom intensity, comorbidity and medication dosage is therefore recommended.

Taken together, an integration of the nascent empirical evidence-base with the outlined conceptual foundations suggests the importance of incorporating techniques for adjusting emotional reactivity, appraisal and behavioural modulation of emotions when intervening with children with ADHD and their parents, whereby relative focuses merit to be tailored to the specificities of the individual family's risk-resiliency balance and challenges. Research-wise there still is a critical need for prospective, follow-up as well as qualitative studies to move towards more fine-grained evidence-based insights into how and under which conditions emotion regulation training with ADHD children and their parents bears fruit.

7. Conclusion

Drawing on the FACE©-model, this chapter has examined ADHD children's emotion regulation skills on a cognitive-emotional adjustment and behavioural expression micro-level, along with parenting and family risks and resources herein on a contextual macro-level. Emotion regulation hereby was operationally conceived as the autonomic and effortful modulation of the transient physiological reactions, the basic and contextualised appraisal, the subjective experience and the overt behavioural expressions involved in emotions.

As far as the extant evidence-base allows concluding, children with ADHD appear vulnerable to some extent to difficulties in modulating each of these emotion regulation components, from adaptively accommodating physiological reactivity through adequately appraising emotions in their context to flexibly modulating experience and behavioural expression of emotions. At the least, children with ADHD as a group seem inclined to process emotions differently compared to peers so that they are in need of extra support in the skill of emotionally adjusting to habitual contextual demands. Throughout the diverse outcomes for this heterogeneous population, it seems that especially children with an externalising pattern of functioning, namely those with the combined ADHD subtype and/or comorbid conduct problems, are most at-risk for demonstrating emotion regulation difficulties at physiological, experiential and behavioural levels. Although as yet scarcely investigated, parental expressed negativity furthermore appears to adversely weigh in on ADHD children's emotion regulation skills at parenting and family-functioning levels.

Given that the research to date predominantly has investigated ADHD children's emotion regulation in cognitive (challenging) situations, findings hereby primarily underscore the importance of considering the impact of ADHD children's emotional functioning on (cognitive) task accomplishments and of acknowledging their non-apparent regulation efforts. These insights call for incorporating mood-management support for children with ADHD in learning conditions. They also call for a paradigm shift so as to value ADHD children's efforts instead of sole outcomes to a much larger extent than is generally the case in academic contexts.

Importantly, the observation that large proportions of investigated children with ADHD do not exhibit the expected emotion regulation difficulties still tends to go unnoticed. This leaves unexploited critical leads for gaining a refined understanding of the impact of ADHD on a child's life and of the resources that may be more or less naturally present in some families to mend its expected adverse effects. Emerging intervention-outcome evidence also points to promising resiliency-building opportunities through the integration of emotion regulation, problem solving, behaviour modification and positive parenting training for those children with ADHD and their parents who confront emotion dysregulation.

The complex field of ADHD children's emotion regulation thus still remains under-explored empirically on several aspects with practical relevance. Children's physiological reactivity, appraisal of emotional cues and modulation of emotional experience and expression hardly have been examined in inherently emotion-driven contexts, such as during parent-child and family interactions. More ecologically valid indices are therefore needed as to which emotion regulation processes underlie ADHD children's observed emotional disruptions in the daily life situations where they matter most in their early years.

In a theory-grounded research utopia, each of the emotion regulation components specified at the micro-level of the FACE©-model would be investigated longitudinally as they develop in children with ADHD while taking into account probable mediating and moderating effects of their macro-level risk and resiliency balance, especially as regards their parenting and family environment. As an added value, ADHD children's emotion regulation trajectories would be compared with those of children with other clinical conditions.

In an evidence-based practice utopia, research would systematically inform about the proportions and specificities of children with ADHD concerned by clinically relevant emotion dysregulation processes. Even more fundamentally, empirical findings would predictively outline the constellation of cognitive-emotional (micro-level) and family environmental (macro-level) characteristics of those ADHD children who are most at-risk for emotion dysregulation so as to direct prevention or intervention efforts toward these children.

While patiently building the empirical evidence-base and advocating shifts toward sustained research policies that stimulate large-scale longitudinal investigations, remembering the final aim of ADHD emotion research may facilitate moving toward the outlined practice utopia. This aim would expectedly consist of significantly contributing to ameliorating ADHD children's outcomes. A strengths-oriented evidence-base consequently deserves to integrate research that also focuses on gaining an understanding of the conditions under which children with ADHD do manage to regulate their emotions in functional ways. The current chapter allows concluding that combining the search for dysfunctional emotion areas with the discovery of individual and contextual characteristics of children with ADHD who fare best emotionally despite their vulnerabilities, offers the strongest leads for durably building ADHD children's resilience.

Acknowledgements

The ongoing research on children with ADHD according to the FACE©-model and -program is supported in part by the OZR VUB Research Grant OZR1075 "ADHD and Bipolar Disorder in Youth". The authors would also like to thank the students who participated in the data collection for the ongoing FACE-ADHD research during the completion of their master thesis.

Author details

Smadar Celestin-Westreich[1*] and Leon-Patrice Celestin[2]

*Address all correspondence to: Smadar.Westreich@vub.ac.be

1 Dept. Clinical & Life Span Psychology, Vrije Universiteit Brussels, Brussels, Belgium

2 Hospital Practitioner Psychiatry & FACE©-program, Paris, France

References

[1] American Psychiatric Association. Rationale for Changes in ADHD in DSM-5. From the ADHD and Disruptive Behavior Disorders Workgroup. 2012. Retrieved from http://www.dsm5.org/ProposedRevisions/Pages/proposedrevision.aspx?rid=383#

[2] Barkley RA. Attention-Deficit Hyperactivity Disorder. A handbook for diagnosis and treatment. Third Edition. New York: The Guilford Press;2006.

[3] Anastopoulos AD, Smith TF, Garrett ME, Morrissey-Kane E, Schatz NK, Sommer JL, et al. Self-Regulation of Emotion, Functional Impairment, and Comorbidity Among ChildrenWith AD/HD. J Atten Disord 2011;15(7):583-92.

[4] Celestin-Westreich S, Celestin LP. [Families' Cognitive-Emotional Adjustments when Facing Attention Deficit Hyperactivity Disorder]. Ann Med Psychol 2008;166(5): 343-49. [Article in French]

[5] Celestin LP, Celestin-Westreich S. The FACE© program: cognitive-emotional adjustment training for children and families with ADHD and Bipolar Disorder. In Stress & Anxiety Research Society ([STAR] Ed.), 26th International Conference of the Stress and Anxiety Research Society (pp.60-61). Halle, Germany: STAR;2005.

[6] Celestin-Westreich S, Celestin LP. [Child, Parenting and Family Assessment in FACE©-perspective]. Leuven/Den Haag: Acco;2010a. [Book in Dutch]

[7] Buschgens CJ, van Aken MA, Swinkels SH, Altink ME, Fliers EA, Rommelse NN, et al. Differential family and peer environmental factors are related to severity and comorbidity in children with ADHD. J Neural Transm 2008;115(2):177-86.

[8] Kepley HO, Ostrander R. Family characteristics of anxious ADHD children: preliminary results. J Atten Disord 2007;10(3):317-23.

[9] Maedgen JW, Carlson CL. Social functioning and emotional regulation in the attention deficit hyperactivity disorder subtypes. J Clin Child Psychol 2000;29(1):30-42.

[10] Mrug S, Molina BS, Hoza B, Gerdes AC, Hinshaw SP, Hechtman L, et al. Peer rejection and friendships in children with Attention-Deficit/Hyperactivity Disorder: contributions to long-term outcomes. J Abnorm Child Psychol 2012;40(6):1013-26.

[11] Bacchini D, Affuso G, Trotta T. Temperament, ADHD and peer relations among schoolchildren: the mediating role of school bullying. Aggress Behav 2008;34(5): 447-59.

[12] Malmberg K, Edbom T, Wargelius HL, Larsson JO. Psychiatric problems associated with subthreshold ADHD and disruptive behaviour diagnoses in teenagers. Acta Paediatr 2011;100(11):1468-75.

[13] Corwin M, Mulsow M, Feng D. Perceived family resources based on number of members with ADHD. J Atten Disord. 2012;16(6):517-29.

[14] Peris TS, Hinshaw SP. Family dynamics and preadolescent girls with ADHD: the relationship between expressed emotion, ADHD symptomatology, and comorbid disruptive behavior. J Child Psychol Psychiatry 2003;44(8):1177-90.

[15] Krauel K, Duzel E, Hinrichs H, Rellum T, Santel S, Baving L. Emotional memory in ADHD patients with and without comorbid ODD/CD. J Neural Transm 2009;116(1): 117-20.

[16] Herpertz SC, Huebner T, Marx I, Vloet TD, Fink GR, Stoecker T, et al. Emotional processing in male adolescents with childhood-onset conduct disorder. J Child Psychol Psychiatry 2008;49(7):781-91.

[17] Humphreys KL, Aguirre VP, Lee SS. Association of anxiety and ODD/CD in children with and without ADHD. J Clin Child Adolesc Psychol 2012;41(3):370-7.

[18] Hinshaw SP, Owens EB, Zalecki C, Huggins SP, Montenegro-Nevado AJ, Schrodek E, et al. Prospective Follow-Up of Girls With Attention-Deficit/Hyperactivity Disorder Into Early Adulthood: Continuing Impairment Includes Elevated Risk for Suicide Attempts and Self-Injury. J Consult Clin Psychol 2012; 80(6):1041-51.

[19] Nigg JT. Future directions in ADHD etiology research. J Clin Child Adolesc Psychol 2012;41(4):524-33.

[20] Seymour KE, Chronis-Tuscano A, Halldorsdottir T, Stupica B, Owens K, Sacks T. Emotion regulation mediates the relationship between ADHD and depressive symptoms in youth. J Abnorm Child Psychol 2012;40(4):595-606.

[21] Edel MA, Juckel G, Brüne M. Interaction of recalled parental ADHD symptoms and rearing behavior with current attachment and emotional dysfunction in adult offspring with ADHD. Psychiatry Res 2010;178(1):137-41.

[22] Thorell LB, Rydell AM, Bohlin G. Parent-child attachment and executive functioning in relation to ADHD symptoms in middle childhood. Attach Hum Dev 2012;14(5): 517-32.

[23] Wagner KD. Associated symptoms of attention-deficit/hyperactivity disorder and posttraumatic stress disorder. J Clin Psychiatry 2012;73(5):709-10.

[24] Arnold LE, Demeter C, Mount K, Frazier TW, Youngstrom EA, Fristad M, et al. Pediatric bipolar spectrum disorder and ADHD: comparison and comorbidity in the LAMS clinical sample. Bipolar Disord 2011;13(5-6):509-21.

[25] Celestin LP, Celestin-Westreich S. (under review). [How to FACE© Pediatric Bipolar Disorder: Diagnostic Challenges]. [Article in French]

[26] West AE, Schenkel LS, Pavuluri MN. Early childhood temperament in pediatric bipolar disorder and attention deficit hyperactivity disorder. J Clin Psychol. 2008;64(4): 402-21.

[27] Davis NO, Kollins SH. Treatment for co-occurring attention deficit/hyperactivity disorder and autism spectrum disorder. Neurotherapeutics. 2012;9(3):518-30.

[28] Sinzig J, Morsch D, Lehmkuhl G. Do hyperactivity, impulsivity and inattention have an impact on the ability of facial affect recognition in children with autism and ADHD? Eur Child Adolesc Psychiatry 2008;17(2):63-72.

[29] Taurines R, Schwenck C, Westerwald E, Sachse M, Siniatchkin M, Freitag C. ADHD and autism: differential diagnosis or overlapping traits? A selective review. Atten Defic Hyperact Disord 2012;4(3):115-39.

[30] Celestin-Westreich S, Celestin LP. ADHD children's emotion recognition skills in FACE©-perspective: initial findings. In Arnaud Destrebecqz, Cécile Colin & Wim Gevers (Eds.), Annual Meeting of the Belgian Association for Psychological Sciences. Brussels: Université Libre de Bruxelles;2010^{b}.

[31] Goldstein S, Rider R. Resilience and the disruptive disorders of childhood. In: Godstein S, Brooks RB [Eds]. Handbook of resilience in children. Second edition. New York: Springer; 2012. p. 183-200.

[32] Lee TY, Cheung CK, Kwong WM. Resilience as a positive youth development construct: a conceptual review. ScientificWorldJournal 2012; doi:10.1100/2012/390450

[33] Celestin LP, Celestin-Westreich S. Enhancing cognitive-emotional adjustment in Bipolar youth and their families: rationale and initial outcome of the FACE© program. J Affect Disorders 2006;91(Supp.1):S74-5.

[34] Celestin LP, Celestin-Westreich S. [How to FACE© Bipolar Disorder in the Elderly]. In: Ferrero F, Aubry JM, eds. Traitements psychologiques des troubles bipolaires; Médecine et psychothérapies. Paris: Elsevier/Masson, 2009:177-90. [Chapter in French]

[35] Celestin-Westreich S, Celestin LP. [Observation and reporting in FACE-perspective. 2nd Edition incl. XTRA]. Amsterdam: Pearson Education;2012. [Book in Dutch]

[36] Ahmadi M, Judi M, Khorrami A, Mahmoudi-Gharaei J, Tehrani-Doost M. Initial Orientation of Attention towards Emotional Faces in Children with Attention Deficit Hyperactivity Disorder. Iran J Psychiatry 2011;6(3):87-91.

[37] Berger A, Kofman O, Livneh U, Henik A. Multidisciplinary perspectives on attention and the development of self-regulation. Prog Neurobiol. 2007 Aug;82(5):256-86.

[38] Kühle HJ, Kinkelbur J, Andes K, Heidorn FM, Zeyer S, Rautzenberg P, et al. Self-regulation of visual attention and facial expression of emotions in ADHD children. J Atten Disord 2007;10(4):350-8.

[39] Shin DW, Lee SJ, Kim BJ, Park Y, Lim SW. Visual attention deficits contribute to impaired facial emotion recognition in boys with attention-deficit/hyperactivity disorder. Neuropediatrics 2008;39(6):323-7.

[40] Cadesky EB, Mota VL, Schachar RJ. Beyond words: how do children with ADHD and/or conduct problems process nonverbal information about affect? J Am Acad Child Adolesc Psychiatry 2000;39(9):1160-7.

[41] Corbett B, Glidden H. Processing affective stimuli in children with attention-deficit hyperactivity disorder. Child Neuropsychol 2000;6(2):144-55.

[42] Eisenberg N, Spinrad TL, Eggum ND. Emotion-related self-regulation and its relation to children's maladjustment. Annu Rev Clin Psychol 2010;6:495-525.

[43] Rapport LJ, Friedman SR, Tzelepis A, Van Voorhis A. Experienced emotion and affect recognition in adult attention-deficit hyperactivity disorder. Neuropsychology. 2002;16(1):102-10.

[44] Arnsten AF, Rubia K. Neurobiological circuits regulating attention, cognitive control, motivation, and emotion: disruptions in neurodevelopmental psychiatric disorders.J Am Acad Child Adolesc Psychiatry 2012;51(4):356-67.

[45] Passarotti AM, Pavuluri MN. Brain functional domains inform therapeutic interventions in attention-deficit/hyperactivity disorder and pediatric bipolar disorder. Expert Rev Neurother 2011;11(6):897-914.

[46] Rinsky JR, Hinshaw SP. Linkages between childhood executive functioning and adolescent social functioning and psychopathology in girls with ADHD. Child Neuropsychol 2011;17(4):368-90.

[47] Barkley RA, Fischer M. The unique contribution of emotional impulsiveness to impairment in major life activities in hyperactive children as adults. J Am Acad Child Adolesc Psychiatry 2010;49(5):503-13.

[48] Musser ED, Backs RW, Schmitt CF, Ablow JC, Measelle JR, & Nigg JT. Emotion Regulation via the Autonomic Nervous System in Children with Attention-Deficit/ Hyperactivity Disorder (ADHD). J Abnorm Child Psych 2011;39(6):841-52.

[49] Plessen KJ, Bansal R, Zhu H, Whiteman R, Amat J, Quackenbush GA, et al. Hippocampus and amygdala morphology in attention-deficit/hyperactivity disorder. Arch Gen Psychiatry 2006;63(7):795-807.

[50] Koole SL, Rothermund K. "I feel better but I don't know why": the psychology of implicit emotion regulation. Cogn Emot 2011;25(3):389-99.

[51] Martel MM. Research review: a new perspective on attention-deficit/hyperactivity disorder: emotion dysregulation and trait models. J Child Psychol Psychiatry 2009;50(9):1042-51.

[52] Sauder CL, Beauchaine TP, Gatzke-Kopp LM, Shannon KE, Aylward E. Neuroanatomical correlates of heterotypic comorbidity in externalizing male adolescents. J Clin Child Adolesc Psychol. 2012;41(3):346-52.

[53] Cummings ME, Davies PT, Campbell SB. Developmental Psychopathology and Family Process: Theory, Research, and Clinical Implications. New York: The Guilford Press; 2002.

[54] Latimer K, Wilson P, Kemp J, Thompson L, Sim F, Gillberg C, et al. Disruptive behaviour disorders: a systematic review of environmental antenatal and early years risk factors. Child Care Health Dev 2012;38(5):611-28.

[55] Listug-Lunde L, Zevenbergen AA, Petros TV. Psychological symptomatology in siblings of children with ADHD. J Atten Disord 2008;12(3):239-47.

[56] Chronis-Tuscano A, O'Brien KA, Johnston C, Jones HA, Clarke TL, Raggi VL, et al. The relation between maternal ADHD symptoms & improvement in child behavior following brief behavioral parent training is mediated by change in negative parenting. J Abnorm Child Psychol 2011;39(7):1047-57.

[57] Johnston C, Mash EJ, Miller N, Ninowski JE. Parenting in adults with attention-deficit/hyperactivity disorder (ADHD). Clin Psychol Rev 2012;32(4):215-28.

[58] Christiansen H, Oades RD, Psychogiou L, Hauffa BP, Sonuga-Barke EJ. Does the cortisol response to stress mediate the link between expressed emotion and oppositional behavior in Attention-Deficit/Hyperactivity-Disorder (ADHD)? Behav Brain Funct 2010;6:45.

[59] Gustafsson P, Hansson K, Eidevall L, Thernlund G, Svedin CG. Treatment of ADHD with amphetamine: short-term effects on family interaction. J Atten Disord 2008;12(1):83-91.

[60] Melnick SM, Hinshaw SP. Emotion regulation and parenting in AD/HD and comparison boys: linkages with social behaviors and peer preference. J Abnorm Child Psychol 2000;28(1):73-86.

[61] Barkley RA. Deficient emotion regulation: a core feature of ADHD. J ADHD Relat Disord 2010;1(2):5–37.

[62] Rosen PJ, Epstein JN. A pilot study of ecological momentary assessment of emotion dysregulation in children. J ADHD Relat Disord 2010;1(4):39–52.

[63] Gross JJ, Thompson RA. Emotion regulation: conceptual foundations. In: Gross JJ. (ed.). Handbook of emotion regulation. New York: The Guilford Press; 2007. p.3-24.

[64] Power M, Dalgleish T. Cognition and emotion. From order to disorder. 2nd Edition. New York: Psychology Press, 2008.

[65] Rash JA, Aguirre-Camacho A. Attention-deficit hyperactivity disorder and cardiac vagal control: a systematic review. Atten Defic Hyperact Disord 2012 Jul 7; 4(4): 167-77.

[66] Scime M, Norvilitis JM. Taks performance and response to frustration in children with Attention Deficit Hyperactivity Disorder. Psychol Sch 2006;43(3):377-86.

[67] Eisenberg N, Spinrad TL. Emotion-related regulation: sharpening the definition. Child Dev. 2004;75:334–39.

[68] Mikami AY, Hinshaw SP, Lee SS, Mullin BC. Relationships between Social Information Processing and Aggression among Adolescent Girls with and without ADHD. J Youth Adolesc 2008;37(7):761-771.

[69] Blaskey LG, Harris LJ, Nigg JT. Are sensation seeking and emotion processing related to or distinct from cognitive control in children with ADHD? Child Neuropsychol 2008;14(4):353-71.

[70] Healey DM, Marks DJ, Halperin JM. Examining the Interplay Among Negative Emotionality, Cognitive Functioning, and Attention Deficit/Hyperactivity Disorder Symptom Severity. J Int Neuropsychol Soc 2011;5:1-9.

[71] Lang van ND, Tulen JH, Kallen VL, Rosbergen B, Dieleman G, Ferdinand RF. Autonomic reactivity in clinically referred children with attention-deficit/hyperactivity disorder versus anxiety disorder. Eur Child Adolesc Psychiatry 2007;16(2):71-8.

[72] Negrao BL, Bipath P, van der Westhuizen D, Viljoen M. Autonomic correlates at rest and during evoked attention in children with attention-deficit/hyperactivity disorder and effects of methylphenidate. Neuropsychobiology 2011;63(2):82-91.

[73] Beauchaine TP, Katkin ES, Strassberg Z, Snarr J. Disinhibitory psychopathology in male adolescents: discriminating conduct disorder from attention-deficit/hyperactivity disorder through concurrent assessment of multiple autonomic states. J Abnorm Psychol 2001;110(4):610-24.

[74] Buchhorn R, Conzelmann A, Willaschek C, Stork D, Taurines R, Renner T. Heart rate variability and methylphenidate in children with ADHD. ADHD Atten Defic Hyperact Disord;4(2):85–91. doi:10.1007/s12402-012-0072-8

[75] Imeraj L, Antrop I, Roeyers H, Deschepper E, Bal S, Deboutte D. Diurnal variations in arousal: a naturalistic heart rate study in children with ADHD. Eur Child Adolesc Psychiatry 2011;20(8):381-92.

[76] Tonhajzerova I, Ondrejka I, Adamik P, Hruby R, Javorka M, Trunkvalterova Z et al. Changes in the cardiac autonomic regulation in children with attention deficit hyperactivity disorder (ADHD). Indian J Med Res 2009;130(1):44-50.

[77] Crowell SE, Beauchaine TP, Gatzke-Kopp L, Sylvers P, Mead H, Chipman-Chacon J. Autonomic correlates of attention-deficit/hyperactivity disorder and oppositional defiant disorder in preschool children. J Abnorm Psychol 2006;115(1):174-8.

[78] Corominas M, Ramos-Quiroga JA, Ferrer M, Sáez-Francàs N, Palomar G, Bosch R, Casas M. Cortisol responses in children and adults with attention deficit hyperactivity disorder (ADHD): a possible marker of inhibition deficits. Atten Defic Hyperact Disord 2012;4(2):63-75.

[79] Fairchild G. Hypothalamic-pituitary-adrenocortical axis function in attention-deficit hyperactivity disorder. Curr Top Behav Neurosci 2012;9:93-111.

[80] van West D, Claes S, Deboutte D. Differences in hypothalamic-pituitary-adrenal axis functioning among children with ADHD predominantly inattentive and combined types. Eur Child Adolesc Psychiatry 2009;18(9):543-53.

[81] Singh SD, Ellis CR, Winton AS, Singh NN, Leung JP, Oswald DP. Recognition of facial expressions of emotion by children with attention-deficit hyperactivity disorder. Behav Modif 1998;22(2):128-42.

[82] Wigal T, Swanson JM, Douglas VI, Wigal SB, Wippler CM, Cavoto KF. Effect of reinforcement on facial responsivity and persistence in children with attention-deficit hyperactivity disorder. Behav Modif 1998;22(2):143-66.

[83] Kats-Gold I, Besser A, Priel B. The role of simple emotion recognition skills among school aged boys at risk of ADHD. J Abnorm Child Psychol 2007;35(3):363-78.

[84] Celestin-Westreich S, Celestin LP. How to FACE ADHD in Children: Facilitating the Adjustment of Cognition and Emotion. Expert Meeting Temperament and Cognitive Vulnerability to Mood Problems in Children and Adolescents, December 16-17th 2010. Leuven: University of Leuven;2010c.

[85] Brotman MA, Rich BA, Guyer AE, Lunsford JR, Horsey SE, Reising MM, et al. Amygdala activation during emotion processing of neutral faces in children with severe mood dysregulation versus ADHD or bipolar disorder. Am J Psychiatry 2010;167(1): 61-9.

[86] Guyer AE, McClure EB, Adler AD, Brotman MA, Rich BA, Kimes AS, et al. Specificity of facial expression labeling deficits in childhood psychopathology. J Child Psychol Psychiatry 2007;48(9):863-71.

[87] Krauel K, Duzel E, Hinrichs H, Lenz D, Herrmann CS, Santel S, et al. Electrophysiological correlates of semantic processing during encoding of neutral and emotional pictures in patients with ADHD. Neuropsychologia 2009;47(8-9):1873-82.

[88] Pelc K, Kornreich C, Foisy ML, Dan B. Recognition of emotional facial expressions in attention-deficit hyperactivity disorder. Pediatr Neurol 2006;35(2):93-7.

[89] Williams LM, Hermens DF, Palmer D, Kohn M, Clarke S, Keage H, et al. Misinterpreting emotional expressions in attention-deficit/hyperactivity disorder: evidence for a neural marker and stimulant effects. Biol Psychiatry 2008;63(10):917-26.

[90] Braaten EB, Rosén LA. Self-regulation of affect in attention deficit-hyperactivity disorder (ADHD) and non-ADHD boys: differences in empathic responding. J Consult Clin Psychol 2000;68(2):313-21.

[91] Da Fonseca D, Seguier V, Santos A, Poinso F, Deruelle C. Emotion understanding in children with ADHD. Child Psychiatry Hum Dev 2009;40(1):111-21.

[92] Yuill N, Lyon J. Selective difficulty in recognising facial expressions of emotion in boys with ADHD. General performance impairments or specific problems in social cognition? Eur Child Adolesc Psychiatry 2007;16(6):398-404.

[93] Sideridis G, Vansteenkiste M, Shiakalli M, Georgiou M, Irakleous I, Tsigourla I, et al. Goal priming and the emotional experience of students with and without attention problems: an application of the emotional stroop task. J Learn Disabil 2009;42(2): 177-89.

[94] Hale TS, Zaidel E, McGough JJ, Phillips JM, McCracken JT. Atypical brain laterality in adults with ADHD during dichotic listening for emotional intonation and words. Neuropsychologia 2006;44(6):896-904.

[95] Walcott CM, Landau S. The relation between disinhibition and emotion regulation in boys with attention deficit hyperactivity disorder. J Clin Child Adolesc Psychol 2004;33(4):772-82.

[96] Beauchaine TP, Webster-Stratton C, Reid MJ. Mediators, moderators, and predictors of 1-year outcomes among children treated for early-onset conduct problems: a latent growth curve analysis. J Consult Clin Psychol 2005;73(3):371-88.

[97] Celestin-Westreich S, Celestin LP, Van Gils Y, Ponjaert-Kristoffersen I. How to FACE© sibling violence: pathways from feud to friend. In A. Dillen (Ed.), When 'Love' Strikes; Social Sciences, Ethics and Theology on Family Violence (pp.259-284). Leuven: Peeters Publishers;2009.

[98] Celestin-Westreich S, Ponjaert-Kristoffersen I, Celestin LP. [The ADHD-child and its family: an explorative study of the ADHD child's perspective]. Revue Canadienne de Psycho-Education 2000;29(2):207-221. [Article in French]

[99] Emeh CC, Mikami AY. The Influence of Parent Behaviors on Positive Illusory Bias in Children With ADHD. J Atten Disord 2012 Apr 16. [Epub ahead of print]

[100] Jones HA, Epstein JN, Hinshaw SP, Owens EB, Chi TC, Arnold LE, Hoza B, Wells KC. Ethnicity as a moderator of treatment effects on parent--child interaction for children with ADHD. J Atten Disord 2010;13(6):592-600.

[101] World Health Organization (WHO). Child and Adolescent Mental Health Policies and Plans (WM 34 2005ME-1). 2005; Retrieved from WHO; http://www.who.int/mental_health/policy/services/essentialpackage1v11/en/index.html

[102] Modesto-Lowe V, Yelunina L, Hanjan K. Attention-deficit/hyperactivity disorder: a shift toward resilience? Clin Pediatr (Phila) 2011;50(6):518-24.

[103] Whalen CK, Henker B, Jamner LD, Ishikawa SS, Floro JN, Swindle R, et al. Toward mapping daily challenges of living with ADHD: maternal and child perspectives using electronic diaries. J Abnorm Child Psychol 2006;34(1):115-30.

[104] Lee PC, Niew WI, Yang HJ, Chen VC, Lin KC. A meta-analysis of behavioral parent training for children with attention deficit hyperactivity disorder. Res Dev Disabil. 2012;33(6):2040-9.

[105] Wagner SM, McNeil CB. Parent-Child Interaction Therapy for ADHD: A Conceptual Overview and Critical Literature Review. Child Fam Behav Ther 2008;30(3):231-56.

[106] Fabiano GA, Pelham WE, Cunningham CE, Yu J, Gangloff B, Buck M, et al. A wait-list-controlled trial of behavioral parent training for fathers of children with ADHD. J Clin Child Adolesc Psychol 2012;41(3):337-45.

[107] Shelleby EC, Shaw DS, Cheong J, Chang H, Gardner F, Dishion TJ, et al. Behavioral control in at-risk toddlers: the influence of the family check-up. J Clin Child Adolesc Psychol 2012;41(3):288-301.

[108] Webster-Stratton C, Reid MJ, Beauchaine TP. One-Year Follow-Up of Combined Parent and Child Intervention for Young Children with ADHD. J Clin Child Adolesc Psychol. 2012 Sep 28; 2013;42(2):251-61.

[109] Perwien AR, Kratochvil CJ, Faries D, Vaughan B, Busner J, Saylor KE, et al. Emotional expression in children treated with ADHD medication: development of a new measure. J Atten Disord 2008;11(5):568-79.

Chapter 13

A Comparison Between Life Quality and Weight-Height Measurements of Patients, Under Stimulant and Non-Stimulant Treatment due to Attention-Deficit and Hyperactivity Disorder, and Healthy Population

Esra Ozdemir Demirci, Merve Cikili Uytun,
Rabia Durmus and Didem Behice Oztop

Additional information is available at the end of the chapter

http://dx.doi.org/10.5772/53790

1. Introduction

Attention Deficit and Hyperactivity Disorder (ADHD) comprises a disorder which is characterized with inattention, hyperactivity and impulsivity, seen in 3-7% of school-age children Boys are two to nine times more often affected than girls [1]. Twin, adoption, and molecular genetic studies show ADHD to be highly heritable. Evidence from animal and human studies implicates the dysregulation of frontal-subcortical-cerebellar catecholaminergic circuits in the pathophysiology of ADHD. Imaging studies suggest that abnormalities of the dopaminergic and adrenergic transmitter systems lead to impaired neurotransmission [2]

The main course of ADHD is a persistent pattern of inattention and/or hyperactivity-impulsivity that may be seen more frequently and/or severely compared to individuals with the same level of development. Its pathophysiology appears to involve different alterations in dopaminergic and noradrenergic pathways related to the control of attention and impulsivity [1,3,4].

ADHD is associated with important deterioration at numerous fields such as developmental, cognitive, emotional, social and academical, and also associated with personal time for parents because of affecting several health risks and academic performance. Deterioration in these fields based on basic sypmtoms of ADHD: hyperactivity, inattention and impulsivity [5]. In case of ADHD, as a result of inadequacies any time in the life of the child, reduction in self-confidence, misery, failure and thus reduced quality of life; deterioration of interpersonal and intra-family relations, being affected adversely of psychological well-being could be seen. Therefore, it is reported that "psychosocial dimension" gains importance gradually besides clinical parameters in multidimensional monitoring of disease and adequacy and inadequacy in this dimension could be explained with "life quality" concept [6]. Because of difficulties in academical, social and emotional fields, the effects of deterioration over life quality came into discussion in the context of the recent literature [7,8,9]. This level of interest is not surprising due to the complexity of the relationships; QoL(Quality of life) is not only influenced by the disorder itself, but also by many proximal (i.e. family, friendship) and distal (socioeconomic and cultural) factors. In addition to its core symptoms of attention deficit, hyperactivity and impulsivity, ADHD is associated with numerous developmental, cognitive, emotional, social and academic impairments [10,11].

The psychostimulants (e.g., methylphenidate) are considered the first-line of therapy for ADHD, relieving symptoms by increasing intrasynaptic dopamine, norepinephrine, and serotonin [12]. Nevertheless, some patients fail to respond to stimulants or are unable to tolerate them, and the stimulants such as methylphenidate are contraindicated for some children and adolescents including those with Tourette's disorder. Nonstimulant agents used in ADHD include tricyclic antidepressants, bupropion, clonidine, guanfacine, selective serotonin reuptake inhibitors, and newer atypical antidepressants [13,14]. But their current use is limited, because these agents do not improve impulsive behavior and cognitive impairments and also they have serious adverse effects [15].

On the other hand, atomoxetine, a highly selective inhibitor of the noradrenergic transporter, is the first non-psychostimulant agent approved by the Food and Drug Administration (FDA) for ADHD. Compared to its effect on the norepinephrine transporter, atomoxetine has very little affinity for the dopamine or serotonin transpoter. As a result of the central role of CYP2D6 in metabolism of atomoxetine, the activity of this enzyme plays a significant role in its pharmachokinetics. The majority of people ([90%), who metabolise atomoxetine and other CYP2D6 substrates relatively rapidly, are designed as CYP2D6 extensive metaboliser. Its efficacy in children with ADHD has been demonstrated in three double-blind, placebo-controlled trials [16].

Commonly used drugs for ADHD are shown in table 1.

Drug	Dosage	Dosage range	Time of Maximum plasma concentraiton (hour)	FDA approval year
Concerta	18,27,36,54,72	18-72	8	2000
Metadate CD	10,20,30	20-60	5	2001
Ritalin LA	10,20,30,40	20-60	5	2002
Adderall XR	10,20,30	10-40	1-4	2001
Ritalin	5,10,20	10-60	0.3-4	2000
Atomoksetin	10,18,25,40,60	10-60	1-2,3-4	2002

Table 1. Commonly used drugs for ADHD

http://dx.doi.org/10.5772/53790

Consequently, methylphenidate for stimulant group and atomoxetine for nonstimulant group are in primer use for ADHD treatment. The use of these medications becomes widespread gradually. It is reported that both medications are effective on treatment of ADHD's basic symptoms in children and adolescents. Thus, significant improvement could be seen in life quality [9,17,18]. When comparing with normal population, difficulties in academical, social and emotional fields could be developed more frequently.

The side effects on weight and height of these medications which are used considerably in child psychiatry are in discussion over a long time. Although a few studies defend inefficiency over weight and height, some studies show arrest in height development and shortness in ultimate height [19]. Current studies in this content on children and adolescents are subjects of only a few studies specially in our country [20].

In our study, we aimed to compare the effect of long acting methylphenidatefor and/or atomoxetine usage due to ADHD, weight-height measurements, and comparison of life quality between children and adolescents, and healthy population.

2. Material and methods

This study was conducted in Department of Child and Adolescent Pscyhiatry, Erciyes University Faculty of Medicine in the period from September 2011 to May 2012. Study population consists of 52 patients with ADHD based on DSM-IV and these patients were pharmacologically treated for at least 12 months and sypmtom severity is consistent with Scanning and Evaluation Scale based on DSM-IV for Behavioral Disorders in Children and Adolescents. Coexisting psychiatric disorders were accepted as exclusion criteria. Children with no previous history of psychopharmalogical treatment except ADHD and simultaneously no previous history of epilepsy and other medical disease was examined. Control group was selected randomly between patients of social pediatric clinical and specified as 25 healthy children in physical and psychological way. Smilarity between control and patient group from the point of gender and age avaragewas noticed. Parents of children with ADHD filled sociodemographic data form, The Pediatric Quality of Life Inventory(PedsQL), Atilla Turgay Scanning and Evaluation Scale based on DSM-IV for Behavioral Disorders in Children and Adolescents. Weight and height measurements were performed by our nurse specialist. Parents of control group also filled the same tests. Parents of both group signed informed consent and ethics committee approval was obtained.

3. Scales used in this study

The Pediatric Quality of Life Inventory(PedsQL): Developed for psychosocial and physcial life quality measurement of children and adolescent between 2-18 age interval by Varni and et all. and adapted into Turkish for 8-18 age interval was carried out by Çakın Memik et al. [21,22]. It is obtained that Cronbach Alfa coefficients vary between 0.80 and 0.88. PedsQL between the ages of 8-18 children / adolescents, there are forms for both self-report and parent and consists of 23 articles. The scale of physical health, emotional functioning, social functioning, and school functioning challenged areas. Scoring, scale total score (CAP), physical health score (FSTP), emotional, social and school functioning scores evaluating the substance of the calculation of the total score of psychosocial health (PSTP) to be carried out in three areas. This is the last month of children and adolescents with the scale in question. Substances "never", "rarely", "sometimes", "often" or "always" in the form of, and in turn responded, 100, 75, 50, 25, 0 points are given. Points total score is obtained by dividing the number of items collected and replenished. As a result the higher the PedsQL total score, the better the perceived health-related quality of life [20].

Thus fields of physical health, emotional functioning, social functioning and shcool functioning as features of well-being, identified by WHO, was examined.

Turgay DSM-IV Based Child and Adolescent Behavior Disorders Screening and Rating Scale: This scale was developed by Turgay [23], based on DSM-IV diagnosis criteria. This scale consists of 41 questions; 9 of them for attention deficit, 9 of them for mobility and impulsivity, 8 of them for comorbid oppositional defiant disorder (ODD), and 15 of them for behavioral disorder. Each question has 4 choices: 0 for strongly disagree, 1 for somewhat, 2 for agree, 3 for strongly agree. For ADHD diagnosis, min 6 of 9 questions that examine attention deficit should have 2 or 3 scoring, min 6 of 9 questions that examine hyperactivity or impulsivity should have 2 or 3 scoring. For ODD, min 4 of 8 questions should have 2 or 3 scoring; for BD diagnosis, min 2 of 25 questions should exist for 6 months or 1 year. Confidence validity test was conducted by Ercan et al. in Turkey [24].

4. Statistical evaluation

The statistics software SPSS 17.0 is utilized in this study. The data obtained through measurement is indicated as arithmetic mean (X) and standard deviation (SD); the data obtained through census is indicated as percentages (%).The significance level in the evaluations is determined as $p<0.05$. One- Sample Kolmogorov- Smirnov Test is used for control if variables are normal distribution or not. The grading differences between the groups (children-adolescents with ADHD diagnoses and healthy children-adolescents) are compared by using the "Student t test" for the measuremental variables that conform to the normal distribution and "Mann Whitney-U test" for the measuremental variables that do not conform to the normal distribution. Tukey and Dunnett post hoc tests are also used for varyans analyze. Sperman correlation test is used for showing correlations.

5. Results

Fourty two of patients who admitted into study were men (80.8%) and ten were women (19.2%). The avarage age of children was 10.42 ±2.136. Control group was smilar to patient

http://dx.doi.org/10.5772/53790

group in terms of avarage age and sex ratio. Socio- demographic characteristics of the group with ADHD and the control group are shown in tables (Table 2 and table 3). Socio-demographic differences between the two groups are outstanding.

	Mean	**Standart deviation/Percent**
Age	10,57	2,17
Mother age	36,03	5,87
Father Age	40,44	6,16
Education	n	%
The First 5 years	32	61,5
6th-10th.years	20	38,5
Number of siblings	n	%
2 and under 2	46	93,9
2- 4 siblings	3	6,1
Mother's Educational level	**n**	**%**
Not education	2	3,8
Primary school	20	38,5
Secondary high school	4	7,7
High school	16	30,8
University	10	19,2
Father'sEducational level	n	%
Not education	0	0
Primary school	15	28,8
Secondary high school	6	11,5
High school	14	26,9
University	17	32,7
Location	n	%
Metropolitan	43	82,7
City	3	5,8
Town	5	9,6
Village	1	1,9
Monthly Income	**n**	**%**
Under 1000 TL	18	34,6
1000-3000 TL	27	51,9
4000-10000 TL	6	11,5
up to 10000	1	1,9
Father Occupation	**n**	**%**
Employee	16	30,8
Civil servant	11	21,2
Tradesman	3	5,8

	Mean	Standart deviation/Percent
Retired	5	9,6
Other	17	32,7
Mother Occupation	n	%
Housewife	41	78,8
Civil servant	6	11,6
Nurse	2	3,8
Other	3	5,8
Psychopathology in family	n	%
Psychopathology in mother	3(ADHD,depression)	5,7
Psychopathology in father	3(ADHD,depression ,psychotic disorder)	5,7
Psychopathology in siblings	5(DEHB)	9,6

Table 2. Socio-demographic characteristics of the group with ADHD

	Mean	Standart deviation/Percent
Age	10,4	2,66
Mother age	37,7	5,28
Father Age	41,8	6,79
Education	n	%
The First 5 years	15	60
6th-10th.years	10	40
Number of siblings	n	%
2 and under 2	22	88
2- 4 siblings	3	12
Mother's Educational level	**n**	**%**
Not education	0	0
Primary school	0	0
Secondary high school	2	8
High school	8	32
University	15	60
Father'sEducational level	n	%
Not education	0	0
Primary school	0	0
Secondary high school	0	0
High school	6	24
University	17	68
Location	n	%
Metropolitan	22	88
City	1	4

	Mean	Standart deviation/Percent
Town	2	8
Village	0	0
Monthly Income	**n**	**%**
Under 1000 TL	0	0
1000-3000 TL	10	40
4000-10000 TL	14	56
up to 10000	1	4
Father Occupation	**n**	**%**
Employee	2	8
Civil servant	4	16
Tradesman	4	16
Retired	1	4
Other	9	36
Mother Occupation	**n**	**%**
Housewife	12	48
Civil servant	7	28
Nurse	6	24
Other	0	0
Psychopathology in family	n	%
Psychopathology in mother	0	0
Psychopathology in father	0	0
Psychopathology in siblings	0	0

Table 3. Socio-demographic characteristics of the control group

33 of patients (63.5%) were under long acting methylphenidate (OROS-MPH) therapy and 19 (36.5%) were under atomoxetine therapy. The medication use duration of first group was 18.54±15.43 months and second group was 18.3±14.8 months. No significant difference was found between these two groups in terms of duration (p=0,958, t=0,52).

Dose rate for OROS-MPH was averagely 29,4±7,88 mg and for atomexetine was averagely 45,42±12,36 mg.

Height average in patient group was 141,4±13,8 cm, weight average was 37,07±11,17 kg and height average for control group was 145,6±17,9cm, weight average was41,1±15,5 kg (p=0,251). In terms of weight and height, there is no significant difference between atomexetine users, MPH-OROS users and control group (Table 4 and 5).

When considered sub-group of life quality scale in patient group, phsycal sub-group was found as 80,8 ±15,27, while emotianol sub-group was 66,05±18,26, life quality social was 76,15±22,28 and sub-group associated with school was 66,25±18,86. In control group, physcal sub-group was found as 96,37±7,02, while emotional sub-group was 90,2±13,5, life quality social 97,4±7,92 and sub-group associated with school was 91,6±10,19. There is significant difference between all fields of life quality in both groups ($p<0.001^*$). When comparing life quality of atomexetine and MPH users, no significant difference was found. But when comparing long acting MPH users and atomexetine users with control group individually, significant difference was examined in life quality sub-groups between control group and other two groups (Table 4).

	Patient group	Control group	Comparement of groups
Mean of ages	10,42 ±2,136	10,4±2,66	p= 0,970 t= 0,041
Mean of height	141,63 ±14,19	145,6±17,9	p= 0,296 t= 1,051
Mean of weight	37,07±11,17	41,12±15,5	p= 0,251 t= 1,166
Mean of physical health field in PedsQL	80,8 ±15,27	96,37±7,02	p< 0,001* z= 4,845
Mean of emotional functioning field in PedsQL	66,05±18,26	90,2±13,5	p< 0,001* t= 5,867
Mean of , social functioning field in PedsQL	76,15±22,28	97,4±7,92	p<0,001* z=5,155
Mean of shcool functioning field in PedsQL	66,25±18,86	91,6±10,19	P<0,001* t= 7,668
(p<0,05*)			

Table 4. Comparement of Socialdemographic datas and life quality

In OROS-MPH user group, while score between age and life quality in school field was found significantly correlated; ($p<0.05^*$, $r=0.443$) in atomexetine user group, no correlation was found. When considering changes in hand-writing and drug use, 20 patients of 52 parents showed recovery in hand writing after drug intake.

26 patients (50%) were applied before any other treatment of ADHD. However, several side effects, and due to non compliance of previously treatment patients couldn't maintain previous treatment is observed. 16 patients of the 26 patients, (20.8%), inability to benefit from treatment, 2 patients (2.6%), insomnia, and 2 (2.6%), loss of appetite, and 2 (2.6%), nervousness, 1 'patients (1.3%) hyperactivity, and 1 (1.3%), treatment noncompliance, and 1 (1.3%) increase in anxiety, and 1 (1.3%) were somnolence. The relationship between these side effects, drugs, the treatment of patients do not benefit from atomoxetine before 4 out, 11 patients are used long-or short-acting MPH, that 1 learned that used risperidone treatment. Insomnia, loss of appetite, and nervousness side effects was seen with all the OROS MPH. Increase in hyperactivity and

http://dx.doi.org/10.5772/53790

	Comparement of patients under OROS-MPH treatment with atomoxetine treatment	Comparement of patients under OROS-MPH with control group	Comparement of patients under atomoxetine treatment with control group
Mean of ages	p= 0,586	p= 0,933	p= 0,806
Mean of height	p= 0,294	p= 0,336	p= 1,00
Mean of weight	p= 0,475	p= 0,225	p= 0,937
Mean of physical health field in PedsQL	p= 0,991	p<0,001*	p<0,005*
MMean of emotional functioning field in PPedsQL	p= 1,00	p<0,001*	p<0,001*
MMean of , social functioning field in PedsQL	p= 0,821	p<0,001*	p<0,005*
MMean of shcool functioning field in PedsQL	p= 0,683	p<0,001*	p<0,001*

(p<0,05*)

Table 5. Comparement of patients under OROS-MPH, atomoxetine treatment with each others and control group

anxiety side effects could be showed with the use of OROS MPH. The side effects of somnolence and non-compliance with the development of atomoxetine (Table 6).

Reason of finishing first treatment / First treatment	MPH	Atomoxetine	Risperidone
Non effective	11	4	1
Insomnia	2	-	-
Loss of appetite	2	-	-
Nervoussness	2	-	-
Non compliance of treatment	-	1	-
Hyperactivity	1	-	-
Increase in anxiety	1	-	-
Somnolence	-	1	-

Table 6. Reason of finishing first treatment and relationship between drugs

6. Discussion — conclusions

Life quality measurement is a method that gains gradually importance in children and adolescent, mental health surveys and clinical practice. Investigators and practioners supposed that important deterioration in psychosocial fields associated with ADHD based on basic symptoms of ADHD.

Children and adolescent with ADHD are at increased risk of academic failure, dropping out of school or college, teenage pregnancy, alcohol and substance use and criminal behaviour. Driving poses an additional risk. The emotional impairments of children and adolescents with ADHD may include poor self-regulation of emotion, greater excessive emotional expression, especially anger and aggression, greater problems coping with frustration, reduced empathy, and decreased arousal to stimulation [25]. Children and adolescents with ADHD have problems with peer relationships lack friendships, or have limitations in their activities with friends if they do have friends. More than half of these children and adolescents have serious problems with peer relationships [26]. Relationships and activities within the family can be impaired and in some cases family relationships can break down, bringing additional social and financial difficulties causing children to feel sad or show oppositional or aggressive behavior [27].

Specific academic difficulties noted in children with ADHD include slower reading fluency weaker reading comprehension (Ghelani and poor penmanship. Mastery of academic skills can also be hampered by the secondary effects (impulsivity, inattention, and disorganization) that ADHD can have upon a child's ability to practice newly learned skills or study recently presented material in the homework setting [28,29].

ADHD affects not only on the child, but also on parents and siblings, causing disturbances to family and marital functioning, increased healthcare costs for patients and their family. Children and their families changes from the preschool years to primary school and adolescence, with varying aspects of the disorder being more prominent at different stages. Also, ADHD had more parent-reported problems in terms of emotional-behavioral role function, behavior, mental health, and self-esteem. In addition, the problems of children with ADHD had a significant impact on the parents' emotional health and parents' time to meet their own needs, and they interfered with family activities and family cohesion[30].

ADHD is one of the most common psychiatric conditions estimated to affect 5-10% of all children and ADHD predisposes children to impaired academic, familial, social, vocational and emotional functioning if untreated. ADHD does not remit with the onset of puberty alone and teenagers and adults continue to have symptoms of the disorder that cause significant problems in their lives[31].

Children with attention-deficit and disruptive behavior disorder had, according to parent ratings, a better emotional functioning score than children with anxiety disorders. Their academic performance was significantly lower than for children with anxiety disorders and other disorders, but school functioning was reported as equal. Clinicians reported more problems in behavior toward others for this group compared to children with anxiety and mood disorders. Comorbidity of attention-deficit disorder or disruptive behavior disorder with other psychiatric diagnoses did not influence overall Quality of Life. Also ıt had been found that children with ADHD were more limited in schoolwork and social functioning[32]. Danckaerts M. et al. showed that a robust negative effect on QoL was reported by the parents of children with ADHD across a broad range of psychopathology symptoms [33].

Because of difficulties in academical, social and emotional fields, the adverse effect of ADHD on life quality is in evidence in current studies. Numerous studies have shown significant recovery in life quality with medication use in case of ADHD [6,7,8]. The results of studies carried out in this content showed adverse effect on all fields of children with ADHD diagnosis and therapy requirement. Also, it is suggested that recovery attempts for children with ADHD diagnosis should include all fields of life [34]. In line with previous studies, our study showed that there is significantly difference in all sub-fields of life quality scale between control group and under ADHD treatment [6,7,8]. Among this, when comparing all sub-fields of life quality scale, there is no significant difference between atomexetine and OROS-MPH users. This result is consistent with Leo Bastiaens's study [35] conducted in 75 children between 6-12 age interval, comparing the effects of atomexetine and stimulant therapy over life quality, and there are further studies that suggests efficiency of OROS-MPH on life quality [36]. Also in another study of Leo Bastiaens, 84 patients (atomoxetine n = 39/stimulants n = 45), between the ages of 5 and18, were treated for approximately 8 months. At end point, there were no significant differences in improvements of quality of life between the two groups [37].

However an interesting study is that; 977 Male and female patients aged 6-17 years seeking treatment for symptoms of ADHD were assessed,they were grouped according to whether they were prescribed psycho- and/or pharmacotherapy (treatment) or not (no/'other' treatment) Although both treatment and no/'other' treatment cohorts showed improvements in mean Quality of Life over 12 months, the difference was small and not statistically significant [38].

In our study, we found that confounding result, although patients with ADHD tent to show a decrease in school success with increase in age, patients who take OROS-MPH treatment show an increase in life quality school sub-score. This increase could be due to enhancement in OROS-MPH usage dose with age. Higher dose levels in OROS-MPH could be asserted as more effective for increase in academical success. Compared with the control group, decrease of life quality sub-areas is supported the view of pharmacotherapy alone not enough. However, further studies are needed to obtain certain data.

İn this point; V A Harpin showed that the primary school children with ADHD frequently begins to be seen as being different as classmates start to develop the skills and maturity that enable them to learn successfully in school. ADHD to succeed, more frequently the child experiences academic failure, rejection by peers, and low self esteem. And This study suggested that assessment by an educational psychologist may help to unravel learning strengths and difficulties, and advise on necessary support in the classroom [39].

50 children and adolescents with ADHD diagnosis, 30 control group and both of their parents are examined. Rosenberg Self-Esteem Scale and Children's Quality of Life Scale are used. The

results of this study suggest that self-esteem in the children and adolescents with ADHD is not significantly high and that their quality of life is significantly low. This is noticeable for it draws attention to the psycho-social dimension in the clinical evaluation of the children with ADHD [40]. İn this way, social support and motivational therapy may needed.

From anoher study Figure 1 shows benefit (dark green bars) or no benefit (light green bars) by outcome group in treated participants with attention deficit hyperactivity disorder (ADHD) versus untreated ADHD. Improvement was reported most often in studies of driving and obesity outcomes (left side), with a greater proportion of outcomes reported to exhibit no benefit following treatment compared with no treatment in studies of occupation (right side). An intermediate proportion of studies of self-esteem, social function, academic, drug use/ addictive behavior,antisocial behavior, and services use outcomes reported benefit with treatment [41].

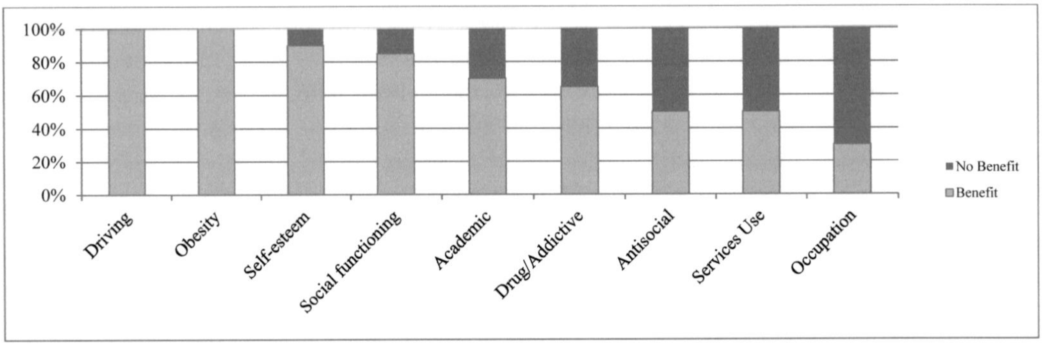

*This figure is taken from" A systematic review and analysis of long-term outcomes in attention deficit hyperactivity disorder: effects of treatment and non-treatment "

Figure 1. Benefit and no benefit with treatment by outcome group

Treatment with OROS-MPH and atomoxsetine also have side effects. Evidence shows that ADHD medications are safe and effective for children ages 6 and older. For children over the age of 6, long-term effectiveness and adverse effects are not well studied. More studies showed that psychostimulants and atomoxetine may cause insomnia, appetite loss, tiredness, social withdrawal, and abdominal pain. Psychostimulants and atomoxetine may also cause a modest increase in average blood pressure and average heart rate in some children and adolescents. Children or adolescents taking atomoxetine may be more likely to think about suicide than children who do not take it. More adverse effects were reported in preschoolers than in elementary school children. Moodiness and irritability often led to discontinuation of treatment with MPH. [42] In our study; 26 patients were applied before any other treatment of ADHD. However, several side effects, and due to non compliance of previously treatment patients couldn't maintain previous treatment is observed. İnsomnia, loss of appetite, nervousness, hyperactivity, increase in anxiety, and somnolence areside effect which cause to stop first treatment. Insomnia, loss of appetite, and nervousness side effects was seen with all the OROS MPH. Increase in hyperactivity and anxiety side effects could be showed with the use of OROS MPH. The side effects of somnolence and non-compliance with the development of atomoxetine. But our datas are limited about relationship of side effects and life quality. Further studies are needed side effects of OROS-MPH and atomoxetine on life quality.

Long-term effects of methylphenidate and atomoxsetine on growth rates of children with ADHD are the other size of the treatment which also effect the Quality of life. The effect of OROS-MPH and atomoxsetine over weight and height is still a subject of discussion. The final results, as to children with attention deficit who take stimulant medication grow slower than children with no treatment, verify the results of previous studies in 1972-1973. Recent study showed a decrease in expected weight and height growing in children who take stimulant therapy. In treatments continuing 2-3 years, the growing speed shows normalization tendency [43,44].

İn the one of the review about effects of stimulants on height and weight; the quantitative analyses showed that treatment with stimulant medication led to statistically significant delays in height and weight. Treatment with stimulants in childhood reduced expected height and weight. This review also found statistically significant evidence of attenuation of these deficits over time. The qualitative review suggested that growth deficits may be dose dependent. Some data suggest that ultimate adult growth parameters are not affected [45].

Prolonged medication (data evaluated at 6 months - 5 years) with short-acting MPH has shown to have minimal impact on height only at the first 6 months; however, catch up growth was detected during adolescent period in 96 cases wo were treated with short-acting MPH 0.41-0.49 mg/kg/day [46]. İn another research about the potential negative influence of methylphenidate on growth; mean value of height was lower than expected mean height for age by 0.42 cm at diagnosis. This difference increased to 2.69 cm (at 30 months of treatment), but it subsequently decreased to 0.83 cm (at 48 months of treatment). The relationship between nutritional status and the negative effects on the height curve in those patients would require nutritional optimization to return anthropometric variables to normal [47].

Two new researches was performed on the effect of amoxetine on growing patients with 5 year follow-up and long- time efficiency and reliability of atomoxetine. After a 5 year follow-up, it is suggested that while atomoxetine has no or a little effect on growing, in some cases could cause reduction in growing. Especially in 18 months, growing could be affected a little, however normal development could proceed in a period of 2-3 years [43,44]. Spencer et al present findings from an ongoing 5-year study of the efficacy and safety of treatment with atomoxetine. After 1 month's treatment,they found patients weighed less than expected from their starting percentiles relative to population norms, with a maximum shortfall at 15 months and a return to expected weight by 36 months. Patients were slightly shorter than expected after 12 months, reaching a maximum shortfall at 18 months and returning to expected height by 24 months. Patients in the top quartile for body mass index (BMI) or weight at baseline, and those in the third quartile for height, showed 5-year decreases from expected values. Those below median height at baseline showed increases relative to expected values.[43]

In our study, we found no significant difference between both control group of OROS-MHP and atomoxetine in terms of weight and height. And also no significant difference were between treatment under OROS-MHP and atomoxetine. This result could be associated with time limitation. Further studies are needed if there are difference effects of between OROS-MPH and atomoxetine treatment on weight-height.

Although one of the research children with ADHD who performed poorly on the neuropsychological battery had greater BMI z-scores, and were more likely to be classified as overweight/obese compared with children with ADHD who performed better on the neuropsychological battery. In addition, children with ADHD who were taking a stimulant medication had significantly lower BMI z-scores compared with children with ADHD who were not taking medication or who were taking a non-stimulant medication. They claimed that EF (Executive Function) is more impaired among children with ADHD and co-occurring weight problems, highlighting the importance of self-regulation as a link between pediatric obesity and ADHD [48].

An intresting point is that last studies reported an association between overweight and ADHD. Although a higher prevalence of overweight/obesity was reported in clinical samples of patients with ADHD, longitudinal studies are needed to better understand the mechanisms underlying the association between ADHD and overweight/obesity [49].

Current data suggests an association between growing and medical effect of stimulants. Also normal growing speeds have been shown in children who take no treatment with attention deficit hyperactivity disorder. Therefore, further studies should focus on fields as detailed definition of growing and development effects of stimulants in children with different ages, determining the growing deficiency mechanism up to stimulant [50].

Gender differences is another variability that may affect the quality of life. Children with high levels of ADHD symptoms have many associated behaviour problems, even in pre-school years, and boys with high levels of ADHD symptoms are more severely affected compared with girls. Datas of researches are not enough in this field.

Data from 5 clinical atomoxetine trials (4 from Europe and 1 from Canada) with similar inclusion and exclusion criteria and similar durations (8- to 12-week follow-up) were included in the pooled analysis. 136 girls and 658 boys were treated with atomoxetine. Atomoxetine was effective in improving some aspects of health-related quality of life (HR-QoL) in both genders without any significant differences across genders.Also, ıt was found that correlations between core symptoms of ADHD and HR-QoL were low to moderate in both boys and girls [51].

Also 6-17 aged of patients were treated with atomoxetine in two studies. ADHD-related difficulties were assessed after 8 and 24 weeks using the Global Impression of Perceived Difficulties (GIPD) instrument, which can be taken to reflect the patient's QoL from the three perspectives. The GIPD scores over time suggest that patients' QoL, as reflected by perceived

http://dx.doi.org/10.5772/53790

ADHD-related difficulties, improved with time on atomoxetine The sexes did not differ significantly in mean GIPD total scores.and also improvement in ADHD-related difficulties did not differ significantly between boys and girls [52]. In the second step of our study; we aimed to compare effects of sex differences on response of treatment with both atomoxetine and OROS-MPH, also correlation with life quality, ıt is our limitation of this study.

Consequently, ADHD, which is a chronic neuropsychiatric disorder, is known as negatively effective on life quality perception in reports about children and it is suggested that evaluation of life quality in follow-up and treatment stages of ADHD and efficiency of pharmacological treatment on life quality of this patients could be a guide for determining the fields that children have difficulty on. Besides, when comparing with normal population, the difficulties in academical, social and emotional fields could be seen more frequently. Medical treatment of attention deficit and hyperactivity disorder alone could cause increasing in conseptualization tendency of problems and nondevelopment on problem solving skills. Therefore, it is suggested that recovery attempts for children with ADHD diagnosis should include all fields of life. Karabekiroğlu K. et al found that more than half of the teachers denoted that the medication used for ADHD would have serious side effects and even with treatment ADHD would not sufficiently improve, and the children diagnosed with ADHD or autism should be trained at separate classes. So that the parents and teachers may benefit from structured educative programs inorder to get rid of wrong assumptions and stigma [53].

One of the importent point is that further study is needed to understand the social and psychological processes that underlie stigmatization, how parents balance perceived benefits of treatment with mental health stigma concerns, and to determine how stigmatization effects quality of life children with ADHD.

Although in our study, patients with ADHD tent to show a decrease in school success with increase in age, patients who take OROS-MPH treatment show an increase in life quality school sub-score. This information could be a guide for examining of detailed determining of OROS-MPH effects.

Limitaton of our study are number of patients and time of treatments. Our datas are not enough effects of socio-demographic differences, side effects, gender and stigma on life quality. Measurement of quality of life in attention-deficit-hyperactivity disorder (ADHD) gives a more complete picture of day-to-day functioning and treatment effects than behavioural rating alone. Quality of life is effected from numerous factors so that new measurement parameters should be developed.

In conclusion; there is significantly difference in all sub-fields of life quality scale between control group and under ADHD treatment. Tretment is increase life quality of ADHD patients but only medical treatment is not enought.There is no significant difference between weight and height when comparing between control groups of OROS-MPH and atomexetine. Further studies are needed to support the effects of OROS-MPH and atomoxetine on life quality and weight-height.

Acknowledgements

PubChem chemical substance (submitted) records that are classified under the same Medical Subject Headings (MeSH) controlled vocabulary as the current articles.

Author details

Esra Ozdemir Demirci, Merve Cikili Uytun, Rabia Durmus and Didem Behice Oztop

Department of Child and Adolescent Psychiatry, Erciyes University Medical Faculty, Kayseri, Turkey

References

[1] American Psychiatric Association. Diagnostic and Statistical Manual of Mental Disorders, 4th edition, Text Revision (DSM-IV-TR). Washington, DC: American Psychiatric Association, 2000.

[2] Biederman J, Faraone SV. Attention-deficit hyperactivity disorder. Lancet 2005;366:237–48.

[3] Biederman J, Spencer TJ (1999) Attention-deficit/hyperactivity disorder (ADHD) as a noradrenergic disorder. Biol Psychiatry 46:1234–1242

[4] Safer DJ (2000) Commentary: stimulant treatment in the community. J Am Acad Child Adolesc Psychiatry 39:989–992

[5] Perwien AR, Faries DE, Kratochvil CJ, et al. Improvement in healthrelated quality of life in children with ADHD: An analysis of placebo controlled studies of atomoxetine. J Dev Behav Pediatr 2004;25:264–71

[6] Güleç C, Köroğlu E. (1998) Psychiatry Text Book. in: Şenol Ü, Şener Ş (eds). Attention deficit hyperactivity disorder. Ankara, 2, 1119-1129.

[7] Escobar R, Soutullo CS, Hervas AH ve ark. Worse quality of life for children with newly diagnosed atention-deficit/hyperactivity disorder, compared with asthmatic and healthy children. Pediatrics 2005; 116:364-9.

[8] Bastiaansen D, Koot HM, Ferdinand RF ve ark. Quality of life in children with psychiatric disorders: self, parent, and clinician report. J Am Acad Child Adolesc Psychiatry 2004; 43:221-30.

[9] Yıldız Ö, Çakın Memik N, Ağaoğlu B. Quality of Life in Children with (Attention-Deficit Hyperactivity Disorder): A Cross-Sectional Study. Neuropsychiatry Archives 2010; 47: 314-8

http://dx.doi.org/10.5772/53790

[10] Raggi VL, Chronis AM (2006) Interventions to address the academic impairment of children and adolescents with ADHD. Clin Child Fam Psychol Rev 9:85–111

[11] Wehmeier PM, Schacht A, Barkley RA (2010) Social and emotional impairment in children and adolescents with ADHD and the impact on quality of life. J Adolesc Health 46:209–217

[12] Popper CW (2000) Pharmacological alternatives to psychostimulants for the treatment of attention deficit/hyperactivity disorder. Child Adolesc Psychiatr Clin N Am 9:605–646

[13] Scahill L, Chappell PB, Kim YS, Katsovich L, Sheperd E et al (2001) A placebo-controlled study of guanfacine in the treatment of children with tic disorders and attention deficit hyperactivity disorder. Am J Psychiatry 158:1067–1074

[14] Silver LB (1999) Alternative (nonstimulant) medications in the treatment of attention-deficit/hyperactivity disorder in children. Pediatr Clin North Am 46:965–975

[15] Wilens TE, Biederman J, Baldessarini RJ, Geller B, Schleifer D, Spencer TJ et al (1996) Cardiovascular effects of therapeutic doses of tricyclic antidepressants in children and adolescents. J Am Acad Child Adolesc Psychiatry 35:1491–1501

[16] Sauer JM, Ponsler GD, Mattiuz EL, Long AJ, Witcher JW, Thomasson HR et al (2003) Disposition and metabolic fate of atomoxetine hydrochloride: the role of CYP2D6 in human disposition and metabolism. Drug Metab Dispos 31:98–107

[17] Hechtman A, Abikoff H, Klein RG, et al. Academic achievement and emotional status of children with ADHD treated with long-term methylphenidate and multimodal psychosocial treatment. J Am Acad Child Adolesc Psychiatry 2004;43:812–9.

[18] Banaschewski T, Coghill D, Santosh P, et al. Long-acting medications for the hyperkinetic disorders. A systematic review and European treatment guidelines. Eur Child Adolesc Psychiatry 2006;15:476–95.

[19] Zhang H, Du M, Zhuang S. Impact of long-term Treatment of Methylphenidate on Height and Weight of School Age Children with ADHD. Neuropediatrics 2010;41:55-59

[20] Yıldız Ö, , Ağaoğlu B., , Karakaya I,Şahika G, Şişmanlar ŞG, Çakın Memik N, Efficiency and tolerability of OROS-methylphenidate in Turkish children and adolescents with attention-deficit/hyperactivity disorder, Anatolian Journal of Psychiatry, 2010; 11:44-50

[21] Çakın Memik N, Ağaoğlu B, Coşkun A, et al. The validity and reliability of pediatric quality of life inventory in 8-12 year old turkısh children. . Turkish Journal of Child Adolesc Psychiatry 2008; 15:87-98.

[22] Çakın Memik N, Ağaoğlu B, Coşkun A ve ark. The validity and reliability of pediatric quality of life inventory in 13-18 year old turkısh adolescents. Turkish Journal of Psychiatry 2007; 18:353-63

[23] Turgay A. Turgay DSM-IV Based Child and Adolescent Behavior Disorders Screening and Rating Scale, Integrative Therapy Institude Toronto, Kanada 1995.

[24] Ercan ES, Amado S, Somer O, et al. Development of A Test Battery for the Assessment of Attention Deficit Hyperactivity Disorder. Turkish Journal of Child Adolesc Psychiatry 2001; 8:132-42.

[25] Barkley RA. Attention-Deficit/Hyperactivity Disorder: A Handbook for Diagnosis and Treatment. 3rd edition. New York, NY: Guilford Press, 2006

[26] Escobar R, Soutullo CA,Hervas A, et al.Worse quality of life for children with newly diagnosed attention-deficit/hyperactivity disorder, compared with asthmatic and healthy children. Pediatrics 2005;116:e364–9.

[27] Schreyer I, Hampel P. (ADHD among boys in childhood: quality of life and parenting behavior)(Article in German). Z Kinder Jugendpsychiatr Psychother 2009;37:69–75.

[28] Ghelani K, Sidhu R, Jain U, Tannock R: Reading comprehension and reading related abilities in adolescents with reading disabilities and attention-deficit/hyperactivity disorder. Dyslexia 10:364–384, 2004.

[29] Racine MB, Majnemer A, Shevell M, Snider L: Handwriting performance in children with attention deficit hyperactivity disorder (ADHD). J Child Neurol 23:399–406, 2008.

[30] Anne F. Klassen, DPhil, Anton Miller, MB, ChB, FRCPC, Stuart Fine, MB, Health-Related Quality of Life in Children and Adolescents Who Have a Diagnosis of Attention-Deficit/Hyperactivity Disorder , PEDIATRICS Vol. 114 No. 5November 1, 2004 pp. e541 -e547)

[31] Pliszka S, AACAP Work Group on Quality Issues. Practice parameter for the assessment and treatment of children and adolescents with attention-deficit/hyperactivity disorder. J Am Acad Child Adolescent Psychiatry 2007; 46:894-921.)

[32] Bastiaansen D, Koot MH, Fedinand FR, Verhulst FR. Quality of Life in Children With Psychiatric Disorders: Self-, Parent, and Clinician Report Journal of the American Academy of Child & Adolescent Psychiatry, Volume 43, Issue 2, Pages 221-230

[33] Danckaerts M, Sonuga-Barke EJ, Banaschewski T, Buitelaar J, Dopfner M, Hollis C, Santosh P, Rothenberger A, Sergeant J, Steinhausen HC, Taylor E, Zuddas A, Coghill D (2010) The quality of life of children with attention deficit/hyperactivity disorder: a systematic review. Eur Child Adolesc Psychiatry 19:83–105

[34] Üneri ÖŞ, Turgut S, Öner P, Bodur Ş, Rezaki B, Quality of life in 8-12 years old children with attention deficit hyperactivity disorder Turkish Journal of Child Adolesc Psychiatry, 2010,17(1):27-31

[35] Bastiaens L. Improvement in global psychopathology increases quality of life during treatment of ADHD withatomoxetine or stimulants. Psychiatr Q. 2011 Dec;82(4):303-8. doi: 10.1007/s11126-011-9172-4.

[36] Niederkirchner K, Slawik L, Wermelskirchen D, Rettig K, Schäuble B. , Transitioning to OROS(®) methylphenidate from atomoxetine is effective in children and adolescents with ADHD. Expert Rev Neurother. 2011 Apr;11(4):499-508.

[37] Leo Bastiaens, Both Atomoxetine and Stimulants Improve Quality of Life in an ADHD Population Treated in a Community Clinic, Psychiatr Q (2008) 79:133–137)

[38] Michal Goetz M. Yeh C.B, Ondrejka I, Akay A, et all A 12-Month Prospective, Observational Study of Treatment Regimen and Quality of Life Associated With ADHD in Central and Eastern Europe and Eastern Asia J Atten Disord 2012; 16:1 44-59

[39] V A Harpin, The effect of ADHD on the life of an individual, their family, and community from preschool to adult life , Arch Dis Child 2005;90(Suppl I):i2–i7. doi: 10.1136/adc.2004.059006)

[40] Zeynep Göker*, Evrim Aktepe**, Sema Kandil Self-esteem and Quality of Life in Children and Adolescents with Attention Deficit Hyperactivity Disorder New/Yeni Symposium Journal 2011 I 49 I 4

[41] Shaw M, Hodgkins P, Caci H, Young S, Kahle J, Woods AG, Amold LE. A systematic review and analysis of long-term outcomes in attention deficit hyperactivity disorder: effects of treatment and non-treatment. BMC Medicine 2012, 10:99

[42] Eisenberg John M. Comparative Effectiveness Review Summary Guides for Clinicians (Internet). Rockville (MD): Agency for Healthcare Research and Quality (US); 2007-.AHRQ Comparative Effectiveness Reviews.2012 Jun 26.

[43] Spencer TJ., Kratochvil JC, Sangal RB, Saylor KE, Bailey CE, Dunn DW, Geller DA, Casat CD, Lipetz RS, Jain R, Newcorn JH, Ruff DD, Feldman PD, Furr JA, and Allen JA. Effects of Atomoxetine on growth in children with Attention Deficit/hyperactivity disorder following up to five years of treatment. J Child Adolesc Psychopharmacol 17 (5): 689-699.

[44] Kratochvil JC, Wilens ET, Greenhill LL ve ark (2006) Effects of long term Atomoxetine treatment for young children with Attention Deficit/hyperactivity disorder. J Child Adolesc Psychiatry 45 (8): 919-927.

[45] Faraone VS,Biederman J, Morley PC, Thomas. Spencer JT, Effect of Stimulants on Height and Weight: A Review of the Literature J. Am. Acad. Child Adolesc. Psychiatry, 2008; 47(9):000–000.

[46] Moungnoi P, Maipang P. Long-term effects of short-acting methylphenidate on growth rates of children with attention deficit hyperactivity disorder at Queen Sirikit National Institute of Child Health.J Med Assoc Thai. 2011 Aug;94 Suppl 3:S158-63.

[47] Durá-Travé T, Yoldi-Petri ME, Gallinas-Victoriano F, Zardoya-Santos P Effects of osmotic-release methylphenidate on height and weight in children with attention-deficit hyperactivity disorder (ADHD) following up to four years of treatment. J Child Neurol. 2012 May;27(5):604-9. Epub 2011 Dec 21.

[48] Graziano PA, Bagner DM, Waxmonsky JG, Reid A, McNamara JP, Geffken GR Co-occurring weight problems among children with attention deficit/hyperactivity disorder: the role of executive functioning. Int J Obes (Lond). 2012 Apr;36(4):567-72. doi: 10.1038/ijo.2011.245. Epub 2011 Dec 13.

[49] Erhart M, Herpertz-Dahlmann B, Wille N, Sawitzky-Rose B, Hölling H, Ravens-Sieberer U.Examining the relationship between attention-deficit/hyperactivity disorder and overweight in children and adolescents. Eur Child Adolesc Psychiatry. 2012 Jan;21(1):39-49. Epub 2011 Nov 26

[50] Poulton A. Growth and maturation in children and adolescents with attention deficit hyperactivity disorder Current Opinion in Pediatrics turkish edition, Vol 1, No 4, 2006.

[51] Wehmeier PM, Schacht A, Escobar R, Hervas A, Dickson R. Health-related quality of life in ADHD: a pooled analysis of gender differences in five atomoxetine trials. Atten Defic Hyperact Disord. 2012 Mar;4(1):25-35.

[52] Wehmeier PM, Schacht A, Dittmann RW, Banaschewski T. Minor differences in ADHD-related difficulties between boys and girls treated with atomoxetine for attention-deficit/hyperactivity disorder. Atten Defic Hyperact Disord. 2010 Jun;2(2):73-85

[53] Karabekiroðlu K, Memik NC, Özel ÖÖ, Toros F, Öztop D, Özbaran B et all.. Stigmatization and Misinterpretations on ADHD andAutism: A Multi-Central Study with Elementary School Teachers and Parents Klinik Psikiyatri 2009;12:79-89

Section 6

Ethical Issues

Chapter 14

Ethical Concerns Raised by Neuroscience, Labeling, and Intervening in the Lives of Individuals with ADHD

Debby Zambo

Additional information is available at the end of the chapter

http://dx.doi.org/10.5772/53004

1. Introduction

Take a moment to consider how individuals with Attention Deficit Hyperactivity Disorder (ADHD) are described. When people talked about these individuals what do they say about their behaviors, bodies, and minds? Do these descriptions vary across individuals, contexts, and time? Now compare your reflections as to how individuals with ADHD are often described. In today's world ADHD is described as a:

- disorder/dysfunction.
- heterogeneous developmental disorder.
- chronic condition with life-span implications.
- brain difference.
- delay or deterioration in their cognitive, social, and emotional functioning.
- universal condition transcending culture, socio-economic, and race.
- social and emotional burden.

These descriptions are common and, as a matter of fact, most of them were drawn from chapters in this book.

My point for using this activity to open this chapter is to make you aware of your personal theories and how the symptoms of ADHD, who has it, and what happens as a result is influenced by our perspectives. Let me clarify what I mean a bit more with a boy name Michael and a role-play for you. Imagine that you are a teacher and Michael is a student in your classroom. You enjoy Michael's humor but he is showing uneven academic progress and is constantly fidgety and out of his seat. Take a few minutes to answer these questions: From where is Michael's lack of progress stemming? Why is he so fidgety and out of his seat? What would you do to help Michael?

Now, let's consider some common answers. If you thought Michael's uneven progress and fidgetiness stemmed from his family's lack of discipline you would likely direct Michael and his family to a counselor, who in turn might place them in some sort of counseling or therapy. If you thought Michael's uneven progress and fidgetiness came from a brain difference you would likely refer Michael to the school psychologist, who in turn might refer him to a physician, who might place Michael on medication. If you thought Michael's uneven progress and fidgetiness stemmed from his environment (your classroom) you might decide to differentiate his instruction and restructure the activities he was given so he could get up and move. Three varied perspectives of Michael with three different outcomes. No perspective was neutral and each set Michael on a different path.

To take the idea of teachers' perspectives about boys like Michael one step further let me explain a study conducted by two colleagues and myself (Zambo, Zambo & Sidlik) in 2009. We wanted to understand what teachers thought about individuals with ADHD and if neuroscience was useful to them so we based on the work of McCabe and Castel (2008) and Weisberg, Keil, Goodstein, Rawson, and Gray (2008). These researchers manipulated information and used an fMRI image, a graph, or no image to understand if neuroscience was persuasive and they found it was both persuasive and misleading. These researchers concluded that fMRI images were persuasive because they appealed to their participants' intuitive reductionist notions of learning and confirmed theories and biases they already possessed (learning boils down to brightly lit areas captured in fMRIs). Instead of thinking of learning as a complex process unable to be reduced to biological functions alone, participants believed colorful images proved learning had occurred.

Based on this work, we set out to understand what a group of preservice teachers knew about ADHD, where they learned this information, and what they thought about medical science and neuroscience being useful to them to educate students with attention challenges. We used a general questionnaire but manipulated the type of information participants received. Half of our participants saw an fMRI image and read about ADHD from a neuroscience perspective (e.g., caused by faulty neuroreceptors responding to the neurotransmitter dopamine) and the other half saw an image of a premature infant and read about ADHD from a medical perspective (e.g., infants being born prematurely and weighing less than 3.3 pounds often develop ADHD).

We found that the participants in both groups knew a lot about the behaviors of students with ADHD. They knew, or at had theories that, students with ADHD were hyperactive, excitable, impulsive, irritable, and seldom tired. They also believed that these characteristics inhibit students' learning and social life. They believed that children with attention challenges were distractible, struggle with concentration, get off task easily, and have social and family problems. When asked where they learned this information they said they had friends or family members with it, heard celebrities on television talk about it, and discussed it in their courses (especially special education courses).

http://dx.doi.org/10.5772/53004

Data from the two conditions (neuroscience and medical science) showed some differences. Participants who saw the fMRI image and read information suggesting ADHD was a biological disorder believed that neuroscience would be useful to them. These participants believed information from neuroscience would help them identify students with ADHD, understand how their brain works, and understand why they behave in certain ways. Participants in the neuroscience condition also thought neuroscience would help them teach these students. They thought neuroscience would show them how to create learning environments and lessons conducive to these students' needs.

In comparison, participants in the medical science condition, who saw the image of the premature infant and read information from medical science also saw it as useful but had different theories about its use. Participants in this group thought medical science would help them understand the cause, signs, and symptoms of ADHD, the importance of medication, and how to manage students' behaviors. Different conditions lead to different perspectives of students with ADHD.

I hope these results help you realize that each of us operates from our own vantage point, or the theories that we construct as we go about our daily lives. The theories we build, in this sense, are not like the grand ideas tested by researchers (e.g., behaviorism, information processing, psychoanalysis) but the mental models or internal maps we use to navigate and make sense of our world and the things and individuals in it. We each construct our own theories based on our observations, but we also build theories based on what we hear or read. Social relationships matter and through dialogue and other means collective theories get built, spread, and get used to determine good and bad and normal and abnormal (Gergen, 2009). Collective theories gain momentum when they are turned into the stories that we tell. Stories become cultural artifacts and when they are repeated they become the norm and influence our values and behaviors. This includes our perceptions of disorders, who has them, and what this means. Consider the following example in which another culture, in this case the Maori of New Zealand, were seen as different simply because of their culture and its' traditions.

Psychology…has created the mass abnormalization of the Maori people by virtue of the fact the Maori people have been…recipients of defined labels and treatments…Clinical psychology is a form of social control…and offers no more "truth" about the realities of the Maori people's lives than a regular reading of a horoscope page in the local newspaper (Lawson-Te, Ano, 1993)

Foucault (1978; 1979) a proponent of helping people to understand their subjugation revealed the power of taken for granted practices. To Foucault, power is a coordinated cluster of relations and the specialized language a discipline develops creates binaries and divides. Instead of being seen as an individual we get placed into categories such as normal or abnormal. Disciplines also produce certain research procedures that privilege certain kinds of methodologies and scrutinize and classify us along their disciplinary lines. In other words, we become the labels that get assigned to us and the labels we acquire are used to control us. Disciplines gain power and influence public policy. Given this, let's look at mental disorders, like ADHD from a historical perspective.

In the United States, the first classification of a mental disorder occurred in 1840 and given its newness there were only a handful of distinctions. In 1930 psychiatry emerged and the perceptions of mental disorders began to grow. By 1938 the number of disturbances rose to approximately forty and since then, the number of disorders has risen to over three hundred and drug treatments have grown into a multi-billion dollar industry. If an individual has ADHD symptoms it is likely that he/she will be offered medication (Gergen, 2009).

Psychiatry has influence but another discipline neuroscience, has also come into play. In today's disorder-focused society neuroscience is influencing perspectives and this trend is likely to continue to grow (Maxwell, 2004). The past fifty years has seen an explosion of information about the brain offered to laypersons (Stamm, 2007; Stein, della Chiesa, Hinton, & Fischer, 2010). More findings are leading to more interest, more treatments, and as these get normalized and incorporated into policies and beliefs, fewer calls for restraint. When it comes to a disorder like ADHD more findings from are leading to more biological theories of it and more standardized treatments aimed at this cause. Neuroscientists are helping us understand how the brain of individuals with ADHD function but like McCabe and Castel (2008) and Weisberg, Keil, Goodstein, Rawson, and Gray (2008) showed these findings can be persuasive and misleading because they are new, diminutive, and alluring even though much of it is being overextended, misinterpreted, and simplified. If interpreted literally, and in isolation, findings from neuroscience will reduce learning, behavior, and emotions to biological processes alone. There are treatments, curricula, and products that purport to utilize findings from neuroscience to promote the learning and behavior of individuals with ADHD without any scientific backing.

Neuroscience is providing new and important information but if we are not careful it can also produce simplified and detached views of individuals, including those with ADHD. A Pygmalion Effect, or self-fulfilling prophecy is a groundless expectation that leads to behaviors that the make the original expectation come true (Merton, 1948). In other words, we see what we expect and expect what we want to see. Remember the opening exercise where you recalled various perspectives of individuals with ADHD and the Maori people who were perceived to be abnormal and defined and perceived as such. Just because a characterization, or label becomes common does not mean it is right, fair, ethical, or just.

2. The ethics of ADHD

Considering ethical questions that arise when an individual is labeled ADHD is important because five million children (most of whom are boys) between the ages of 3 and 17 years and 8 million adults are diagnosed with it and this number is growing each year (U.S. Department of Health and Human Services, 2010). Thanks to better diagnosis and the spread of information, more and more children, adolescents, and adults are being diagnosed and as a result of identification more and more are being treated with pharmaceutical, social, and behavioral interventions (Barkley, 2005). Unfortunately, and too often, medication is often the only treatment many individuals receive. Medications like methyphenidate (Ritalin) and amphet-

http://dx.doi.org/10.5772/53004

amine (Adderall) slow the reuptake of dopamine in the brain and decrease the impulsivity and agitation of ADHD in 70-90% of cases. This quick and easy removal of symptoms is leading to more and more children at younger ages, and more and more adolescents and adults to be prescribed medication. But too often, medication is the only treatment many individuals receive despite the fact that absolute proof of its benefits is not available and little is known about its long-term effects (Farah, 2005). While there is no doubt medication helps many individuals with ADHD there is also no doubt that, for some, there are unintended consequences and side effects like weight loss, sleeplessness, and cloudy minds (Chau, 2007). Neuroscientists, physicians, psychiatrists, psychologists, and social workers warn that medication needs to be coupled with behavioral, social, and emotional support because alone it is not enough. In other words, medicine is a part of the puzzle but it is not a panacea. Locating an attention problem solely in an individual's brain and treating her/his brain with medication gets results but it does not offer a cure or help an individual truly understand him/herself. Medication focuses on changing behaviors. It does not increase self-awareness or heal a body or mind (Farah, 2005; Morse, 2006; Stein, della Chiesa, Hinton, & Fischer, 2010).

Medicating children can also lead to misuse of medication if they are not instructed as to its proper use. Current sales figures indicate that Ritalin and Adderall are not only being used by individuals with ADHD but by high school and college students without it. A survey by McCabe, Knight, Teter, and Wechsler (2005) discovered that as many as 10% of high school students and 20% of college students say that they have used prescription stimulant medications to increase their performance on a test and this use varies by ethnicity, gender, achievement, and location. White males who receive low grades, and are going to Ivy League colleges in the northeast with high standards, are the most likely to abuse stimulant medication. Interestingly, the stimulants they abuse often come from their peers who have been diagnosed with ADHD. Purchasing Ritalin is so prevalent among young adults it is referred as " kiddy coke" and "study buddies." While my intent is not to criticize or condone the use of medication, I realize medication helps many individuals, but I want to once again point out that of we do not slow our thinking down and become aware of our beliefs we will miss ethical questions like:

- How might the use of this stimulant cause psychological harm (e.g., lower esteem and motivation)? Will an individual on medication be robbed of his/her identity?
- When it comes to medication, what responsibilities are there and who is accountable for these?
- Does the label of ADHD promote standardized, quick and easy treatments?
- Is the label of ADHD promoting biases and stereotypes?
- How can we better the lives and learning of individuals with ADHD?
- How can individuals with ADHD be supported so they know how to compensate, navigate, and fit into the world?

- Do individuals with ADHD really need to change? How can characteristics and relational styles be respected rather than modified? How can individuals with ADHD become their own advocates?

Habermas (2003) notes that the careless use of biomedical advances can undermine the behaviors and passions of individuals, or change individuals so much they lose the ability to understand and take responsibility for their own lives. In the wake of neuroscience and biotechnologies it is important to step back, reflect, make good ethical decisions, and take action to ensure that individuals with ADHD are allowed to be themselves and have a voice in their development and lives (Stein, della Chiesa, Hinton, & Fischer, 2010).

3. Making ethical decisions

Now, the Star-Bell Sneetches had bellies with stars.

The Plain-Belly Sneetches had none upon thars.

Those stars weren't so big. They were really so small.

You might think such a thing wouldn't matter at all.

But, because they had stars, all the Star-Belly Sneetches

Would brag, "We're the best kind of Sneetch on the beaches."

With their snoots in the air, they would sniff and they'd snort

"We'll have nothing to do with the Plain-Belly sort!"

And, whenever they met some, when they were out walking,

They'd hike right on past them without even talking.

Dr. Seuss (1961)

The quote from *The Sneeches* by Dr. Seuss (1961) was written to oppose anti-Semitism and remind us about discrimination. As science moves forward the ethical challenges we will face will continue to grow and change. Neuroscience is seeping into all of our lives and changing what we know and think, including what we think about ADHD. However, making ethical decisions is often perplexing and sometimes stars on bellies become so common we fail to see them. When it comes to neuroscience how do we decide what to believe? How do we know what is right and wrong, what is just and unfair? Where can we find reliable information? Who's ideas matter? Neuroethics brings questions like these into focus and this is important because of the power of our beliefs. Neuroethics sits at the intersection between neuroscience and the ethical, legal and social implications it brings. To Racine and Illes (2006), neuroethics

http://dx.doi.org/10.5772/53004

focuses on the right and wrong, good and bad treatment of, perfection of, or unwelcome invasion of and worrisome manipulation of the human brain. Gazzaniga (2005, 2011) furthered this idea to include "the examination of how we as humans, want to deal with the social issues of disease, normality, mortality, lifestyle, and the philosophy of living informed by our understanding of underlying brain mechanisms." To Gazzaniga, neuroscience should help everyone develop a brain-based philosophy of life. But this is not easy because we tend to focus on ideas that align with our beliefs and allow our beliefs and emotions to cloud our judgment. To develop a brain-based philosophy we will need valid information and time for deep and reflective thought. Beliefs are not easy to change and neuroscience and ethics do not mix easily. Some findings from neuroscience are difficult to understand because they make us question the very fabric of who we are, who we can become, and how is best to live our lives. Moral questions have been around for centuries and after years of debate a human rights approach focuses on ensuring that everyone, including individuals with ADHD receive truthful information, a voice in their lives, the right not to be harmed, and the right to develop and grow. Now look back at the questions posed in the previous section and consider how these positions relate to individuals with ADHD.

In closing. I hope this chapter has made you reflect on your beliefs and ask questions as to how findings from neuroscience, medical science, psychiatry, and all of the other disciplines used to influence the lives of individuals with ADHD can be used fairly, for their good, and for the betterment of individuals with ADHD. Reason (1988) used the term "critical subjectivity" to explain the balance we should strive to achieve. To him we should critically reflect on what we learn and disregard what seems harmful and unjust. Gergan (2009) makes a similar point and reminds us to consider how beliefs stem from dominant disciplines, become obvious, bestow power, and cause some voices to be silenced. Kahneman (2011) notes the importance of slowing down and reflecting on our thinking and how information we focus on influences our thoughts and behaviors. Realizing that neuroscience can be persuasive and influence our beliefs opens the door for us to re-interpret and re-envision our perspectives of it. Moral questions arise when science's findings are applied to lives and we need to examine and change our theories, methodologies, and beliefs if they are wrong (Gopnik, 2009).

Questioning, of course, does not always provide automatic answers to moral issues but it does bring into focus the need to seek valid information and keep a critical eye on the facts we receive and trust. Findings and treatments from neuroscience can have positive or negative effects. Interventions can help individuals focus and behave. But if we are not careful they can also place stars on their bellies and rob individuals of their identities (Racine & Illes, 2006). The limits of methodology and the complexity of relations between research and practice take center stage in the challenges we face (Stein, della Chiesa, Hinton, & Fischer, 2010).

Progress is being made as the many chapters in this volume note, but we have much work ahead. To use neuroscience appropriately a causal chain of evidence needs to be clear and it is important to realize that when it comes to labeling, treating, and caring for individuals with ADHD we must realize:

- The best information from neuroscience is gathered with reliable and valid tools, replicated, and combined with personal insights.

- We need to become better consumers of information from neuroscience.
- We need to understand that the tools neuroscientists use are new, popular, rapidly changing, and persuasive. We need to understand these tools, the level of analysis they are able to perform, the reliability/validity of results, and what this all means to us in understandable and useable terms.
- Neuroscience cannot tell us how to treat individuals. However, it can be used to confirm, enrich, and refine theories and models of learning and behavior. Different vantage points or a consilience of disciplines (e.g., human development, cognitive science, neuroscience, behavioral science) are best (Wilson, 1998). A multi-voiced perspective leads to interventions that work.
- Even though information from neuroscience has grown, given insight, and become part of daily conversations we must not lose sight of the fact that it is an evolving and quickly changing field. We need to be fascinated but remain skeptical at the same time.

This chapter is full of questions, perhaps more than answers, but this is where I see us. Gains are being made and beliefs are being formed. Fortunately the Sneetches came to realize they were wrong.

But Mc Bean was quite wrong. I'm quite happy to say That the Sneetches got really quite smart on that day, The day they decided that Sneetches are Sneetches.

And no kind of Sneetch is best on the beaches, that day all the Sneetches forgot about the stars.

And whether they had one, or not, upon thars.

Dr. Seuss (1961)

Author details

Debby Zambo

Mary Lou Fulton Teachers College, Arizona State University, Phoenix

References

[1] Barkley, R. A. (2001). The executive functions and self-regulation: An evolutionary neuropsychological perspective. *Neuropsychology Review, 11*, 1-29.

[2] Chau, V. (2007). Popping pills to study: Neuroethics in education, *Stanford Journal of Neuroscience, 1*(1), 18-20.

http://dx.doi.org/10.5772/53004

[3] Farah, M. (2005). Neuroethics: The practical and the philosophical. *Trends in Cognitive Science, 9*, 34-40.

[4] Gazzania, M. (2005): *The ethical brain*. New York: Dana Press.

[5] Gazzaniga, M.S. (2011). *Who's in charge: Free will and the science of the brain.* New York: Harper Collins.

[6] Gergen, K.J. (2009). *An invitation to social construction* (2nd ed.). Los Angeles, CA: Sage.

[7] Gopnik, A. (2009). *The philosophical baby*. New York: Farrar, Straus and Giroux.

[8] Habermas, J. (2003). *The future of human nature*. (Cambridge, UK: Polity Press).

[9] Kahneman, D. (2011). *Thinking fast and slow.* New York, NY" Farrar, Strauss, and Giroux.

[10] Lawson-Te, A. (1993). The socially constructed nature of psychology and the abnormation of the Maori, New Zealand Psychological Bulletin, 76, 25030.

[11] McCabe, D.P., & Castel, A.D. (2008). Seeing is believing: The effect of brain images on judgments of scientific reasoning. *Cognition, 107*(1), 343-352. doi:10.1016/j.cognition.2007.07.017

[12] McCabe, S.E., Knight, J.R., Teter, C.J., & Wechsler, H. (2005). Non-medical use of prescription stimulants among US college students: prevalence and correlates from a national survey. *Addiction, 100*, 96-106.

[13] Merton, R.K. (1948). The self-fulfilling prophecy. *Antioch Review,* 8, 193-210.

[14] Morse, S. (2006). Moral and legal responsibility and the new neuroscience. In Illes, J. (Ed.), *Neuroethics: Defining the issues in theory, practice, and policy* (51-61). New York: Oxford University Press.

[15] Reason, P. (1988). Introduction. In P. Reason (Ed.), *Human inquiry in action: Developments in new paradigm research* (pp. 1–17). Newbury Park, CA: Sage.

[16] Seuss, Dr. (1961). *The Sneeeches and other stories*. New York: Random House.

[17] Stamm, J. (2007). *Bright from the start: The simple science-backed way to nurture your child's developing mind, from birth to age 3*. New York: Gotham Books.

[18] Stein, Z., della Chiesa, B. Hinton, C., Fischer, K.W. (f2010). Ethical issues in educational neuroscience: Raising children in a brave new world (p 1-32). *Boston, Oxford* University Press.

[19] U.S. Department of Health and Human Services, (2010). *Summary health statistics for U.S. children: National health interview survey.* Washington, DC: U.S. Government Printing Office.

[20] Weisberg, D.S., Keil, F.C., Goodstein, E.R., Rawson, & Gray, J.R. (2008). The seductive allure of neuroscience explanations. *Journal of Cognitive Neuroscience, 20*(3), 470-477.

[21] Wilson, E.O. (1998). Consilience: The unity of knowledge. New York: Random House.